Williams
Hematology
Fif[...]

Comp[...]

EDITORS

William J. Williams, M.D.

Edward C. Reifenstein Professor of Medicine, State University of New York Health Science Center at Syracuse

Thomas E. Coyle, M.D.

Associate Professor of Medicine; Director, Adult Hemophilia Center, State University of New York Health Science Center at Syracuse

Stephen L. Graziano, M.D.

Associate Professor of Medicine, State University of New York Health Science Center at Syracuse; Chief of Oncology, Veterans Administration Medical Center at Syracuse

Stephen A. Landaw, M.D., Ph.D.

Professor of Medicine, State University of New York Health Science Center and Veterans Administration Medical Center at Syracuse

Thomas P. Loughran, Jr., M.D.

Professor of Medicine and Microbiology/Immunology, State University of New York Health Science Center at Syracuse; Chief of Hematology, Veterans Administration Medical Center at Syracuse

Douglas A. Nelson, M.D.

Professor of Pathology Emeritus, Consultant in Hematopathology, Department of Pathology, State University of New York Health Science Center at Syracuse

Jonathan Wright, M.D.

Professor of Medicine; Director, Hematology/Oncology Fellowship Program and Clinical Track Program, State University of New York Health Science Center at Syracuse

Kenneth Zamkoff, M.D.

Professor of Medicine; Director, Bone Marrow Transplant Program, State University of New York Health Science Center at Syracuse

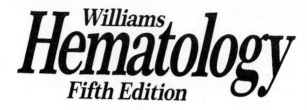

Williams Hematology
Fifth Edition

Companion Handbook

Editor-in-Chief

William J. Williams, M.D.

Associate Editors

Thomas E. Coyle, M.D.

Stephen L. Graziano, M.D.

Stephen A. Landaw, M.D., Ph.D.

Thomas P. Loughran, Jr., M.D.

Douglas A. Nelson, M.D.

Jonathan Wright, M.D.

Kenneth Zamkoff, M.D.

McGraw-Hill

Health Professions Division

New York • St. Louis • San Francisco • Auckland • Bogotá •
Caracas • Lisbon • London • Madrid • Mexico City • Milan •
Montreal • New Delhi • San Juan • Singapore • Sydney •
Tokyo • Toronto

Williams Hematology, 5/e, Companion Handbook

234567890   DOC DOC   98765

ISBN 0-07-070394-9

This book was set in Times Roman by Monotype Composition Company, Inc. The editors were J. Dereck Jeffers and Mariapaz Ramos Englis; the production supervisor was Clare Stanley; the cover designer was Edward Schultheis; the index was prepared by Irving Conde Tullar. R.R. Donnelley and Sons was printer and binder.

This book is printed on acid-free paper.

Library of Congress Cataloging-in-Publication Data

Williams hematology companion handbook / editor-in-chief, William J.
  Williams ; associate editors, Thomas E. Coyle . . . [et al.].
      p.   cm.
  "Companion handbook for the fifth edition of Williams
hematology"—Pref.
  Includes bibliographical references and index.
  ISBN 0-07-070394-9 (alk. paper)
  1. Blood—Diseases.   2. Hematology.   I. Williams, William J.
(William Joseph), (date) . II. Hematology companion handbook.
  [DNLM: 1. Hematologic Diseases—handbooks.   WH 39
RC633.H43 1995 Suppl.   W721 1995]
  616.1′5—dc20
  DNLM/DLC
  for Library of Congress   95-4630

CONTENTS

CONTRIBUTORS

Numbers in parentheses indicate the chapters for which each editor is responsible.

Thomas E. Coyle, M.D.   (51, 52, 73, 76, 78, 79, 81–84)

Associate Professor of Medicine; Director, Adult Hemophilia Center, State University of New York Health Science Center at Syracuse

Stephen L. Graziano, M.D.   (27, 32, 35, 42, 43, 46, 65–68)

Associate Professor of Medicine, State University of New York Health Science Center at Syracuse; Chief of Oncology, Veterans Administration Medical Center at Syracuse

Stephen A. Landaw, M.D., Ph.D.   (9–11, 17, 18, 21, 24, 38–40)

Professor of Medicine, State University of New York Health Science Center and Veterans Administration Medical Center at Syracuse

Thomas P. Loughran, Jr., M.D.   (4, 5, 53–59)

Professor of Medicine and Microbiology/Immunology, State University of New York Health Science Center at Syracuse; Chief of Hematology, Veterans Administration Medical Center at Syracuse

Douglas A. Nelson, M.D.   (6, 20, 25, 29, 30, 41, 47, 48, 50)

Professor of Pathology Emeritus, Consultant in Hematopathology, Department of Pathology, State University of New York Health Science Center at Syracuse

William J. Williams, M.D.   (1, 7, 8, 12–16, 19, 31, 37, 49, 69–72, 74, 75, 77, 80, 85)

Edward C. Reifenstein Professor of Medicine, State University of New York Health Science Center at Syracuse

Jonathan Wright, M.D.   (22, 23, 26, 28, 33, 34, 36, 44)

Professor of Medicine; Director, Hematology/Oncology Fellowship Program and Clinical Track Program, State University of New York Health Science Center at Syracuse

Kenneth Zamkoff, M.D.   (2, 3, 60–64, 86, 87)

Professor of Medicine; Director, Bone Marrow Transplant Program, State University of New York Health Science Center at Syracuse

ix

PREFACE

This *Companion Handbook* for the fifth edition of *Williams HEMATOL-OGY* provides a concise, operationally effective summary of the clinically applicable current information that is presented in detail in the complete text. The *Companion Handbook* is thus designed for convenient, ready access to the basics of clinical hematology so that a rational approach to a patient's problem may be initiated in the clinic or on the hospital floor under circumstances where in-depth review of the presumptive disorder is precluded by constraints of time or availability of a two-thousand page, three-kilogram book. Full consideration of a diagnostic possibility or rationalization of a clinical decision may require the information in the complete text, but a start can be made from the *Companion Handbook,* and that is its sole purpose. To that end information is presented in abbreviated, sometimes skeletal, form, using a "bullet" format. The location of the detailed discussions in the full textbook is presented at the end of each chapter in the *Handbook.*

The *Companion Handbook* was prepared by members of the Hematology faculty of the Departments of Medicine and Pathology of the State University of New York Health Science Center and the Veterans Administration Medical Center at Syracuse. It is based on information presented in the fifth edition of *Williams HEMATOLOGY.* Each chapter was prepared by one of us, reviewed in depth by each of us, and included after approval by all of us. This consensus approach was selected as most likely to lead to accurate, pertinent, and understandable summaries of the complex subjects that comprise modern hematology.

THE EDITORS

NOTICE

Medicine is an ever-changing science. As new research and clinical experience broaden our knowledge, changes in treatment and drug therapy are required. The editors and the publisher of this work have checked with sources believed to be reliable in their efforts to provide information that is complete and generally in accord with the standards accepted at the time of publication. However, in view of the possibility of human error or changes in medical sciences, neither the editors nor the publisher nor any other party who has been involved in the preparation or publication of this work warrants that the information contained herein is in every respect accurate or complete, and they are not responsible for any errors or omissions or for the results obtained from use of such information. Readers are encouraged to confirm the information contained herein with other sources. For example and in particular, readers are advised to check the product information sheet included in the package of each drug they plan to administer to be certain that the information contained in this book is accurate and that changes have not been made in the recommended dose or in the contraindications for administration. This recommendation is of particular importance in connection with new or infrequently used drugs.

Williams Hematology
Fifth Edition

Companion Handbook

1 APPROACH TO THE PATIENT

The care of a patient with a hematologic disorder begins with eliciting an extensive medical history and performing a thorough physical examination. Certain parts of the history and physical examination that are of particular interest to the hematologist are presented here.

HISTORY OF THE PRESENT ILLNESS

- Estimation of the ''performance status'' helps establish the degree of disability and permits assessment of the effects of therapy (Table 1-1).
- Drugs and chemicals often induce or aggravate hematologic diseases, and drug use or chemical exposure, intentional or inadvertent, must be carefully evaluated.
- Fever is a frequent symptom due to hematologic disease itself or, more often, to associated infection. Night sweats suggest the presence of fever.
- Weight loss may occur in some hematologic diseases.

TABLE 1-1 Criteria of Performance Status

Able to carry on normal activity; no special care is needed.	100%	Normal; no complaints, no evidence of disease
	90%	Able to carry on normal activity; minor signs or symptoms of disease
	80%	Normal activity with effort; some signs or symptoms of disease
Unable to work; able to live at home; care for most personal needs; a varying amount of assistance is needed.	70%	Cares for self; unable to carry on normal activity or to do active work
	60%	Requires occasional assistance but is able to care for most personal needs
	50%	Requires considerable assistance and frequent medical care
Unable to care for self; requires equivalent of institutional or hospital care; disease may be progressing rapidly.	40%	Disabled; requires special care and assistance
	30%	Severely disabled; hospitalization is indicated though death not imminent
	20%	Very sick; hospitalization necessary; active supportive treatment necessary
	10%	Moribund; fatal processes progressing rapidly.
	0%	Dead

Source: Table 1-1 of *Williams Hematology,* 5/e, p. 4.

- Fatigue, malaise, lassitude, and weakness are common but nonspecific symptoms and may be due to anemia, fever, muscle wasting associated with hematologic malignancy, or neurologic complications of hematologic disease.
- Symptoms related to specific organ systems or regions of the body may arise because of involvement in the basic disease process, such as spinal cord compression from an epidural tumor, or complications thereof, such as hyperviscosity.

FAMILY HISTORY

- Hematologic disorders may be inherited as autosomal dominant, autosomal recessive, or sex-linked traits. The family history is crucial in such cases and must include information relevant to the disease in question in grandparents, parents, siblings, children, maternal uncles, and nephews. Careful questioning is often necessary because some important details, such as the death of a sibling in infancy, may be forgotten years later.

SEXUAL HISTORY

- It is very important to obtain the history of the sexual preferences and practices of the patient.

PHYSICAL EXAMINATION

- Special attention should be paid to the following aspects of the physical examination
  - *Skin:* pallor, flushing, cyanosis, jaundice, petechiae, ecchymoses, telangiectases, excoriation, leg ulcers.
  - *Eyes:* jaundice, pallor, plethora, retinal hemorrhages and/or exudates, engorgement of retinal veins.
  - *Mouth:* pallor, jaundice, mucosal ulceration, smooth tongue.
  - *Lymph nodes:* enlargement in normal people occurs in the inguinal region in adults, and in the cervical region in children. Enlargement elsewhere, or marked enlargement in these regions, is considered abnormal.
  - *Chest:* sternal and/or rib tenderness.
  - *Liver:* enlargement.
  - *Spleen:* enlargement.

TABLE 1-2 Blood Cell Values in a Normal Population

	Men	Women
White cell count,* $\times 10^3/\mu l$ blood	7.8 (4.4–11.3)[†]	
Red cell count, $\times 10^6/\mu l$ blood	5.21 (4.52–5.90)	4.60 (4.10–5.10)
Hemoglobin, g/dl blood	15.7 (14.0–17.5)[‡]	13.8 (12.3–15.3)[‡]
Hematocrit, ratio	0.46 (0.42–0.50)	0.40 (0.36–0.45)
Mean corpuscular volume, fl/red cell	88.0 (80.0–96.1)	
Mean corpuscular hemoglobin, pg/red cell	30.4 (27.5–33.2)	
Mean corpuscular hemoglobin concentration, g/dl red cell	34.4 (33.4–35.5)	
Red cell distribution width, CV (%)	13.1 (11.5–14.5)	
Platelet count, $\times 10^3/\mu l$ blood	311 (172–450)	

*The International Committee for Standardization in Hematology has recommended that the following units be used (SI units): white cell count, number $\times 10^9$/liter; red cell count, number $\times 10^{12}$/liter; and hemoglobin, g/dl (dl = deciliter). The hematocrit (packed cell volume) is given as a number, for example, 0.41, without adjusted units. Units of liter per liter are implied. Mean corpuscular volume is given as fl (femtoliters), mean corpuscular hemoglobin as pg (picograms), and mean corpuscular hemoglobin concentration as g/dl. Platelets are reported as number $\times 10^9$/liter.
[†]The mean and reference intervals (normal range) are given. Because the distribution curves may be nongaussian, the reference interval is the nonparametric central 95 percent confidence interval. Results are based on 426 normal adult men and 212 normal adult women, with studies performed on the Coulter Model S-Plus IV.
[‡]The mean hemoglobin level of blacks of both sexes and all ages has been reported to be 0.5 to 1.0 g/dl below the mean for comparable whites.
Source: Table 2-1 of *Williams Hematology,* 5/e, p. 9.

LABORATORY EVALUATION

- The blood itself must also be evaluated, both quantitatively and qualitatively. This is frequently achieved using automated equipment.
  - Normal blood cell values are presented in Table 1-2, and normal total leukocyte and differential leukocyte counts and hemoglobin levels at different ages are presented in Table 1-3.

TABLE 1-3 Normal Leukocyte Count, Differential Count, and Hemoglobin Concentration at Various Ages

Age	Leukocytes, total	Neutrophils			Eosinophils	Basophils	Lymphocytes	Monocytes	Hemoglobin g/dl blood
		Total	Band	Segmented					
12 mo	11.4(6.0–17.5)	3.5(1.5–8.5) *31*	0.35 *3.1*	3.2(1.0–8.5) *28*	0.30(0.05–0.70) *2.6*	0.05(0–0.20) *0.4*	7.0(4.0–10.5) *61*	0.55(0.05–1.1) *4.8*	12.6(11.1–14.1)
4 y	9.1(5.5–15.5)	3.8(1.5–8.5) *42*	0.27(0–1.0) *3.0*	3.5(1.5–7.5) *39*	0.25(0.02–0.65) *2.8*	0.05(0–2.0) *0.6*	4.5(2.0–8.0) *50*	0.45(0–0.8) *5.0*	12.7(11.2–14.3)
6 y	8.5(5.0–14.5)	4.3(1.5–8.0) *51*	0.25(0–1.0) *3.0*	4.0(1.5–7.0) *48*	0.23(0–0.65) *2.7*	0.05(0–0.2) *0.6*	3.5(1.5–7.0) *42*	0.40(0–0.8) *4.7*	13.0(11.4–14.5)
10 y	8.1(4.5–13.5)	4.4(1.8–8.0) *54*	0.24(0–1.0) *3.0*	4.2(1.8–7.0) *51*	0.20(0–0.60) *2.4*	0.04(0–0.2) *0.5*	3.1(1.5–6.5) *38*	0.35(0–0.8) *4.3*	13.4(11.8–15.0)
21 y	7.4(4.5–11.0)	4.4(1.8–7.7) *59*	0.22(0–0.7) *3.0*	4.2(1.8–7.0) *56*	0.20(0–0.45) *2.7*	0.04(0–0.2) *0.5*	2.5(1.0–4.8) *34*	0.30(0–0.8) *4.0*	♂15.5(13.5–17.5) ♀13.8(12.0–15.6)

NOTE: Values are expressed as cells × $10^3/\mu l$. The numbers in italic type are mean percentages.
Source: Table 2-2 of *Williams Hematology, 5/e*, p. 12.

- Hemoglobin concentration is measured photometrically after conversion to a stable derivative, usually cyanmethemoglobin.
- Packed cell volume (*hematocrit*) may be measured directly by centrifugation of anticoagulated blood. Automated instruments calculate hematocrit as the product of erythrocyte count and the measured mean corpuscular volume.
- Mean corpuscular volume (MCV) is determined directly in automated counters, or may be calculated using the formula:

$$MCV = \frac{\text{hematocrit (\%)}}{\text{erythrocyte count } (\times 10^6/\mu l)} \times 10$$

The units are femtoliters (fl) or cubic micrometers per cell.
- Mean corpuscular hemoglobin (MCH) is calculated as follows:

$$MCH = \frac{\text{Hb (g/dl)}}{\text{erythrocyte count } (\times 10^6/\mu l)} \times 10$$

The units are picograms per cell.
- Mean corpuscular hemoglobin concentration (MCHC) is calculated as follows:

$$MCHC = \frac{\text{hemoglobin (g/dl)}}{\text{hematocrit (\%)}} \times 100$$

The units are grams of hemoglobin per deciliter (dl) of erythrocytes, or a percentage.
- Red cell distribution width (RDW) is calculated by some automatic counters and reflects variability in red cell size (anisocytosis).
- Enumeration of erythrocytes, leukocytes, and platelets may be done by manual methods utilizing a specially designed counting chamber, but electronic methods provide much more precise data and are now widely used for routine blood counts.
- Similarly, leukocyte differential count can be obtained from properly stained blood films prepared on glass slides. Normal values for patients at different ages are given in Table 1-2. The identifying features of the various types of leukocytes are summarized in Chaps. 2, 73, 86, and 93 of *Williams Hematology, 5/e.*
- Electronic methods which provide for rapid and accurate classification of leukocyte types based largely on the physical properties of the cells have been developed and are in general use. For example, one system classifies cells based on size and peroxidase activity, while other systems classify the cells on the basis of volume, or a combination of volume, conductivity, and light scattering.

TABLE 1-4 Diseases in which the Blood Cell Count May Be Normal but Examination of the Blood Film Will Suggest or Confirm the Disorder

Disease	Findings on blood film
Compensated acquired hemolytic anemia	Sphereocytosis, polychromatophilia, erythrocyte agglutination
Hereditary spherocytosis	Spherocytosis, polychromatophilia
Hemoglobin C disease	Target cells
Elliptocytosis	Elliptocytes
Lead poisoning	Basophilic stippling
Incipient pernicious anemia or folic acid deficiency	Macrocytosis, with oval macrocytes, hypersegmented neutrophils
Multiple myeloma, macroglobulinemia	Rouleaux formation
Malaria, babesiosis	Parasites in the erythrocytes
Consumptive coagulopathy	Schizocytes
Mechanical hemolysis	Schizocytes
Severe infection	Relative increase in neutrophils; increased band forms, left shift, Döhle bodies, neutrophil vacuoles*
Infectious mononucleosis	Atypical lymphocytes*
Agranulocytosis	Decreased neutrophils; relative increase in lymphocytes*
Allergic reactions	Eosinophilia*
Chronic lymphocytic leukemia (early)	Relative lymphocytosis*
Acute leukemia (early)	Blast forms*

* Likely to be identified as suspicious by automated three-part differential.
Source: Table 2-3 of *Williams Hematology*, 5/e, p. 14.

- Properly stained blood films also provide important information on the morphology of erythrocytes and platelets as well as leukocytes. Examination of the blood film may suggest the presence of a number of diseases in which the blood count may be normal. These are listed in Table 1-4.
- Some components of the blood count in infancy and childhood differ significantly from those in adults.
  - Hemoglobin levels are high at birth but fall over the first 12 weeks of life to reach levels which persist throughout childhood. Adult levels in males are only achieved with puberty (Tables 1-3 and 1-5).
  - The leukocyte count is high at birth, with neutrophils comprising more than half the cells. The leukocyte count falls over the next 2 weeks or so, to reach levels that persist throughout childhood. Lymphocytes are the predominant cell for the remainder of the first 4 years of life (Table 1-3).

TABLE 1-5 Red Cell Values for Term Infants During the First 12 Weeks of Life*

Age	Hb, g/dl ± SD	RBC × 10⁶/μl ± SD	Hematocrit, % ± SD	MCV, fl ± SD	MCHC, g/dl ± SD	Reticulocytes, % ± SD
Days:						
1	19.3 ± 2.2	5.14 ± 0.7	61 ± 7.4	119 ± 9.4	31.6 ± 1.9	3.2 ± 1.4
3	18.8 ± 2.0	5.11 ± 0.7	62 ± 9.3	116 ± 5.3	31.1 ± 2.8	2.8 ± 1.7
5	17.6 ± 1.1	4.97 ± 0.4	57 ± 7.3	114 ± 8.9	30.9 ± 2.2	1.2 ± 0.2
7	17.9 ± 2.5	4.86 ± 0.6	56 ± 9.4	118 ± 11.2	32.0 ± 1.6	0.5 ± 0.4
Weeks:						
1–2	17.3 ± 2.3	4.80 ± 0.8	54 ± 8.3	112 ± 19.0	32.1 ± 2.9	0.5 ± 0.3
3–4	14.2 ± 2.1	4.00 ± 0.6	43 ± 5.7	105 ± 7.5	33.5 ± 1.6	0.6 ± 0.3
5–6	11.9 ± 1.5	3.55 ± 0.2	36 ± 6.2	102 ± 10.2	34.1 ± 2.9	1.0 ± 0.7
7–8	11.1 ± 1.1	3.40 ± 0.4	33 ± 3.7	100 ± 13.0	33.7 ± 2.6	1.5 ± 0.7
9–10	11.2 ± 0.9	3.60 ± 0.3	32 ± 2.7	91 ± 9.3	34.3 ± 2.9	1.2 ± 0.6
11–12	11.3 ± 0.9	3.70 ± 0.3	33 ± 3.3	88 ± 7.9	34.8 ± 2.2	0.7 ± 0.3

*Capillary blood samples. The RBC and MCV measurements were made on an electronic counter.
Source: Table 8-3 of Williams Hematology, 5/e, p. 60.

- Platelet counts are at adult levels throughout childhood.
- Leukocyte function may be depressed in normal infants in the newborn period.
- Blood count and cell function may also vary with advanced age.
  - The hemoglobin levels of men over 60 years of age are statistically lower than those of younger men even in the absence of a demonstrable cause for anemia, but are not sufficiently lower to warrant use of specific normal values for older men.
  - The hemoglobin level for women does not change significantly with advancing age.
  - Total and differential leukocyte counts also do not change significantly with advancing age.
  - Leukocytosis in response to infection (e.g., appendicitis or pneumonia) is the same in older individuals as in people below the age of 60, but special studies indicate that the marrow granulocyte reserve may be reduced in the elderly.
  - Both cellular and humoral immune responses are reduced in older patients.
  - The erythrocyte sedimentation rate increases significantly with age.
- Examination of the marrow is critically important in the study and management of a wide variety of hematologic disorders.
  - All bones contain hemopoietic marrow at birth.
  - Fat cells begin to replace hemopoietic marrow in the extremities in the fifth to sixth year of life.
  - In adults hemopoietic marrow is limited to the axial skeleton and the proximal quarter of the humeri and femora.
  - Hemopoietic marrow cellularity is reduced in the elderly, falling after age 65 from about 50 percent to 30 percent, roughly in inverse proportion to age.
  - Marrow is obtained by aspiration and/or needle biopsy. The most frequently utilized site is the iliac crest at the posterior superior iliac spine. The Jamshidi needle is most often used for biopsy, and provides excellent material for study.
  - Aspirated marrow may be evaluated after preparation of thin or thick films on glass slides and appropriate staining.
  - Marrow biopsies are examined after fixation, sectioning, and staining. Touch preparations provide useful information and should be made for all biopsies.
  - Interpretation of marrow films and biopsy sections is discussed in Chap. 3 of *Williams Hematology*, 5/e, and under specific diseases.

For a more detailed discussion, see William J. Williams: Approach to the patient, Chap. 1, p. 1; Williams et al: Examination of the blood,

Chap. 2, p. 8; William J. Williams, Douglas A. Nelson; Examination of the marrow, Chap. 3, p. 15; George B. Segel: Hematology of the newborn, Chap. 8, p. 57; William J. Williams: Hematology in the aged, Chap. 9, p. 72; Michael W. Morris et al: Automated blood cell counting, Chap. L1, p. L3; Stephen A. Landaw: Tissue imaging and cell survival studies for evaluating patients with hematologic disorders, Chap. L2, p. L12 in *Williams Hematology*, 5/e, 1995.

2 SUPPORTIVE CARE

TREATMENT OF INFECTION IN THE IMMUNOCOMPROMISED HOST

- Cytoreductive chemotherapy can induce profound pancytopenia. *Neutropenia* is often severe and results in infection in many patients. Patients with lymphoid neoplasms have additional risk factors for infection, i.e., *altered humoral* and *cell-mediated immunity.*

Risk Factors and Infecting Organisms

- Absolute neutrophil count below 500/μl
- Duration of neutropenia
- Rate of decline of the neutrophil count
- Breaks in the integumental barriers; e.g., indwelling catheters
- Gram-negative aerobic bacilli frequently involved are
  - *Pseudomonas*
  - *Klebsiella*
  - *E. coli*
  - *Proteus*
- The most common causes of infection are gram-positive organisms:
  - staphylococcal species
  - enterococcus
  - *Corynebacterium*
- Lymphoid malignancy often is associated with infection with encapsulated organisms, i.e., pneumococcus or *Hemophilus,* or with *Listeria* or *Nocardia.*
- Fungal infections arise in the setting of prolonged neutropenia, impaired cell-mediated immunity, glucocorticoid use, and indwelling catheters.
- Herpes simplex, varicella-zoster, cytomegalovirus, and adenoviruses are the most important causes of viral infections, and these occur with impaired cell-mediated immunity.
- *Pneumocystis carinii* produces pneumonia and arises in setting of impaired cell-mediated immunity and glucocorticoid use.
- Parasitic infestations with *Toxoplasma gondii* and *Strongyloides* occur with lymphoid neoplasms and glucocorticoid use.

Recognition and Diagnosis of Infection

- Clinical manifestations of infections may include
  - shaking chills
  - fever
  - hypothermia
  - altered mental status
  - myalgias

- The following are frequent sites of infection in neutropenic patients, and should be carefully examined:
  - mouth
  - skin
  - perianal and perirectal areas (include rectal and pelvic exams if indicated)
- Chest x-ray initially
- Chest CT if clinically indicated
- Sinus x-rays if symptoms are present
- Blood cultures from peripheral veins and from indwelling venous access catheter(s) and urine culture in all patients
- Biopsy and culture suspicious skin lesion(s)
- Nasal culture may help diagnose pulmonary aspergillosis
- Invasive pulmonary procedures (open lung biopsy, transbronchial biopsy) are of limited value for the risks taken
- Bronchial brushing with lavage may be of benefit with lower risk than open lung or transbronchial biopsy

Initial Treatment

- Bacterial infections
  - Prompt initiation of antibiotics is imperative.
  - For initial empiric therapy, select antibiotics that treat a broad spectrum of aerobic gram-negative bacilli.
  - Brief delays in initiating therapy specifically for gram-positive organisms may not increase mortality rates.
  - The best antibiotic therapy is not known for febrile neutropenic patients.
  - For antibiotic programs frequently used, with doses, see Tables 17-1 and 17-2 of *Williams Hematology*, 5/e.
  - Single-drug therapy with third generation cephalosporins or imipenam is not recommended for routine use in profoundly neutropenic patients, i.e., neutrophils less than $100/\mu l$.
  - Therapeutic granulocyte transfusions are rarely, if ever, necessary.
- Fungal infections
  - Amphotericin B is agent of choice for most fungal infections in neutropenic patients: Prescribe full dose by second day. Monitor serum potassium, magnesium, and creatinine levels daily.
  - Meperidine, acetaminophen, diphenhydramine, and/or hydrocortisone should be administered concomitantly to reduce the severity of fevers and chills.
  - Flucytosine not routinely used.
  - Fluconazole is used in patients with fluconazole-sensitive fungal infection unable to tolerate amphotericin B. May be used alone in hepatosplenic candidiasis.
  - Itraconazole is not approved for use in candidiasis or *Aspergillus* infection.

- Viral infections
  - Acyclovir is active against herpes simplex and against varicella-zoster at higher doses. Not useful for cytomegalovirus or Epstein-Barr virus.
  - Ganciclovir has efficacy against cytomegalovirus and Herpes simplex but produces significant neutropenia.
  - Foscarnet has efficacy against cytomegalovirus but may produce renal insufficiency.
- Parasitic infections
  - *Pneumocystis carinii* treated with either trimethoprim/sulfamethoxazole or pentamidine.

Adjusting Therapy

- Culture results may indicate that other antibiotics would be more effective or that less toxic agents could be substituted.
- If initial empiric therapy is unsuccessful, broaden coverage to include gram-positive organisms and consider adding antifungal therapy.
- Recurrence of fever suggests superinfection.

Duration of Therapy

- Treatment may be stopped with resolution of neutropenia (absolute neutrophil count greater than $500/\mu l$) and no clinical evidence of infection.
- It is acceptable to stop antibiotics while the patient is still neutropenic, if there has been a prompt and complete clinical response.
- Duration of antifungal therapy very variable.
- *Pneumocystis* therapy should be continued for 2 to 3 weeks.
- Herpes infections are treated for 7 days.

Fever after Recovery from Chemotherapy-Induced Neutropenia

- Consider:
  - drug fever
  - fungal infections of liver or lung
  - indwelling catheter infections
- Catheter infections
  - *S. epidermidis* infection may be cured without catheter removal by antibiotic treatment for at least 2 weeks.
  - Tunnel infections, or infections with *S. aureus,* gram-negative, or fungal infections, require catheter removal in addition to antimicrobial therapy.

PREVENTION OF INFECTIONS

- Bacterial infection
  - Oral nonabsorbable antibiotics are poorly tolerated.

- Trimethoprim/sulfamethoxazole and the fluoroquinolones both may be beneficial in preventing bacterial infection in neutropenic patients.
- Strict hand-washing policies, attention to sterile technique, and avoiding invasive procedures reduce bacterial colonization and infection.
- Careful attention to indwelling intravenous lines.
- Parasitic infections
  - Trimethoprim/sulfamethoxazole effective as *Pneumocystis* prophylaxis.
  - Monthly aerosolized pentamidine has not been studied for prophylaxis in non-HIV–infected patients.
  - Need for prophylaxis varies with the intensity of chemotherapy.
- Viral infections
  - Acyclovir is useful in prevention of herpes simplex infection.
  - Varicella-zoster immune globulin is useful in susceptible patients after exposure.
  - Chances of cytomegalovirus infection can be reduced by avoiding blood products from CMV-seropositive donors, if the recipient is seronegative for CMV.
  - Acyclovir and ganciclovir may be useful as prophylactic agents against CMV infection.
- Fungal infections
  - Most oral antifungal drugs reduce colonization.
  - Fluconazole was shown to reduce systemic fungal infection in one study.
  - Superinfection may become problematic with extensive prophylaxis.
  - Earlier initiation of empiric systemic antifungal therapy may be preferred to prophylaxis.

USE OF VENOUS ACCESS DEVICES

- Long-term venous access devices are frequently necessary in patients with malignant disease. Currently available models made of silicone rubber have low potential for thrombosis.
- Long-term venous access devices may be:
  - external catheters
  - implantable subcutaneous ports
- External devices
  - may be pulled out accidentally
  - are more easily monitored for infection
  - can be removed in office or clinic
  - provide excellent venous access for drawing blood and for fluid administration
  - require frequent flushing

- are best suited for intensive treatment with lengthy or toxic infusions, multiple blood sampling, frequent fluid or blood administration
- Implanted devices
  - may be dislodged in the subcutaneous pocket
  - are difficult to monitor for infection
  - require surgical removal
  - limit flow of fluid because of the narrow 20 or 22 g Huber access needle
  - require careful monitoring during prolonged infusions as Huber needles can dislodge, resulting in extravasation
  - require only monthly flushing when not in use
  - best suited for long-term intermittent use
- Number of lumens
  - single, double, or triple lumen external devices
  - single or double lumen implanted devices
  - additional lumens provide greater flexibility, but at greater risk of infection and thrombosis
- Complications due to infections:
  - Exit site infection, tunnel or pocket infection, line sepsis.
  - Exit, tunnel, and pocket infection are usually due to organisms colonizing the skin, e.g., *S. epidermidis.*
  - Exit site infection usually responds to local wound care and appropriate systemic antibiotics.
  - Tunnel or pocket infections usually track along the catheter from the exit site or are tracked into the pocket by the access needle.
  - Treatment of tunnel or pocket infections requires removal of the catheter, surgical drainage and debridement, and systemic antibiotics.
  - Catheter-related bacteremia requires systemic antibiotics and often removal of the catheter.
  - Indications for catheter removal include (1) quantitative blood cultures consistent with a line infection, (2) systemic symptoms temporally related to catheter manipulation, (3) worsening clinical status while receiving systemic antibiotics, and (4) line infection with difficult-to-eradicate organisms, e.g., *S. aureus, Bacillus* sp., gram-negative bacilli, fungal organisms, *Mycobacterium fortuitum.*
- Complications due to catheter occlusion and/or thrombosis
  - If fluid cannot be infused or blood aspirated, obtain plain film and contrast study to ascertain catheter position.
  - Occlusion treated with intraluminal urokinase, 2500 to 10,000 U for 30 min to 2 h.
  - Venous thrombosis usually managed by catheter removal and systemic anticoagulation.

- Systemic urokinase can be used to induce clot resolution and salvage catheter.

PAIN MANAGEMENT

- Pain is defined as an unpleasant sensory and emotional experience associated with actual or potential tissue damage.
- Pain may be acute or chronic
  - Acute pain is of recent onset, and is often associated with sympathetic nervous system overactivity.
  - Pain is chronic when symptoms persist after investigation of the cause. Chronic pain implies that the cause cannot be quickly eliminated.
- Cancer pain
  - Two-thirds of cancer patients have significant pain.
  - 80 percent of patients experience durable pain relief with effective oral medication.
  - Parenteral opioids can provide adequate analgesia when oral medications do not.
  - Pain associated with diagnostic interventions is underappreciated, especially in children with cancer.
- Pain assessment
  - Elicit a pain history to determine possible causes and intensity.
  - Rate pain intensity on a self-reporting numeric scale, e.g., 0 through 4, with 0 indicating absence of pain and 4 the worst pain imaginable.
- Mechanisms of pain
  - Somatic pain arises in skin, bone, muscle, soft tissue. It is described as dull, or aching, and responds to nonsteroidal anti-inflammatory drugs (NSAIDs) or opioids.
  - Visceral pain is less well localized, and responds to NSAIDS or opioids.
  - Neuropathic pain is less responsive to NSAIDs or opioids and may require coanalgesics, e.g., heterocyclic antidepressants.

Treatment of Cancer Pain

- NSAIDs
  - inhibit prostaglandin synthesis
  - have significant potential for toxicity (gastrointestinal, renal, hematologic)
  - show ceiling effect, e.g., no additional analgesia with dose escalation
  - offer better analgesia with regular, rather than intermittent, use
- Mild opioids
  - can be added if NSAIDs inadequate

TABLE 2-1 Comparison of Potent Opioid Agonists Used in Cancer Pain Management*

Generic name	Trade name	Dose, mg	Route	Duration, h
Morphine sulfate		10	IM	2–4
Morphine sulfate, immediate release	MSIR, Roxanol	20–30	Oral	2–4
Controlled-release morphine	MS Contin, Oromorph	30	Oral	8–12
Morphine		20	Rectal	3–4
Hydromorphone	Dilaudid	7.5	Oral	2–4
		1.5	IM	2–4
		6	Rectal	3–4
Oxymorphone	Numorphan	1	IM	3–6
		5–10	Rectal	4–6
Meperidine	Demerol	300	Oral	2–3
		75–100	IM	2–3
Heroin	Diamorphine	5	IM	4–5
		60	Oral	4–5
Methadone	Dolophine	10	IM	4–12
		20	Oral	4–12
Levorphanol	Levodromoran	4	Oral	4–8
		2	IM	4–8
Oxycodone	Roxycodone	30	Oral	2–4
Transdermal fentanyl	Duragesic	†	TD	60–72

*Relative potencies and a guide for initiating treatment or converting from drug to drug. The correct dose is variable and should be individualized.
†Usual starting dose ranges from 20 to 50 μg/h; refer to package insert for recommended conversions.
Source: Table 21-1 of *Williams Hematology*, 5/e, p. 204.

- should not be continued if pain control inadequate; advance to potent opioids (Table 2-1)
- Potent opioids: dosing guide
  - correct dose is that which relieves pain without inducing intolerable side effects
- Potent opioids: adverse effects
  - constipation: use prophylactic laxatives to prevent fecal impaction
  - nausea and sedation, often transient at start of therapy
  - intractable side effects require a different potent opioid
  - reassess treatment program often for adequacy and toxicity
- Scheduling potent opioids around the clock more effective than as needed for pain
  - long-acting analgesic used for maintenance, with short-acting agents for breakthrough pain
  - if breakthrough pain occurs > 2 to 3 times per 12-h period, increase dose of long-acting agent

- Adjuvants to potent opioids
  - tricyclic antidepressants, helpful with pain of neuropathic origin
  - anticonvulsants—carbamazepine, phenytoin, valproic acid, clonazepam—for pain of neuropathic origin
  - mexilitene, second line for neuropathic pain
- Route of administration
  - orally or transdermally if possible
  - parenteral if inability to swallow, nausea, vomiting, malabsorption, obstruction
- Specific potent opioids
  - controlled-release morphine sulfate is given orally every 8 to 12 h. Tablets should not be broken, crushed, or chewed.
  - transdermal fentanyl peak level not reached for 12 to 18 h, and short-acting supplemental analgesics needed during this time. Fentanyl patch provides analgesia for up to 72 h and forms a skin depot of active drug which lasts for 12 to 18 h after removal of the patch.

Pain in Sickle Cell Disease

- Accept patient's history of pain intensity.
- Incidence of opioid addiction is low in sickle cell patients.
- Meperdine is poor choice for repetitive administration.
- For acute sickle cell pain, morphine sulfate elixir 15 mg q 20 min until analgesia or sedation.
- Once analgesia obtained, give 30 to 60 mg morphine sulfate elixir q 2 h plus aspirin or other NSAID with hydration.
- Continuous intravenous morphine or meperidine in children with acute chest syndrome (respiratory arrest) is contraindicated.
- Patient controlled analgesia (PCA) has been used successfully in hospitalized patients with sickle cell pain.

Pain in HIV Disease

- High incidence of pain in patients with AIDS.
- 30 percent of hospital admissions in AIDS patients related to pain.
- Heterogeneous pain syndromes, with variants of neuropathic pain predominant.
- Manage as for cancer pain.

For a more detailed discussion, see Steven M. Beutler: Treatment of infections in the immunocompromised host, Chap. 17, p. 166; Elizabeth Steinhouser, H. Richard Alexander: The use of venous access devices, Chap. 20, p. 200; and Richard B. Patt, Richard Payne: Pain management, Chap. 21, p. 203, in *Williams Hematology*, 5/e, 1995.

3 PHARMACOLOGY AND TOXICITY OF ANTINEOPLASTIC DRUGS AND THERAPEUTIC USE OF CYTOKINES

BASIC PRINCIPLES OF CANCER CHEMOTHERAPY

- Knowledge of drug actions, clinical toxicities, pharmacokinetics, and drug interactions is essential.
- Utilize proven regimens.
- Choice of a particular protocol should depend on the disease, histology, and stage of the disease and on an assessment of individual patient tolerance to the drug program chosen.
- High-dose chemotherapy programs used in stem cell transplantation result in additional organ toxicities not seen at conventional doses.
- Chemotherapy usually targets process of DNA replication.

COMBINATION CHEMOTHERAPY

- Combination chemotherapy utilizes several drugs simultaneously based on certain empiric principles:
  - Each drug selected has demonstrable antitumor activity against the neoplasm for which it is used.
  - Each drug should have a different mechanism of action.
  - The drugs should not have a common mechanism of resistance.
  - Drug toxicities should not overlap.
  - Specific combinations chosen should be based on preclinical evidence of synergistic activity.

CELL KINETICS AND CANCER CHEMOTHERAPY

- Cell cycle specific agents, such as antimetabolites, kill cells as they traverse the DNA synthetic phase (S phase) of the cell cycle.
- Non-cell cycle dependent agents do not require cells to be exposed during a specific phase of the cell cycle.

DRUG RESISTANCE

- Basis for drug resistance is spontaneous occurrence of resistant mutants and selection of drug resistant cells under pressure of chemotherapy (*clonal selection hypothesis*).
- Theory implies:
  - use of multiple drugs not sharing resistance mechanisms should be more effective than single agents.
  - multiple agents should be used simultaneously, as probability of double or triple resistant cells is the product of the probabilities of

the independent drug resistant mutations occurring simultaneously in the same cell.

DRUGS USED TO TREAT HEMATOLOGIC MALIGNANCIES

Cell Cycle-Active Agents

Methotrexate

- Methotrexate is used for maintenance therapy of acute lymphocytic leukemia, combination chemotherapy of lymphomas, and treatment and prophylaxis of meningeal leukemia.
- Inhibits dihydrofolate reductase, which leads to depletion of cellular folate coenzymes and to inhibition of DNA synthesis and cessation of cell replication.
- Acquired resistance is due to increased levels of dihydrofolate reductase via gene amplification, defective polyglutamylation, and impaired cellular uptake.
- Is well absorbed orally in doses of 5 to 10 mg, but doses of more than 25 mg must be given intravenously.
- Excreted primarily unchanged by the kidney.
- Renal impairment is contradiction to methotrexate therapy.
- Dose limiting toxicities are myelosuppression and gastrointestinal (mucositis, diarrhea, bleeding).
- Intrathecal methotrexate may produce acute arachnoiditis, dementia, motor deficits, seizures, and coma. Leucovorin cannot prevent or reverse CNS toxicities.
- Leucovorin intravenously will reverse acute toxicity of methotrexate, except for CNS toxicity.

Cytosine Arabinoside (Ara-C)

- Used primarily to treat acute myelogenous leukemia, in combination with an anthracycline drug.
- Ara-C triphosphate (Ara-CTP) formed intracellularly, inhibits DNA polymerase, and also causes termination of strand elongation.
- Acquired resistance is due to loss of deoxycytidine kinase, the initial activating enzyme of Ara-C, decreased drug uptake or increased deamination.
- Ara-C is not active orally and must be given parenterally.
- High CSF concentration achieved (50 percent of plasma level).
- Ara-C may be given intrathecally.
- At usual doses (100 to 150 mg/m^2/day for 5 to 10 days) myelosuppression is dose-limiting toxicity.
- At higher doses (g/m^2), neurologic, hepatic, and gastrointestinal toxicities may occur. Patients over 50 years of age may develop cerebellar toxicity (ataxia, slurred speech), which can progress to confusion, dementia, and death. Severe conjunctivitis may also

occur, but may be prevented or reduced by glucocorticoid eye drops.

5-Azacytidine

- A cytidine analog that has cytotoxic activity and may induce differentiation at low doses.
- Main clinical toxicities are reversible myelosuppression, severe nausea and vomiting, hepatic dysfunction, myalgias, fever, and rash

Purine Analogs: 6-Mercaptopurine (6-MP) and 6-Thioguanine (6-TG)

- Both 6-MP and 6-TG are converted to nucleotides by the enzyme hypoxanthine-guanine phosphoribosyl transferase (HPRT). Cell death correlates with incorporation of the 6-MP or 6-TG nucleotides into DNA.
- Both 6-MP and 6-TG are given orally.
- Equivalent myelosuppression occurs with either 6-MP or 6-TG.
- Metabolism of 6-MP is inhibited by allopurinol; 6-TG metabolism is not affected.

Fludarabine Phosphate

- A purine analog active in chronic lymphocytic leukemia (CLL) and low-grade lymphomas.
- Administered intravenously, and eliminated mainly by renal excretion.
- At recommended doses, moderate myelosuppression and opportunistic infection are major toxicities. Peripheral sensory and motor neuropathy may also occur.
- Tumor lysis syndrome may occur with treatment of patients with large tumor burdens.

2-Chlorodeoxyadenosine (2-CDA; Cladribine)

- A purine analog active in hairy cell leukemia, CLL, and low-grade lymphomas.
- Administered intravenously, and eliminted mainly by renal excretion.
- Myelosuppression, fever, and opportunistic infection are major toxicities.
- Repeated doses produces cumulative thrombocytopenia.

2-Deoxycoformycin (DCF)

- A purine analog that inhibits adenosine deaminase, resulting in accumulation of intracellular adenosine and deoxyadenosine nucleotides, which are probably responsible for the cytotoxicity.

- Severe depletion of T cells occurs and opportunistic infections are common.
- DCF is eliminated entirely by the kidney.

Hydroxyurea

- Hydroxyurea inhibits ribonucleotide reductase, which converts ribonucleotide diphosphates to deoxyribonucleotides.
- Hydroxyurea is used to treat polycythemia vera, the chronic phase of chronic myelogenous leukemia (CML), and to reduce rapidly rising blast counts in the acute phase of CML.
- Resistance occurs as a result of increases in ribonucleotide reductase activity, or from development of a mutant enzyme that binds the drug less avidly.
- Well absorbed when administered orally.
- Renal excretion is major source of elimination.
- Major toxicities are leukopenia and induction of megaloblastic changes in blood and bone marrow.

Vinca Alkaloids (Vincristine and Vinblastine)

- Vinca alkaloids bind to microtubules and inhibit mitotic spindle formation.
- Resistance occurs by acquistion of multidrug resistance phenotype or development of microtubules with decreased vinca alkaloid binding.
- Vincristine and vinblastine are both administered intravenously. About 70 percent of vincristine is metabolized in the liver. The site of vinblastine metabolism is unidentified.
- The dose-limiting toxicity of vincristine is neurotoxicity, which begins with paresthesias of fingers and lower legs and loss of deep tendon reflexes.
- Severe weakness of extensor muscles of hands and feet may occur with continued use.
- Bone marrow suppression is not a common side effect.
- Primary toxicity of vinblastine is leukopenia.
- Both vincristine and vinblastine are potent vesicants upon extravasation during administration.
- Neither vincristine nor vinblastine can be given intrathecally.

Epipodophyllotoxins

- Etoposide (VP-16) is used in Hodgkin disease, aggressive lymphomas, leukemias, and as a component of high-dose chemotherapy programs.
- Binds to DNA and induces double-stranded breaks.
- Resistance is a result of expression of multidrug resistance phenotype or diminished drug binding.
- May be given orally or intravenously.

- Clinical activity is schedule dependent. Single conventional doses are ineffective; daily doses for 3 to 5 days are required.
- Hypotension may occur with intravenous administration.
- Major toxicity is leukopenia; thrombocytopenia is less common.
  - In high-dose protocols, mucositis is common and hepatic damage may occur.
  - Etoposide may induce secondary acute myelogenous leukemias.

Bleomycin

- Bleomycin is used in combination chemotherapy programs for Hodgkin disease, aggressive lymphomas, or germ cell tumors.
- Antitumor activity is due to formation of single and double-stranded DNA breaks.
- Resistance is due to accelerated drug inactivation, enhanced DNA repair capacity, or decreased drug accumulation.
- Administered intravenously or intramuscularly for systemic effects, and may be instilled intrapleurally or intraperitoneally to control malignant effusions.
- Eliminated largely by renal excretion. May need dose reduction with renal dysfunction.
- Has little effect on normal marrow.
- A major toxicity is pulmonary fibrosis which is dose related and usually is irreversible.
- Skin changes, also a major toxicity, are dose related, and include erythema, hyperpigmentation, hyperkeratosis, and ulceration.
- Fever and malaise commonly occur.

Non-Cell-Cycle Active Agents

Alkylating Drugs

- Used as single agents or in combination with other drugs to treat hematologic neoplasms.
- All form covalent bonds with electron-rich sites on DNA.
- Myelosuppression and mucositis are the major acute toxicities.
- Pulmonary fibrosis and secondary leukemias are the major delayed toxicities.
- Clinical basis of resistance to alkylating drugs is not fully understood.
- Rapidly eliminated by chemical conjugation to sulfhydryl groups or by oxidative metabolism.
- Cyclophosphamide and ifosfamide produce a toxic metabolite (acrolein) that is excreted in the urine and can cause hemorrhagic cystitis. Acrolein may be detoxified by sodium 2-mercaptoethane sulfonate (mesna) given simultaneously.
- Nitrogen mustard is a potent vesicant.
- Marrow toxicity is cumulative and is a function of the total dose.

- The incidence of secondary leukemias is related to total dose administered and to the drugs used. Procarbazine is especially potent in inducing secondary leukemia.
- Dose-limiting toxicity of dacarbazine is nausea and vomiting.
- Nitrosoureas produce delayed myelosuppression, with nadir of blood counts 4 to 6 weeks after the dose, and can also cause nephrotoxicity.
- All alkylating agents can produce pulmonary fibrosis. Busulfan and nitrosoureas are the most likely to do so.

High-Dose Alkylating Agent Therapy

- High-dose chemotherapy programs use one or several alkylating agents because of the strong relationship between dose and cytotoxicity of these drugs.
- With hemopoietic stem cell support doses of alkylating agents can be increased 2 to 18-fold, until extramedullary toxicities become limiting.

Anthracycline Antibiotics

- Doxorubicin is used in acute leukemias, Hodgkin disease, and lymphomas.
- Daunorubicin and idarubicin are used in combination with Ara-C for acute myelogenous leukemia.
- Mitoxantrone is used for acute myelogenous leukemia and breast cancer.
- Anthracyclines act by forming a complex with both DNA and the DNA repair enzyme topoisomerase II, resulting in double-stranded DNA breaks.
- Anthracyclines generate free radicals, which may cause cardiac toxicity.
- Resistance occurs with increased activity of the P-glycoprotein transport system in multidrug resistance cells and with altered topoisomerase II activity.
- Doxorubicin and daunorubicin are metabolized in the liver.
- Doxorubicin is usually given every 3 to 4 weeks. Schedules that avoid high peak plasma levels may reduce cardiac toxicity.
- Myelosuppression is the major acute toxicity. When doxorubicin is combined with other myelotoxic agents the dose is usually reduced by one-third to one-half.
- Doxorubicin may produce mucositis.
- All these drugs can produce reaction in previously irradiated tissues.
- All can produce tissue necrosis if extravasated.
- Dose-related cardiac toxicity is a major side effect of doxorubicin and daunorubicin.
- Acute cardiac effects are arrhythmias, conduction disturbances, pericarditis-myocarditis syndrome.

- Chronic cardiac effects are diminished ejection fraction and clinical congestive heart failure, with high mortality.
- Children receiving anthracyclines may show abnormal cardiac development and late congestive heart failure as teenagers.

Asparaginase

- L-Asparaginase is used in the treatment of lymphoid neoplasms.
- Neoplastic lymphoid cells require exogenous L-asparagine for growth. L-Asparaginase destroys this essential nutrient.
- L-Asparaginase is given either intravenously or intramuscularly.
- Hypersensitivity reactions vary from urticaria to anaphylaxis.
- Hypoalbuminemia may result from inhibition of hepatic protein synthesis.
- Decreased AT III, protein C, and protein S levels may result in arterial or venous thrombosis.
- Decreased levels of fibrinogen, factors II, VII, IX and X may result in bleeding.
- Inhibition of insulin production may result in hyperglycemia.
- High doses of L-asparaginase may cause cerebral dysfunction manifested by confusion, stupor, and coma and may also cause nonhemorrhagic pancreatitis.
- L-Asparaginase can be used to prevent marrow suppression if given after high-dose methotrexate.

Differentiating Agents

- Chemical agents such as carotenes, retinoids, vitamin D, and some cytotoxic drugs can cause differentiation of neoplastic cells.
- All-*trans*-retinoic acid (tRA) may induce a complete response in acute promyelocytic leukemia (APL) for reasons that are incompletely understood.
- tRA is given orally.
- Toxicities are dry skin, cheilitis, mild but reversible hepatic dysfunction, bone tenderness, hyperostosis on x-ray, and occasionally pseudotumor cerebri.
- The "retinoic acid syndrome" may occur, with respiratory failure, pleural and pericardial effusions, and peripheral edema associated with a rapid increase in the number of leukemic cells in the blood.
- High-dose glucocorticoid therapy may reverse the syndrome if the white blood cell count is rising rapidly. Otherwise, prompt administration of cytotoxic chemotherapy may prevent the syndrome.

THERAPEUTIC USE OF CYTOKINES

- Hemopoietic growth factors, also known as cytokines, are hormones that regulate the proliferation, differentiation, and maturation of hemo-

poietic progenitors and the survival and function of mature blood cells.
- Recombinant DNA technology has allowed the rapid introduction of these molecules into clinical practice.
- Hemopoietic growth factors are named for the type of colonies they stimulate when added to semisolid cultures of bone marrow cells, e.g., granulocyte, macrophage, erythroid.
- The term *interleukin* is derived from the concept that the source and target of these molecules are both leukocytes. However, interleukins are produced by cells other than leukocytes.

Erythropoietin (EPO)

- The primary cytokine that regulates erythropoiesis. It stimulates production and terminal maturation of erythroid colony and burst forming cells, i.e., CFU-E and BFU-E. Its clinical uses are as follows.

Anemia of Chronic Renal Disease

- EPO therapy results in significant elevation of the hematocrit in patients with end-stage renal disease, whether or not they are on dialysis.
- Hematocrit rises promptly and patients become transfusion independent in about 8 weeks.
- Adverse effects are
  - diastolic hypertension (occurs in 33 percent of patients) due to increased blood volume.
  - iron deficiency (in 50 percent of patients) requires iron supplementation.
  - seizures (in 5 percent of patients)

Anemia of AIDS Treated with Zidovudine

- Moderate to severe anemia is frequent.
- EPO therapy will produce a rise in reticulocyte count and hematocrit after up to 8 weeks of therapy.
- Responses occur in patients who are receiving standard zidovudine doses and have a serum EPO level of less than 500 U/liter.
- Patients with EPO levels greater than 500 U/liter may respond to larger doses.

Anemia of Cancer

- EPO may be of benefit, whether or not patients are receiving chemotherapy, and in patients with marrow infiltration due to lymphoma or myeloma.
- Optimal timing for administering EPO in relation to chemotherapy is not known.
- EPO given to patients with cancer has no important side effects.

Granulocyte-Macrophage Colony-Stimulating Factor (GM-CSF)

- Stimulates growth and maturation of bone marrow progenitors, including granulocyte, erythrocyte, macrophage, and megakaryocyte colony forming units.
- Enhances the function of mature granulocyte and monocyte effector cells.
- Increases the synthesis and secretion of other cytokines.
- Prolongs the survival of neutrophils and eosinophils in vitro.
- May act as a growth factor for leukemic myeloblasts in some patients.

Patients with Normal Hemopoiesis

- Dose dependent increases in neutrophil count occur with GM-CSF administration.
- No consistent changes occur in platelet or reticulocyte counts or hemoglobin levels.
- Monocytes and eosinophils are often increased in number late in the treatment cycle.
- Within minutes of administration, GM-CSF produces transient neutropenia, monocytopenia, and eosinopenia, due to sequestration of cells in the lung, that resolve within 2 h.
- Lowers serum cholesterol, independent of effect on neutrophil count.

Patients with AIDS and Neutropenia

- GM-SCF produces a dose dependent increase in neutrophil count, eosinophil count, and monocyte count.
- Elevated leukocyte count peaks after the first week of therapy and returns to baseline within a week after GM-CSF is stopped.
- GM-CSF administration results in increased HIV production in mononuclear phagocytes. Consequently, should be administered with an antiviral agent in AIDS patients.

Myelodysplastic Syndrome and Neutropenia

- GM-CSF increases the neutrophil, platelet, and red cell count in one-third or fewer of patients with myelodysplastic syndromes.
- In patients with oligoblastic leukemia, it produces a dose dependent increase in neutrophilis and, in some, an increase in marrow myeloblasts.

Chemotherapy and Radiotherapy-Induced Neutropenia

- GM-CSF administered after chemotherapy does not eliminate severe neutropenia, but does produce an earlier and less profound nadir of the neutrophil count, and a shortened duration of neutropenia.
- Allows for more frequent dosing in chemotherapy and for higher doses.

- Has little or no effect on platelet count recovery after chemotherapy.
- When administered after autologous stem cell reinfusion in stem cell transplantation, produces earlier neutrophil recovery, fewer infections, fewer days of antibiotic administration, and fewer days of hospitalization compared to a placebo control.

Blood Progenitor Procurement

- GM-CSF administered after chemotherapy increases the number of blood CFU-GM 60-fold compared to baseline.
- Blood progenitor cells mobilized in this fashion and collected for autologous blood stem cell transplantation shorten the duration of neutropenia and reduce transplant-associated morbidity compared to historical controls.

Adverse Effects of GM-CSF

- Closely correlated with dose.
- Serious side effects include
  - capillary leak syndrome with fluid retention
  - large vessel thrombosis
  - first dose reaction with flushing, hypotension, hypoxia, and tachycardia (may occur in patients receiving nonglycosylated GM-CSF)
- Mild-to-moderate side effects are
  - bone pain, fever, rash, myalgias, local reactions at the injection site, mild transaminase elevations

Granulocyte Colony-Stimulating Factor (G-CSF)

- G-CSF regulates proliferation and maturation of neutrophilic precursors. It may be the primary endogenous regulator of neutrophil production.

Chemotherapy-Induced Neutropenia

- G-CSF produces a dose-dependent increase in blood neutrophils when given 24 h after the last dose of chemotherapy.
- Administration after standard dose chemotherapy may reduce the degree of mucositis and increase the proportion of patients eligible for further doses of chemotherapy. It also reduces the number of days of febrile neutropenia, reduces intravenous antibiotic use, and decreases the incidence of documented infection, all by approximately 50 percent.
- When administered after dose intensive therapy, allows for dose escalation and for drug administration to occur on schedule.
- G-CSF–mobilized blood progenitors when collected and transplanted in autologous stem cell transplants shorten the period of neutropenia and thrombocytopenia compared to marrow transplants alone.

Hereditary, Cyclic, or Chronic Neutropenia

- G-CSF increases the neutrophil count in patients with either congenital, cyclic, or idiopathic neutropenia. This reduces the incidence and duration of infections and decreases the duration of antibiotic use.

Neutropenia Associated with Myeloma, Aplastic Anemia, Hairy Cell Leukemia, Acute Myelogenous Leukemia, or Myelodysplasia

- G-CSF may improve the neutrophil count and reduce the incidence of infection in neutropenic patients with multiple myeloma, moderate severity aplastic anemia, hairy cell leukemia, or myelodysplastic syndrome
- Can accelerate neutrophil recovery in patients with acute myelogenous leukemia with hypocellular marrows induced by chemotherapy.

Adverse Effects of G-CSF

- Most common side effect is bone pain in the sternum, lower back, sacrum, ribs, and lower extremities.
- Mild splenomegaly may occur with chronic use.
- Patients with autoimmune disease may experience a flare of their disease.
- Cutaneous vasculitis is a rare association with G-CSF administration.
- Transient laboratory abnormalities are associated with its use, including increase in serum levels of uric acid, LDH, and alkaline phosphatase, and leukocyte alkaline phosphatase activity.

For a more detailed discussion, see Bruce A. Chabner, Wyndham Wilson: Pharmacology and toxicity of antineoplastic drugs, Chap. 15, p. 143; and Ann A. Jakobowski, David W. Golde: Therapeutic use of cytokines, Chap. 16, p. 155, in *Williams Hematology,* 5/e, 1995.

---

4 APLASTIC ANEMIA

DEFINITION

- Pancytopenia with markedly hypocellular marrow.
- Incidence world wide is 2 to 5 cases/million population/year.
- Severe aplastic anemia has been defined as marrow of less than 25 percent cellularity or less than 50 percent cellularity with less than 30 percent hemopoietic cells, with at least two of the following:
  - absolute neutrophil count of less than 500/μl
  - platelet count of less than 20,000/μl
  - corrected reticulocyte index of less than 1

ETIOLOGY AND PATHOGENESIS

- Mechanisms of pathogenesis:
  - intrinsic stem cell defect
  - failure of stromal microenvironment
  - growth factor defect or deficiency
  - immune suppression of marrow
- Etiologic classification
  - Acquired
    - chemicals, e.g., benzene and related compounds
    - drugs, e.g., chloramphenicol (see Table 4-1 for most frequent offenders; Table 24-2 in *Williams Hematology*, 5/e, provides a more complete list)
    - radiation
    - viruses, e.g., EBV, hepatitis
    - miscellaneous, e.g., connective tissue diseases, pregnancy
  - Hereditary
    - Fanconi anemia
      - autosomal recessive
      - abnormal skin pigmentation, skeletal abnormalities, renal anomalies, microcephaly

TABLE 4-1 Drugs Associated with Moderate Risk of Aplastic Anemia*

Gold salts
Penicillamine
Phenylbutazone
Oxyphenbutazone
Carbamazepine
Hydantoins
Chloramphenicol
Quinacrine
Acetazolamide

*Drugs with 30 or more reported cases.
Source: Adapted from Table 24-2 of *Williams Hematology*, p. 241.

- chromosome fragility, especially after exposure to DNA cross-linking agents such as diepoxybutane (used as a diagnostic test)
- Dyskeratosis congenita may evolve into aplastic anemia.
- Schwachman-Diamond syndrome may evolve into aplastic anemia.
- Idiopathic (about 65 percent of patients)

CLINICAL FEATURES

- Fatigue, bleeding, or infections as a consequence of cytopenias.
- Physical examination generally is unrevealing except for signs of anemia, bleeding, or infection.

LABORATORY FEATURES

- Pancytopenia
- Low reticulocyte index; red cells may be macrocytic.
- Markedly hypocellular marrow.
- Absolute neutrophil count low (if <200, prognosis is extremely poor).
- Abnormal cytogenetic findings suggest hypoplastic myelodysplastic syndrome rather than aplastic anemia.
- Negative sucrose hemolysis test to rule out PNH.

DIFFERENTIAL DIAGNOSIS OF PANCYTOPENIA AND HYPOPLASTIC MARROW

- Hypoplastic myelodysplastic syndrome
- Paroxysmal nocturnal hemoglobinuria
- Hypoplastic acute lymphocytic leukemia
- Hairy cell leukemia

CLINICAL COURSE

- Median survival of untreated severe aplastic anemia is 3 to 6 months (20 percent survive longer than 1 year).

TREATMENT

- Marrow transplantation is curative:
- Indicated in patients less than 40 years of age with an HLA-related matched or 1 antigen mismatched donor.
- Only one-third of patients have a suitable donor.
- 75 to 85 percent of previously untransfused patients achieve cure with appropriate donor.
- 55 to 60 percent of multiply transfused patients achieve cure with appropriate donor.
- Immunosuppressive therapy: not curative.
  - Antithymocyte globulin (ATG)

- 50 percent response rate
- dose: 15 to 40 mg/kg daily intravenously for 4 to 10 days
- fever, chills common on first day of treatment
- accelerated platelet destruction with thrombocytopenia frequent
- serum sickness common with fever, rash, and arthralgias occurring 7 to 10 days after beginning treatment
- Cyclosporine (CSP)
  - primary treatment or in patients refractory to ATG
  - dose: 3 to 7 mg/kg daily orally for at least 4 to 6 months
  - dose adjusted to maintain proper blood levels
  - renal impairment common side effect
  - 25 percent of patients respond overall (range of response is 0 to 80 percent)
- Combinations
  - ATG + CSP may yield an improved response rate.
  - As high as 57 percent of patients in one series showed long term sequelae of immunosuppressive therapy after 8 years, such as:
    - recurrent aplasia
    - PNH
    - acute myelogenous leukemia
    - myelodysplastic syndrome
- Androgen as primary therapy has not been efficacious in severe or moderate aplastic anemia.
- Hemopoietic growth factors have been used to treat neutropenia.
  - Temporary improvement in neutrophil counts has been observed with GM-CSF or G-CSF treatment in some patients.
  - IL-3 gave temporary improvement in the absolute neutrophil count in a few patients.
  - IL-1 was not effective in a small group of patients.
- Supportive care
  - Immediate HLA typing of patient and siblings as possible marrow donors.
  - Minimal or no transfusions in potential transplant recipients.
  - If transfusions are needed, do not use family donors in a potential transplant recipient.
  - Transfuse platelets based on assessment of risk of bleeding, and not solely on platelet count.
  - Single donor platelets should be used to minimize HLA sensitization and subsequent refractoriness.
  - Use of leukocyte-depleted blood products helps to reduce sensitization.
  - Transfuse packed RBC's (irradiated, leukocyte-depleted) when hemoglobin level is less than 7 to 8 g/dl.
  - Obtain CMV serology for prospective transplant recipients; transfuse only CMV-negative blood products until these results are known. If the patient is CMV⁺, can discontinue these precautions.

Use of leukocyte depletion filters also decreases risk of CMV acquisition.

- Neutropenic precautions for hospitalized patients with absolute neutrophil counts of less than 500.
- Prompt institution of broad spectrum IV antibiotics for fever after appropriate cultures have been obtained.

For a more detailed discussion, see Richard A. Shadduck: Aplastic anemia, Chap. 24, p. 238, in *Williams Hematology,* 5/e, 1995.

---

5 PAROXYSMAL NOCTURNAL HEMOGLOBINURIA (PNH)

DEFINITION

- An acquired hemopoietic stem cell disorder.
- Central diagnostic feature is increased sensitivity of red blood cells to the hemolytic action of complement.

ETIOLOGY AND PATHOGENESIS

- Appears to arise as a clonal abnormality of stem cells.
- The classic abnormality is increased sensitivity to complement-mediated lysis of erythrocytes, detected by different tests:
  - acid hemolysis test
  - sucrose hemolysis test
- Several populations of cells of different sensitivity to complement have been identified in some patients.
- The disorder appears to be a consequence of somatic mutations which cause an error in synthesis of the glycosylphosphatidylinositol (GPI) anchor.
- Deficiencies in several GPI-anchored membrane proteins, such as decay accelerating factor (DAF), CD59, CD58, CD16, and CD14, have been identified.
- Absence of CD59 antigen (membrane inhibitor of reactive lysis; MIRL) identified. This absence plays the most critical role.

CLINICAL FEATURES

- Nocturnal hemoglobinuria is uncommon.
- Hemoglobinuria occurs irregularly in most patients, precipitated by a variety of events including infection, surgery, or contrast dye injection.
- Patients have chronic hemolytic anemia, which may be severe.
- Modest splenomegaly in some patients.
- Iron deficiency due to iron loss in the urine.
- Bleeding may occur secondary to thrombocytopenia.
- Thrombosis is a prominent feature.
  - Venous thromboses occur frequently.
  - Arterial thromboses also occur.
  - Budd-Chiari syndrome often observed.
  - Pulmonary hypertension may develop secondary to thromboses in the pulmonary microvasculature.
- Pregnancy in PNH patients may be associated with abortion and venous thromboembolism.
- Renal manifestations include:
  - hyposthenuria

- abnormal tubular function
- acute and chronic renal failure
- Neurologic manifestations:
  - headaches
  - cerebral venous thrombosis uncommon

LABORATORY FEATURES

- Anemia may be severe with hemoglobin levels of less than 5 g/dl.
- Macrocytosis may be present due to mild to moderate reticulocytosis.
- May be hypochromic and microcytic due to iron deficiency.
- Low leukocyte count is characteristic.
- Low platelet count common; normal in about 20 percent.
- Marrow examination usually shows erthroid hyperplasia; marrow cellularity is not greatly increased, and marrow may be aplastic.
- Urine:
  - hemoglobin sometimes present
  - hemosiderinuria a constant feature and of diagnostic importance
- Decreased leukocyte alkaline phosphatase activity.
- Sucrose hemolysis test and Ham acid hemolysis test positive.

DIFFERENTIAL DIAGNOSIS

- Consider PNH in patients with pancytopenia, particularly when accompanied by reticulocytosis.
- Screening tests:
  - urine for hemosiderinuria
  - sucrose hemolysis test (Ham acid hemolysis test to confirm positive result)

TREATMENT

- Transfusion for anemia: washed red cells (avoids transfusing complement in plasma)
- Oral iron therapy for iron deficiency
- Steroids:
  - androgens of some benefit in increasing hemoglobin level: Fluoxymesterone 20 to 30 mg orally daily
  - prednisone useful in some patients to reduce transfusion requirement: 20 to 60 mg orally every other day
- Anticoagulants:
  - no role for prophylactic anticoagulation
  - useful in management of thrombotic complications, e.g., Budd-Chiari syndrome

- Splenectomy not indicated.
- Marrow transplantation is curative.

COURSE

- Variable, but most patients succumb to complications.
- Acute leukemia, aplastic anemia, or myelodysplastic syndrome may develop in a small number of patients.

For a more detailed discussion, see Ernest Beutler: Paroxysmal nocturnal hemoglobinuria, Chap. 25, p. 252; and Sucrose hemolysis and acidified-serum lysis test, Chap. L15, p. 248, in *Williams Hematology,* 5/e, 1995.

---

6 MYELODYSPLASTIC DISORDERS

DEFINITION

- An abnormal, clonal proliferation of marrow cells characterized clinically by varying degrees of cytopenia and pathologically by maturation defects in one or more cell lines. It merges into acute leukemia and includes "preleukemia" and "oligoblastic leukemia."
- "Preleukemia" (refractory anemia, see FAB classification, below) refers to clonal proliferation of marrow pluripotential stem cells without blast cells in the marrow or blood. The manifestations vary from isolated anemia with a nearly normal marrow to severe pancytopenia with hypercellular marrow.
- "Oligoblastic leukemia" (refractory anemia with excess blasts, see FAB classification, below) refers to clonal proliferation of marrow stem cells with greater than 3 percent blast cells in the marrow.
- Classification is difficult because of the numerous clinical syndromes which comprise the myelodysplastic disorders. The French-American-British (FAB) classification recognizes five subsets:

  1. Refractory anemia (RA)
  2. Refractory anemia with ringed sideroblasts (RARS)
  3. Refractory anemia with excess blasts (RAEB)
  4. Refractory anemia with excess blasts in transformation (RAEBT)
  5. Chronic myelomonocytic leukemia (CMML)

ETIOLOGY AND PATHOGENESIS

- May be due to retroviral action and/or mutation of cellular protooncogenes.
- Exposure to benzene, chemotherapeutic agents, or radiation can cause myelodysplastic disorders.
- Pathophysiology is defective maturation coupled with enhanced proliferation of precursor cells.

CLINICAL FEATURES

- Onset usually after age 50; earlier if preceded by chemotherapy or irradiation.
- May be asymptomatic, or have symptoms due to anemia, granulocytopenia, and/or thrombocytopenia.

LABORATORY FEATURES

- Anemia in more than 85 percent, may be macrocytic, with circulating nucleated red cells. Hemoglobin F levels may be increased, hemoglobin H may be present, and red cell enzymes may be abnormal.
- Neutropenia occurs in about 50 percent. Coarse chromatin and nuclear

38

hyposegmentation (acquired Pelger-Huët abnormality) and decreased cytoplasmic granules commonly occur.

- Monocytosis often found and may be the only abnormality.
- Thrombocytopenia or mild thrombocytosis may be present. Platelets may be large, with decreased or fused granules. Platelet aggregation tests may be abnormal.
- Marrow abnormalities include hypercellularity, delayed nuclear maturation, abnormal cytoplasmic maturation, abnormal sideroblasts, including ringed sideroblasts, megakaryocytes with uni- or bilobed nuclei, micromegakaryocytes, and increased numbers of myeloblasts. The following blast counts have been proposed for the FAB classification:

1. Refractory anemia (RA): marrow blasts <5 percent; no blasts in blood
2. Refractory anemia with ringed sideroblasts (RARS): marrow blasts <5 percent; >15 percent of marrow erythroid precursors are ringed sideroblasts
3. Refractory anemia with excess blasts (RAEB): marrow blasts 5 to 19 percent; <5 percent blasts in blood
4. Refractory anemia with excess blasts in transition (RAEBT): marrow blasts 20 to 29 percent, or 5 to 29 percent blasts in blood, or Auer rods present
5. Chronic myelomonocytic leukemia (CMML): marrow blasts <20 percent; <5 percent blasts in blood; monocytes >1000/μl in blood

- Chromosomal abnormalities occur in up to 80 percent. Common abnormalities are +8; loss of long arm of 5, 7, 9, 20, or 21; and monosomy 7 or 9.

SPECIFIC PRELEUKEMIC SYNDROMES

Acquired Refractory Sideroblastic Anemia *(FAB: RARS)*

- Predominant abnormalities are ineffective erythropoiesis with impaired heme synthesis and mitochondrial iron overload.
- Most patients are over 50 years of age and have signs and symptoms of anemia.
- Anemia may be mild to severe, macrocytic, with dimorphic red cells (hypochromic and normochromic) on blood film, and no appropriate reticulocyte response.
- Serum iron levels and ferritin levels, as well as saturation of transferrin, are increased. Marrow storage iron is increased.
- Marrow cellularity is increased, with defective cytoplasmic maturation of erythroblasts, and many ringed sideroblasts are present.
- Therapeutic trial with folic acid and pyridoxine should be attempted, but success is unlikely. Transfusion may be necessary.
- Disorder may not progress for many years. Some patients develop

hemochromatosis and about 10 percent develop acute myelogenous leukemia.

Acquired Refractory Nonsideroblastic Anemia *(FAB: RA)*

- Similar to sideroblastic anemia but without a significant number of sideroblasts in the marrow.

Pancytopenia with Hypercellular Marrow

- About two-thirds of patients with preleukemia present with neutropenia and/or thrombocytopenia as well as anemia.
- The blood and marrow findings are as described for acquired refractory nonsideroblastic anemia, above.
- May be seen in patients with AIDS, but progression to acute leukemia has not been reported.
- Blood component transfusions as needed are mainstays of treatment. Therapeutic trials with erythropoietin, GM-CSF, G-CSF, or IL-3 may be beneficial, but these could enhance leukemic progression and do not prolong survival.
- Median survival is about 20 months. AML develops in about 50 percent, and about 25 percent die of infection or hemorrhage.

The 5q-Syndrome

- Patients have refractory anemia, with marrow abnormalities of dyserythropoiesis, erythroid multinuclearity, and hypolobulated small megakaryocytes.
- Marrow cells have deletion of long arm of chromosome 5, the locus of several genes that encode for hemopoietic growth factors.
- Clinical course as for other patients with refractory anemia, including risk of developing leukemia.

OLIGOBLASTIC LEUKEMIAS

Definition

- Patients have 5 to 30 percent leukemic blasts in the marrow and 0 to 10 percent in the blood and survive for months or years without specific antileukemic therapy. Also known as "smouldering acute leukemia."

Refractory Anemia with Excess Myeloblasts *(FAB: RAEB)*

- Patients are usually over 50 years of age, with cytopenias or qualitative cellular abnormalities, as in preleukemia.
- Subclassified by FAB group as RAEB (5 to 19 percent blasts in marrow) and RAEB in transition (20 to 29 percent marrow blasts).

- Evolves into overt acute myelogenous leukemia in 30 to 50 percent of cases. Median survival is 5 to 10 months.

Chronic Myelomonocytic Leukemia *(FAB: CMML)*

- About 75 percent of cases are over 60 years of age.
- Hepatomegaly and splenomegaly occur in about 40 percent.
- Usually anemia and monocytosis ($>1000/\mu l$) are present. Less than 10 percent myeloblasts in blood.
- Marrow is hypercellular, with granulomonocytic hyperplasia.
- Myeloblasts and promyelocytes are increased but are less than 30 percent of cells in marrow.
- Plasma and urine lysozyme concentrations are nearly always elevated.
- *RAS* gene mutations are frequent. Includes most cases of so-called Philadelphia chromosome–negative, breakpoint cluster region–negative chronic myelogenous leukemia.

Median survival is 20 months.

Treatment

- Therapy is complex and is presented in detail in Chap. 26 of *Williams Hematology*, 5/e.
- Low-dose cytosine arabinoside, which may induce maturation of cells, induces remission in about 20 percent of cases, with median duration of 10 months.
- Other cytotoxic drugs, maturation-enhancing agents, interferons, and growth factors have been used.
- Marrow transplantation has yielded more favorable results than other therapies.

Prodromal Syndromes Antedating Lymphocytic Leukemia

- Aplastic marrow may rarely be a prodrome of acute lymphocytic leukemia.
- More likely to occur in females.
- Marrow shows fibrosis and lymphocytosis.
- Spontaneous, temporary recovery is frequent.

For a more detailed discussion, see Marshall A. Lichtman, James K. Brennan: Myelodysplastic disorders, Chap. 26, p. 257, in *Williams Hematology*, 5/e, 1995.

---

7 ACUTE MYELOGENOUS LEUKEMIA

Acute myelogenous leukemia (AML) is a clonal malignancy of hemopoietic tissue characterized by proliferation of abnormal blast cells in the marrow and impaired production of normal blood cells, resulting in anemia and thrombocytopenia. It occurs in several morphologic variants, each with characteristic clinical and laboratory features.

ETIOLOGY AND PATHOGENESIS

- Three environmental factors—high-dose radiation, chronic benzene exposure, and treatment with alkylating agents or other cytotoxic drugs—have been established as causative agents. Other possible environmental factors remain unproven.
- The chronic myeloproliferative disorders (see Chaps. 8 to 11) and the preleukemic syndromes (see Chap. 6) may progress to AML.
- AML may develop in patients with AIDS, Down or Bloom syndrome, or Fanconi anemia.
- Genetic alterations, reflected in chromosome abnormalities, occur in many patients with AML. Familial occurrence has been reported, but its significance is unknown.

EPIDEMIOLOGY

- AML accounts for 80 percent of acute leukemias in adults and 15 to 20 percent in children.
- AML is the most frequent leukemia in neonates.

CLINICAL FEATURES

- Frequent presenting symptoms and signs are those of anemia: pallor, fatigue, weakness, palpitations, and dyspnea on exertion; or of thrombocytopenia; bruising, petechiae, epistaxis, gingival bleeding, conjunctival hemorrhages, and prolonged bleeding after minor cuts.
- Minor pyogenic infections of the skin are common.
- Anorexia and weight loss may occur.
- Fever may be present at onset.
- Splenomegaly or hepatomegaly are present in about one-third of patients. Lymph node enlargement is uncommon, except with the monocytic variant.
- Leukemic cells may infiltrate any organ in the body, but consequent organ dysfunction is unusual. Occasionally large accumulations of myeloblasts or monoblasts (*granulocytic sarcoma*) may develop.

LABORATORY FEATURES

- Anemia and thrombocytopenia are nearly always present.
- Total leukocyte count is below 5000/μl in about one-half of patients,

and the absolute neutrophil count is less than 1000/μl in over one-half of patients at diagnosis. Mature neutrophils may be hyper- or hyposegmented, or hypogranular.

- Myeloblasts comprise from 3 to 95 percent of the leukocytes in the blood, and from 1 to 10 percent of the blast cells contain Auer rods in about one-third of patients.
- Marrow contains leukemic blast cells, identified by reactivity with cytochemical stains, presence of Auer rods, or reactivity with antibodies to epitopes specific for myeloblasts.
- Cytogenetic abnormalities are present in about one-half of patients.
- Serum uric acid and lactic dehydrogenase levels are frequently elevated.
- Electrolyte abnormalities are infrequent, but severe hypokalemia may occur, and spurious hyperkalemia may be found in patients with very high leukocyte counts.
- Patients with very high leukocyte counts may also have spurious hypoglycemia and hypoxia due to consumption by the blast cells after the specimen was obtained.
- Hypercalcemia and hypophosphatemia may be present.

HYPERLEUKOCYTOSIS

- Signs and symptoms due to extreme elevations of the leukocyte count, usually to greater than 100,000/μl, appear in about 5 percent of patients.
- Leukostasis is most likely to occur in the circulation of the central nervous system, leading to intracerebral hemorrhage; in the lungs, resulting in pulmonary insufficiency; or in the penis, causing priapism.

UNUSUAL PRESENTATIONS OF AML

- Hypoplastic leukemia. AML may present with pancytopenia and a hypoplastic marrow.
- Oligoblastic (smoldering) leukemia. The disease may present with anemia and thrombocytopenia and a few blast cells in the blood and marrow. This disorder is often considered a myelodysplastic syndrome and is discussed in Chap. 6.
- Transient myeloproliferation, i.e., markedly elevated leukocyte count with blast cells in the blood and marrow, present at birth or appearing shortly thereafter and resolving slowly over weeks or months without treatment.
- Similar cases with a transient cytogenetic abnormality may resolve and then appear as acute leukemia. Such disorders are referred to as *transient leukemia.*
- Apparently normal newborns may have congenital or neonatal leukemia, but the syndrome is 10 times more common in babies with Down syndrome.

TABLE 7-1 Morphologic Variants of AML

Variant	FAB classification	Cytologic features
Acute myeloblastic leukemia	M1—myeloblastic M2—myeloblastic with differentiation	1. Myeloblasts are usually large, with moderate nuclear cyto-plasmic ratio. Cytoplasm usually contains granules and occasion-ally Auer rods. Nucleus shows fine reticular pattern and dis-tinct nucleoli. 2. Leukemic cells are sudanophi-lic. They are positive for myelo-peroxidase and chloracetate es-terase, negative for nonspecific esterase, and negative or dif-fusely positive for PAS (no clumps or blocks). 3. Electron microscope (EM) shows primary cytoplasmic granules. 4. Differentiation is neutrophilic, rarely basophilic.
Acute promyelocytic leukemia	M3	1. Leukemic cells resemble promy-elocytes. They have large atypi-cal primary granules and a kid-ney-shaped nucleus. Branched or multiple Auer rods are common. 2. Histochemical features similar to those in AML. Peroxidase in-tensely positive. 3. A variant has microgranules, otherwise the same course and prognosis.
Acute myelomonocytic leukemia	M4	1. Both myeloblastic and mono-blastic leukemic cells in blood and marrow. 2. Peroxidase-, Sudan-, chloroace-tate esterase-, and nonspecific esterase-positive cells. 3. Variant has marrow eosinophilia with abnormal eosinophils present.

(cont.)

Source: Table 27-4 of Williams Hematology, 5/e, p. 278.

Special clinical features	Special laboratory features
1. Most common in adults and most frequent variety in infants 2. About 50% of cases	1. Chromosomes +8, −5, −7, common 2. AML with maturation often associated with t(8;21) karyotype
1. Usually in adults 2. Fibrinolysis common 3. Leukemic cells mature in response to all-*trans* retinoic acid 4. About 10% of cases	1. t(15;17) karyotype 2. HLA-DR-negative
1. Similar to myeloblastic leukemia but with more frequent extramedullary disease 2. Slightly elevated serum and urine muramidase 3. About 15% of cases	1. Eosinophilic variant has inversion or other abnormalities of chromosome 16.

(*cont.*)

TABLE 7-1 Morphologic Variants of AML (*Continued*)

Variant	FAB classification	Cytologic features
Acute monocytic leukemia	M5	1. Leukemic cells are large and often bizarre; low nuclear cytoplasmic ratio. Cytoplasm contains fine granules. Auer rods are rare. Nucleus is often convoluted and contains 1 to 4 large nucleoli. 2. Histochemically, nonspecific esterase-positive inhibited by NaF; Sudan-, peroxidase-, and chloro-acetate esterase negative. PAS occurs in granules and blocks. 3. Cytoplasmic microfibrils demonstrable by EM.
Acute erythroleukemia	M6	1. Abnormal erythroblasts are in abundance initially in marrow and often in blood. Later the morphologic findings are indistinguishable from those of AML. 2. Erythroblasts are often strongly PAS-positive
Acute megakaryocytic leukemia	M7	1. Large and small megakaryoblasts with high nuclear cytoplasmic ratio, cytoplasm agranular or containing fine pink granules. 2. Peroxidase-negative, platelet peroxidase-positive, occasionally strongly PAS-positive.

- Hybrid (biphenotypic) leukemias are those in which individual cells may have both myeloid and lymphoid markers (chimeric), or in which individual cells may have either myeloid or lymphoid markers but appear to arise from the same clone (mosaic). In some cases, individual cells may have markers for two or more myeloid lineages, such as granulocytic and megakaryocytic.
- Mixed leukemias have myeloid and lymphoid cells present simultaneously, each derived from a separate clone.
- Mediastinal germ cell tumors and AML may coexist, and there is

Special clinical features	Special laboratory features
1. Usually in children or young adults 2. Gum, CNS, lymph node, and extramedullary infiltrations are common. 3. DIC occurs. 4. Plasma and urine muramidase moderately elevated. 5. About 10% of cases	1. t(4;11) common in infants
1. May have long prodromal period. 2. About 5% of cases	
1. High blood blast counts and organ infiltration are rare. 2. Markedly elevated serum lactic dehydrogenase levels 3. Marrow aspirates are usually "dry taps" because of the invariable presence of myelofibrosis. 4. Common phenotype in the AML of Down syndrome 5. About 5% of cases	1. Antigens of von Willebrand factor, and glycoprotein Ib, IIb/IIIa, IIIa on blast cells

evidence for a clonal relationship between the neoplastic cells of the two diseases.

MORPHOLOGICAL VARIANTS OF AML

- Features of the morphological variants of AML are presented in Table 7-1.
- Eosinophilic leukemia, a rare form of AML with large numbers of eosinophilic cells in the blood and marrow.

- Basophilic leukemia, also rare, may evolve from chronic myelogenous leukemia or arise *de novo*.
- Mast cell leukemia, rare, may arise from systemic mastocytosis (see Chap. 46).

DIFFERENTIAL DIAGNOSIS

- Extensive proliferation of promyelocytes in the marrow may occur upon recovery from agranulocytosis induced by drugs or bacterial infection and may mimic acute promyelocytic leukemia. This condition resolves spontaneously and has been called *pseudoleukemia*.
- In patients with hypoplastic marrows it may be difficult to differentiate acute leukemia, aplastic anemia, and preleukemia. Careful evaluation of marrow cytology should permit correct diagnosis.
- Leukemoid reactions and nonleukemic pancytopenias do not have leukemic myeloblasts in the marrow.

THERAPY, COURSE, AND PROGNOSIS

- Patient and the family must be fully informed about the nature of the disease, the treatment, and all the potential side effects of the treatment.
- Treatment should be initiated as soon as possible after diagnosis, unless the patients is too sick from unrelated illnesses.
- Associated problems such as hemorrhage, infection, or anemia should be treated concurrently.
- Pretreatment laboratory studies must be obtained to establish a specific diagnosis and to evaluate the general condition of the patient, including blood chemistry tests, radiographic examinations, and cardiac studies. Hemostasis must also be evaluated, in detail if screening tests show any abnormalities, if severe thrombocytopenia is present, or if the patient has acute promyelocytic or monocytic leukemia.
- An indwelling central venous catheter should be inserted surgically prior to beginning treatment.
- Treatment with allopurinol, 300 to 600 mg daily, orally or intravenously, should be given if the serum uric acid level is greater than 7 mg/dl, if the marrow is hypercellular with increased blast cells, or if the blood blast cell count is moderately or markedly elevated. Therapy may be discontinued after cytoreduction.
- Exposure to pathogenic infectious agents should be minimized by handwashing by attendants, meticulous care of the intravenous catheter, assignment to an unshared room, and avoidance of fresh fruits, vegetables, and flowers.

Remission Induction Therapy

- Cytotoxic chemotherapy is based on the concept that the marrow contains two competing populations of cells (leukemic and normal) and that profound suppression of the leukemic cells such that they can no longer be detected morphologically in marrow aspirates or biopsies is necessary in order to permit recovery of normal hemopoiesis.

- Therapy is usually initiated with two or more drugs, including an anthracycline or anthraquinone antibiotic and cytosine arabinoside (see Table 27-5 in *Williams Hematology*, 5/e, p. 283).
- Response is less likely to occur in older patients or in those who have AML induced by prior chemo- or radiotherapy, or in patients who had an antecedent preleukemia syndrome.
- Patients with leukocyte counts of $100,000/\mu l$ or more should be treated to achieve rapid cytoreduction using hydroxyurea 1.5 to 2.5 g orally every 6 h for about 36 h. Leukapheresis can accelerate reduction of the white count (see Chap. 87). Hydration sufficient to maintain urine flow of at least 100 ml/h/m^2 is necessary during the first few days.
- About 80 percent of patients with acute promyelocytic leukemia will develop complete remissions when treated with all-*trans* retinoic acid, but require subsequent cytotoxic therapy for sustained remission.
- Neutropenic fever is an expected complication of cytotoxic therapy and requires antibiotic therapy (see Chap. 2).
- Red cell and platelet transfusions are regularly required. Patients who are candidates for allogeneic marrow transplantation should receive cytomegalovirus-negative blood products unless they are known to be positive carriers.
- Patients with evidence of intravascular coagulation or excessive fibrinolysis should be treated for those conditions (see Chaps. 79 and 80).

Remission Maintenance Therapy

- Intensive cytotoxic chemotherapy after remission (consolidation) results in longer duration of remission. A proportion of patients remain in remission for more than 2 years.
- A combination of intensive chemotherapy and autologous marrow transplantation is currently under investigation.
- Allogeneic marrow transplantation for patients with AML in remission is also under investigation. Using current criteria, only about 10 percent of patients with AML are of appropriate age for transplantation and have a sibling donor available. A high proportion of patients have disease-free survival of 4 years or longer after transplantation, but about one-third of the patients die in the immediate posttransplant period of complications of the transplantation procedure.
- Allogeneic marrow transplantation in patients with AML in second remission can induce long-term survival in about 25 percent. Treatment with chemotherapy alone in this group is unlikely to be successful.

Relapsed or Refractory Patients

- Patients who relapse more than 6 months after initial treatment can be given the same treatment again.
- Another therapy for relapsed patients is high-dose cytosine arabinoside with or without additional drug(s).
- Marrow transplantation may be done in relapsed or refractory patients. About 10 percent of such AML patients can be cured, and about 25 percent achieve remissions of at least 3 years with marrow transplantation.

Special Therapeutic Considerations

- It may be necessary to reduce the dose of cytotoxic drugs administered to patients over 60 years of age.
- Treatment of pregnant patients in the first trimester with antimetabolites increases the risk of congenital anomalies in the infant. However, babies born after intensive chemotherapy in the second and third trimesters appear to develop normally.
- Intensive chemotherapy has been used successfully in patients less than 17 years of age. Children under 2 do not respond well to chemotherapy and should be considered for marrow transplantation.

Special Nonhemopoietic Adverse Effects of Treatment

- Skin rashes develop in over 50 percent of the patients with AML during chemotherapy, often due to one of the following drugs: allopurinol, β-lactam antibiotics, cytosine arabinoside, trimethoprim-sulfamethoxazole, miconazole, and ketoconozole.
- Cardiomyopathy may develop in patients receiving anthracycline antibiotics (see Chap. 2).
- Systemic candidiasis syndrome presents with fever, abdominal pain, and hepatomegaly and is associated with multiple hepatic candidiasis lesions detected radiographically or by ultrasound. Responds to prolonged therapy with amphotericin B.
- Patients receiving intensive cytotoxic therapy may develop necrotizing inflammation of the cecum (typhlitis) which may require surgical intervention.
- Thrombotic thrombocytopenic purpura has developed in patients with AML during consolidation therapy.
- Fertility may be sustained in both men and women undergoing intensive cytotoxic therapy.

Results of Treatment

- Using current therapeutic approaches remission rates approach 90 percent in children, 70 percent in young adults, 50 percent in the middle aged, and 25 percent in the elderly.

- Median survival is about 12 months. If remission is obtained, about 25 percent of patients will survive for at least 2 years, and about 10 percent for at least 5 years.
- Relapse or development of a new leukemia has occurred after 8 years in adults and 16 years in children.

Features Influencing the Outcome of Therapy

- Both the probability of remission and the duration of response decrease with increased age at the time of diagnosis.
- Cytogenetic abnormalities such as inv(16), t(8;21), or trisomy 21 may indicate better prognosis, while $5-$, $7-$, $5q-$, $7q-$, etc. indicate a poorer prognosis.
- AML that develops after prior cytotoxic therapy for another disease, or after a myelodysplastic (preleukemia) syndrome, has a significantly lower remission rate and shorter remission duration.
- A leukocyte count of greater than 30,000/μl or a blast cell count above 15,000/μl decreases the probability and the duration of remission.
- Many other laboratory findings are correlated with decreased remission rate or duration.

For a more detailed discussion, see Marshall A. Lichtman: Acute myelogenous leukemia, Chap. 27, p. 272, in *Williams Hematology,* 5/e, 1995.

8 CHRONIC MYELOGENOUS LEUKEMIA AND RELATED DISORDERS

Chronic myelogenous leukemia (CML) is a hemopoietic stem cell disorder characterized by granulocytic leukocytosis and immaturity, basophilia, anemia, thrombocytosis, and splenomegaly. The disease frequently develops an accelerated phase that resembles acute myelogenous leukemia.

ETIOLOGY

- Exposure to ionizing radiation increases the incidence of CML, after a latent period which ranges from 4 to 11 years in different populations.
- Chemical agents have not been implicated.

PATHOGENESIS

- CML, an acquired disorder, is due to malignant transformation of a single stem cell. The Philadelphia chromosome (see below) is present in erythroid, neutrophilic, eosinophilic, basophilic, monocytic, megakaryocytic, and probably B lymphocytic cells, suggesting the cell of origin may be a pluripotential stem cell.
- Over 90 percent of patients with CML have a reciprocal translocation between chromosomes 9 and 22 that results in visible shortening of the long arms of one of the no. 22 chromosome pair (22,22q−). The abnormal chromosome is referred to as the *Philadelphia (Ph) chromosome* [t (9,22)(q 34; q 11)].
- Probably all patients with CML have a rearrangement of the breakpoint cluster region on the long arm of chromosome 22, even those who do not have a detectable Ph chromosome.
- The translocation from chromosome 9 leads to fusion between a portion of the *BCR* gene on chromosome 22 with a segment of the *ABL* gene from chromosome 9. This chimeric gene directs the synthesis of a novel 210-kD tyrosine phosphoprotein kinase that has been postulated to be responsible for the transformation to CML.
- In CML there is a marked expansion of granulocytic progenitors and a decreased sensitivity of the progenitors to regulation. The enlargement of the blood granulocyte pool is primarily due to increased granulopoiesis.

EPIDEMIOLOGY

- CML accounts for about 20 percent of all cases of leukemia and about 3 percent of childhood leukemia.

CLINICAL FEATURES

- Symptoms are gradual in onset and include easy fatigability, malaise, anorexia, abdominal discomfort and early satiety, weight loss, and excessive sweating.
- Less frequent symptoms are those of hypermetabolism, such as night sweats, heat intolerance, and weight loss, mimicking hyperthyroidism; gouty arthritis; priapism, tinnitus, or stupor from leukostasis due to hyperleukocytosis; left upper quadrant and left shoulder pain due to splenic infarction; diabetes insipidus; and urticaria due to histamine release.
- Physical signs may be pallor, splenomegaly, and sternal tenderness.
- The disease is sometimes discovered incidentally when a blood count is done for a routine evaluation.

LABORATORY FEATURES

- The leukocyte count is elevated, usually above $25,000/\mu l$, and often above $100,000/\mu l$. Granulocytes at all stages of development are present in the blood, but mature neutrophils and bands predominate. Hypersegmented neutrophils are often present.
- An increase in the absolute basophil count is found in virtually all patients. Basophils usually comprise less than 10 to 15 percent of leukocytes in the chronic phase but occasionally make up a much higher proportion. The absolute eosinophil count may also be increased.
- The hematocrit is decreased in most patients at the time of diagnosis. Nucleated red cells are often seen on the stained blood film.
- The platelet count is normal or increased at diagnosis but may increase during the course of the chronic phase, often reaching $1,000,000/\mu l$ and sometimes as much as $5,000,000$ to $7,000,000/\mu l$.
- Neutrophil alkaline phosphatase activity is low or absent in over 90 percent of patients. It may also be low in paroxysmal nocturnal hemoglobinuria, hypophosphatasia, with androgen therapy, and in about 25 percent of patients with myelofibrosis.
- The marrow is markedly hypercellular, primarily due to granulocytic hyperplasia. Megakaryocytes may be increased in number. Sea-blue histiocytes and cells which look like Gaucher cells may be present.
- Reticulin fibrosis may be prominent in the marrow and is correlated with the number of megakaryocytes.
- The Ph chromosome is present in about 90 to 95 percent of patients. The remaining patients have variant translocations or molecular abnormalities of the long arm of chromosome 22.
- Hyperuricemia and hyperuricosuria are frequent.
- Serum vitamin B_{12} binding protein and serum vitamin B_{12} levels are increased in proportion to the total leukocyte count.
- Serum lactic dehydrogenase activity is elevated.

- Pseudohyperkalemia may be due to release of potassium from granulo-cytes, and spurious hypoxemia and hypoglycemia may result from cellular utilization.
- Serum cholesterol levels are reduced in CML.

HYPERLEUKOCYTOSIS

- About 15 percent of patients will present with leukocyte counts of $300,000/\mu l$ or higher and signs and symptoms of leukostasis from impaired microcirculation in the lungs, brain, eyes, ears, or penis. Patients may have tachypnea, dyspnea, cyanosis, dizziness, slurred speech, delirium, stupor, visual blurring, diplopia, retinal vein disten-sion, retinal hemorrhages, papilledema, tinnitus, impaired hearing, or priapism.
- Hyperleukocytosis usually responds rapidly to leukapheresis and hy-droxyurea therapy.

DIFFERENTIAL DIAGNOSIS

- The diagnosis of CML is made on the basis of granulocytosis with immaturity of the cells, basophilia, and splenomegaly, coupled with demonstration of the Ph chromosome or a *BCR* rearrangement on the long arm of chromosome 22.
- Closely overlapping clinical features may be found in polycythemia vera, idiopathic myelofibrosis, and primary thrombocythemia, but the diagnosis can usually be made from associated findings, and particularly by the absence in the other diseases of the characteristic chromosomal abnormalities of CML.
- Some patients who appear to have essential (primary) thrombocy-themia may have the Ph chromosome and *BCR-ABL* rearrangement and only later develop clinical CML or blast crisis.
- Extreme reactive leukocytosis (leukemoid reaction) may occur in patients with an inflammatory disease, cancer, or infection and is not associated with basophilia, granulocytic immaturity, or splenomegaly. The neutrophil alkaline phosphatase activity is elevated in the leukem-oid reactions, and the chromosomal abnormalities of CML are absent.

TREATMENT

- Patients should receive allopurinol, 300 mg/day orally and adequate hydration before and during therapy to minimize the possibility of hyperuricemia and its complications.
- Hematological improvement may be obtained in nearly all patients with oral therapy with hydroxyurea or busulfan. Hydroxyurea is pre-ferred because it is less toxic, provides longer median survival than busulfan, and may permit greater success with subsequent transplanta-tion therapy.

- Busulfan is given at a dose of 4 to 6 mg/day orally until the leukocyte count falls to 30,000/μl. The effects of the drug persist for some time, and a further decrease in the count may occur. After reaching the nadir, the leukocyte count will again increase, and maintenance therapy will be required, often as little as 2 mg orally twice weekly. Therapy must be monitored with blood counts at appropriate intervals.
- Toxic effects of busulfan are prolonged aplasia of the marrow, pulmonary fibrosis, and a syndrome simulating adrenal insufficiency, with skin pigmentation, weakness, fever, and diarrhea.
- Hydroxyurea is given orally at a dose of 1 to 6 g/day, depending on the height of the white count. The dose is decreased as the count decreases, and is usually 1 to 2 g/day when the leukocyte count reaches 20,000/μl. Maintenance doses should be adjusted to keep the total white count at about 25,000/μl. Blood counts must be obtained frequently when therapy is initiated and at longer intervals as stability is achieved. The drug should be stopped if the white count falls to 5000/μl or less.
- The major side effect is suppression of hemopoiesis, often with megaloblastic erythropoiesis.
- Intensive chemotherapy regimens have been employed in attempts to eliminate cells containing the Ph chromosome, but this approach does not appear to increase survival.
- Interferon-α at a daily dose of 3 to 9 million units subcutaneously or intramuscularly will produce hematologic improvement in about 75 percent of patients in the chronic phase of CML. Maintenance therapy, usually at a daily dose of 3 to 9 million units intramuscularly 4 to 7 days a week, is required.
- Intensive treatment with interferon-α over several months leads to a significant decrease in the number of Ph chromosome–containing cells, and about 15 percent of patients have less than 5 percent Ph chromosome–positive cells.
- Interferon-α may be particularly useful in patients with markedly elevated platelet counts.
- Interferon-α may be more effective than hydroxyurea in prolonging the chronic phase of CML.
- Initial side effects of interferon-α are fever, fatigue, sweats, anorexia, headache, muscle pain, nausea, and bone pain. These occur in about 50 percent of patients.
- Later effects are apathy, agitation, insomnia, or depression; bone and muscle pain; hepatic, renal, or cardiac dysfunction; and immune-mediated anemia, thrombocytopenia, or hypothyroidism.
- Hypertriglyceridemia occurs in nearly all patients, and elevation of serum transaminase levels is common.
- Irradiation of the spleen may be beneficial in patients with marked splenomegaly and splenic pain or encroachment on the gastrointestinal tract.

- Radiotherapy may also be useful for extramedullary granulocytic tumors.
- Splenectomy is of limited value but may be helpful in some situations, such as thrombocytopenia and massive splenomegaly refractory to therapy. Postoperative complications are frequent.
- Autologous marrow transplantation to "rescue" patients after intensive chemotherapy is under investigation.
- Allogeneic marrow transplantation can be carried out after intensive cytotoxic therapy in patients under 55 years of age with a histocompatible donor.
- Engraftment and long-term survival can be achieved in 45 to 70 percent of patients, and some patients appear to have been cured.
- Transplanted T lymphocytes may play an important role in successful suppression of the leukemia by initiating a graft-versus-leukemia reaction.
- Early posttransplantation mortality has been 20 to 40 percent, largely due to graft-versus-host disease, but also to infection or the adult respiratory distress syndrome.
- Leukapheresis may be useful in patients with hyperleukocytosis, or in early pregnancy when it is necessary to control the disease without chemotherapy.

COURSE AND PROGNOSIS

- Median survival of patients receiving standard therapy for the chronic phase of CML is at least 39 to 47 months. Survival appears to be longer if hydroxyurea is used rather than busulfan, and it may be even longer with interferon-α.
- The percentage of blast cells in the blood, the total basophil plus eosinophil count, and the size of the spleen, all at the time of diagnosis, are most closely associated with the duration of the chronic phase.
- Most patients die as a result of conversion to the accelerated phase of the disease (see below).

ACCELERATED PHASE OF CML

- Most patients eventually become resistant to standard therapy and the disease enters a more aggressive phase characterized by severe dyshemopoiesis, refractory splenomegaly, extramedullary tumors, and, most often, development of a clinical picture of acute leukemia—the *blast crisis.*
- The Ph chromosome persists in both myeloid and lymphoid blasts in the accelerated phase, but additional chromosomal abnormalities often develop, such as trisomy 8, trisomy 19, isochromosome 17, or gain of a second Ph, and characteristic molecular genetic changes have been identified.

- Clinical features that may signal onset of the accelerated phase are unexplained fever, night sweats, weight loss, malaise, arthralgias, development of new extramedullary sites of disease containing blast cells, or diminished responsiveness to previously successful therapy.
- Laboratory findings may be progressive anemia with increasing aniso- and poikilocytosis, increased numbers of nucleated red cells, an increasing proportion of blasts in the blood or marrow (which may reach 50 to 90 percent at the time of blastic crisis), increase in the percentage of basophils (occasionally to levels of 30 to 80 percent), appearance of hyposegmented neutrophils (Pelger-Huët anomaly), and thrombocytopenia.
- Marrow findings are highly variable. Marked dysplastic changes may be seen in any or all cell lineages, or florid blastic transformation may occur.
- Extramedullary blast crisis is the first sign of the accelerated phase in about 10 percent of patients. Lymph nodes, serosal surfaces, skin, breast, gastrointestinal or genitourinary tracts, bone, and the central nervous system are most often involved. Central nervous system involvement is usually meningeal. Symptoms and signs are headache, vomiting, stupor, cranial nerve palsies, and papilledema. The spinal fluid contains cells, including blasts, and the protein level is elevated.
- Acute leukemia develops in most patients in the accelerated phase. It is usually myeloblastic or myelomonocytic, but may be of any cell type.
- About one-third of patients develop acute lymphoblastic leukemia (ALL), with blast cells that contain terminal deoxynucleotidyl transferase, an enzyme characteristic of acute lymphoblastic leukemia; and surface markers typical of B cells.
- Treatment of patients with myeloid phenotype is similar to that given for AML (see Chap. 7).
- Treatment of patients with lymphoid phenotype is with vincristine sulfate, 1.4 mg/m^2 (to a maximum of 2 mg) intravenously once per week, and prednisone, 60 mg/m^2/day orally. A minimum of 2 weeks of therapy should be given to judge responsiveness. About one-third of patients will reenter the chronic phase with this treatment, but the median duration of remission is about 4 months, and relapse should be expected. The response rate may be improved by more intensive therapy, similar to that used in *de novo* ALL. Most patients do not respond to repeat therapy.
- Allogeneic marrow transplantation from a histocompatible donor may lead to prolonged remission in blast crisis.
- Patients with myeloid blast crisis have a median survival of about 2 months, and those with lymphoid blast crisis a median survival of about 6 months. Death is usually due to infection, hemorrhage, and hepatic or renal dysfunction.

ACUTE LEUKEMIAS WITH THE PHILADELPHIA CHROMOSOME

- *Philadelphia chromosome–positive AML* appears in some cases to be instances of CML presenting in myeloid blast crisis, while other cases appear to be unrelated to CML.
- *Philadelphia chromosome–positive ALL* represents about 3 percent of cases of childhood ALL and 20 percent of adult ALL. In both adults and children the prognosis is worse for those with the Ph chromosome. Some Ph chromosome–positive ALL patients have the same genetic abnormalities that characterize CML and are believed to be patients with CML presenting in lymphoid blast crisis. The remaining patients appear to have *de novo* ALL.

RELATED DISEASES WITHOUT THE Ph CHROMOSOME

- *Chronic neutrophilic leukemia* is characterized by a leukocyte count of 25,000 to 50,000/µl, with about 90 to 95 percent mature neutrophils. Neutrophil alkaline phosphatase activity is increased. Marrow shows granulocytic hyperplasia with a normal proportion of blasts. Ph chromosome is absent. Liver and spleen are enlarged and are infiltrated with immature myeloid cells and megakaryocytes. There have been no systematic studies of treatment. Busulfan and hydroxyurea have been used with transient benefit. Median survival is 2 to 3 years.
- *Chronic monocytic leukemia* is a rare disease with hepatomegaly and splenomegaly, mild anemia, and elevation in the percentage of monocytes in the blood. After splenectomy, leukocytosis (up to 100,000/µl) and monocytosis (up to 75,000/µl) develop, and the marrow becomes heavily infiltrated with monocytes. Treatment has not been successful, and the median survival is about 25 months. Death is usually due to septicemia or acute monocytic leukemia.
- *Juvenile chronic myelomonocytic leukemia* occurs most often in children under 4 years of age. Nearly all patients have splenomegaly, and about half have eczematoid or maculopapular skin lesions. Anemia, thrombocytopenia, and leukocytosis are common. The blood contains monocytes up to 100,000/µl, immature granulocytes, including blast cells, and nucleated red cells. Fetal hemoglobin concentration is increased in about two-thirds of the patients. The marrow shows granulocytic hyperplasia, with an increase in monocytes and leukemic blast cells. The disease has been refractory to chemotherapy, and the median survival is less than 2 years. Successful marrow transplantation has been reported.
- *Chronic myelomonocytic leukemia* is discussed in Chap. 8, Myelodysplastic syndromes.

- *Philadelphia chromosome–negative CML* is a rare disorder of clonal origin that can undergo lymphoid or myeloid transformation. Most cases resemble chronic myelomonocytic leukemia (see Chap. 6).

For a more detailed discussion, see Marshall F. Lichtman: Chronic myelogenous leukemia and related disorders, Chap. 28, p. 298, in *Williams Hematology,* 5/e, 1995.

---

9 POLYCYTHEMIA VERA

Polycythemia vera is a clonal disorder of the hemopoietic stem cell with proliferation of erythrocytic, granulocytic, and megakaryocytic cells. It may evolve into idiopathic myelofibrosis, myelodysplasia, and/or acute leukemia.

ETIOLOGY AND PATHOGENESIS

- Marrow-derived erythroid colonies develop in vitro in the absence of added erythropoietin.
- 25 percent of patients have karyotypic abnormalities at diagnosis.
- Karyotypic abnormalities developing later in the disease may signify transformation into idiopathic myelofibrosis, myelodysplasia, or acute leukemia.
- Familial incidence has been occasionally reported.
- More common in Eastern European Jews.
- Incidence ranges from 5 to 26 per 1,000,000 population, depending on the reporting country.

CLINICAL MANIFESTATIONS

- The onset is insidious, at average age of 60.
- May occur in children or young adults.
- Symptoms occurring in at least 30 percent of patients are headache, weakness, pruritus, dizziness, and sweating.
  - Pruritus after bathing occurs in 40 percent of patients and is a specific complaint, which should suggest the diagnosis.
  - Neurologic complaints include vertigo, diplopia, scotomata, and transient ischemic events.
  - Associated disorders include peptic ulcer disease (due to increased histamine levels) and gout (due to increased nucleic acid turnover).
- Thrombosis and hemorrhage
  - Thrombotic events occur in about one-third of patients prior to diagnosis and in 40 to 60 percent over the first 10 years.
  - These may be severe, sometimes fatal, and include stroke, myocardial infarction, deep venous thrombosis, hepatic vein thrombosis, and pulmonary embolism.
  - Bleeding and bruising occur in one-fourth of patients and are usually minor, but prolonged gastrointestinal bleeding may be severe enough to mask the polycythemic state ("bled-down" polycythemia vera).
  - Patients with uncontrolled polycythemia vera undergoing surgery have a high risk of bleeding and/or thrombosis.
  - Splenectomy early in the disease leads to uncontrolled, often fatal thrombocytosis and is contraindicated.

LABORATORY FINDINGS

- Erythrocyte count is usually elevated, and in patients who have had gastrointestinal blood loss or have been treated with phlebotomy may

be out of proportion to the hemoglobin level and the hematocrit, with hypochromia and microcytosis and other evidence of iron deficiency.
- Red cell mass is usually elevated in proportion to the hematocrit.
- Nucleated red cells are not present in the blood early in disease.
- The reticulocyte percentage is usually slightly increased.
- Arterial P_{O_2} is often slightly low, with low-normal O_2 saturation on initial presentation, increasing to normal following therapeutic reduction in the hematocrit, and correspondingly decreased blood viscosity.
- Absolute neutrophilia occurs in about two-thirds of patients, with occasional myelocytes and metamyelocytes. Basophilia also occurs in about two-thirds of patients.
- The platelet count is increased in over 50 percent of patients and exceeds 1 million in about 10 percent.
- Platelets have a characteristic functional defect in the primary wave of aggregation induced by epinephrine.
- Prothrombin time and partial thromboplastin time may be spuriously prolonged if the amount of anticoagulant used in the test is not adjusted for the increased hematocrit.

DIAGNOSIS

- The most important diagnostic features of polycythemia vera are
  - erythrocytosis
  - leukocytosis
  - thrombocytosis
  - splenomegaly
- Other helpful clinical features are
  - elevated serum vitamin B_{12} level
  - elevated serum uric acid level
  - normal or near-normal arterial oxygen saturation
  - pruritus
- Measurement of red cell mass is considered by some to be the *sine qua non* for diagnosis of polycythemia vera, but others believe this study should be reserved for special circumstances such as erythrocytosis existing without leukocytosis, thrombocytosis, or splenomegaly.
- Other tests which may be of value are
  - erythropoietin assay
  - erythroid colony growth in vitro

DIFFERENTIAL DIAGNOSIS

- Table 9-1 compares clinical and laboratory findings in patients with polycythemia vera, secondary polycythemia, and apparent polycythemia.
- In patients with hypoxia and/or elevated erythropoietin levels, cardiopulmonary causes should be immediately obvious. Less obvious

TABLE 9-1 Typical Laboratory Findings in Patients with Polycythemia Vera, Secondary Polycythemia, and Apparent Polycythemia*

Findings	Polycythemia vera	Secondary polycythemia	Apparent polycythemia
Splenomegaly	Present	Absent	Absent
Leukocytosis	Present	Absent	Absent
Thrombocytosis	Present	Absent	Absent
Abnormal primary wave of epinephrine-induced platelet aggregation	Present	Absent	Absent
Red blood cell volume	Increased	Increased	Normal
Arterial oxygen saturation	Normal	Decreased or normal	Normal
Serum vitamin B_{12} level	Increased	Normal	Normal
Leukocyte alkaline phosphatase	Increased	Normal	Normal
Marrow	Panhyperplasia	Erythroid hyperplasia	Normal
Erythropoietin level	Decreased	Increased	Normal
Endogenous CFU-E growth	Present	Absent	Absent

*The differences listed are not present in all patients.
Source: Table 29-1 of *Williams Hematology*, 5/e, p. 326.

would be nonhypoxic patients in whom renal cysts, hydronephrosis, and carcinoma of the liver or kidney must be ruled out.
- Familial cases should suggest the presence of a high-affinity hemoglobin.
- All smokers should have a blood carboxyhemoglobin determination.
- Differential diagnosis may be difficult in the following situations:
  - Polycythemia vera with concomitant chronic lung disease.
  - Pure erythrocytosis, which may be familial.
  - Patients who abuse both cigarettes and alcohol. The former may cause absolute polycythemia, while the latter can be associated with leukocytosis, splenomegaly, thrombocytosis, elevated vitamin B_{12} levels, and increased leukocyte alkaline phosphatase activity.

THERAPY

Early (Plethoric) Phase

- Emphasis should be on control of symptoms, decreasing risk of hemorrhagic and/or thrombotic events, and minimizing complications attributable to therapy.

Phlebotomy

- Best initial therapy for most patients.
- Most patients of average size can tolerate phlebotomy of 450 to 500 ml every 4 days.
- Induces iron deficiency. Iron supplementation is counterproductive and may result in rapid reappearance of polycythemia.
- Target hematocrit should be less than 50 percent. Some studies have suggested levels below 46 percent.
- Phlebotomy alone is associated with a higher incidence of fatal thrombotic events in older patients, those with a high phlebotomy requirement, and those with a prior thrombotic event. Such patients should be treated with myelosuppressive agents.

Myelosuppressive Agents

- Should be considered in patients with
  - advanced age
  - extreme thrombocytosis
  - thrombotic or bleeding complications
  - severe systemic complaints not responding to phlebotomy, low-dose aspirin, etc.

Hydroxyurea

- The usual initial dose is 15 to 30 mg/kg/day orally
- The effects of the drug are of short duration and require continuous monitoring and excellent patient compliance.
- The leukemic potential of the drug is probably higher than for phlebotomy alone.

Busulfan

- Has long-lasting myelosuppressive effects which make long-term control possible, but has the potential for long-term toxicity as well.
- The leukemogenic potential of busulfan in U.S. studies appears high.

Radioactive Phosphorus (^{32}P)

- Usual initial dose is 2.7 mCi/m^2 intravenously.
- Long-lasting control is possible with a single dose, making it an option for older, less compliant patients unable to obtain frequent follow-up.
- Use of ^{32}P is limited by its high leukemogenic potential.

Interferon-α

- The initial dose is 3 to 10 million units subcutaneously, 3 to 5 times weekly.

- Limited experience to date indicates this agent can control early disease quite effectively.
- The potential for long-term complications is unknown.

Other Agents

- Pipobroman, cyclophosphamide, and chlorambucil are capable of producing clinical response in most patients, but all of these agents have high leukemogenic potential.
- Anagrelide may be helpful in patients with symptomatic thrombocytosis.

Treatment of Pruritus

- Patients with pruritus induced by bathing should be advised to take cooler showers or baths and to avoid vigorous rubbing of skin.
- Phlebotomy alone may control pruritus. H-1 and/or H-2 blockers may also give relief.
- Photochemotherapy with psoralens and UV light may be beneficial.
- Myelosuppression or interferon therapy should be given if pruritus is intractable to other therapies.

Late (Spent) Phase

- 10 percent of all patients, independent of the treatment chosen, develop anemia, progressive splenomegaly, and signs of myelofibrosis and myeloid metaplasia. Some patients may have leukocytosis, thrombocytopenia, and immature leukocytes, including blasts, in the blood.
- Treatment is symptomatic/supportive only
  - Transfusions are given as needed
  - Painful splenomegaly may require
    - adequate narcotics for pain relief
    - splenic irradiation, which usually provides short-term relief only
    - careful myelosuppression with hydroxyurea
    - splenectomy

PROGNOSIS

- Overall survival is generally quite long and similar for patients treated with phlebotomy or myelosuppression. However, early thrombotic events are more common for the former and leukemo- and carcinogenicity for the latter.
- A reasonable program would be phlebotomy for younger patients, while older patients should receive myelosuppression for the first 2 to 4 years, switching to phlebotomy alone after that time. Interferon merits consideration, especially if long-term complications are minimal.

For a more detailed discussion, see Ernest Beutler: Polycythemia vera, Chap. 29, p. 324, in *Williams Hematology,* 5/e, 1995.

10 IDIOPATHIC MYELOFIBROSIS (AGNOGENIC MYELOID METAPLASIA)

Idiopathic myelofibrosis, or agnogenic myeloid metaplasia, is a clonal disorder of the totipotent hemopoietic stem cell characterized by immature granulocytes, erythroid precursors, and teardrop-shaped red cells in the blood, and varying degrees of marrow fibrosis and splenomegaly.

FIBROPLASIA

- Fine reticulin fibers are increased in number in the marrow, as detected by silver staining. Fibrosis may progress to thick collagen bands identified with the trichrome stain, primarily involving type III collagen.
- Increased concentrations of procollagen III amino-terminal peptide, prolylhydroxylase, and fibronectin are present in the plasma.
- The extent of fibrosis is correlated with the number of dysplastic megakaryocytes and release of fibroblast growth factors.
- The fibroblastic proliferation in the marrow is not an intrinsic part of the clonal expansion of hemopoietic cells.

EXTRAMEDULLARY HEMOPOIESIS

- Always present in liver and spleen in this disorder, and contributes to the organomegaly.
- Extramedullary hemopoiesis is rarely effective.
- Hemopoietic foci are often present in adrenals, kidneys, lymph nodes, bowel, breast, lungs, and other sites.
- Central nervous system sites of extramedullary hemopoiesis can be associated with subdural hemorrhage, delirium, increased cerebrospinal fluid pressure, papilledema, coma, motor and sensory impairment, and paralysis.
- Hemopoietic foci on serosal surfaces can cause effusions in the thorax, abdomen, or pericardial spaces.
- Extramedullary hemopoiesis may be worsened after splenectomy and lead to hepatic failure.

CLINICAL FEATURES

- The median age at diagnosis is 60, but the disorder may occur at any age.
- The sex incidence is equal in adults, but twice as many females as males in young children.
- The disease may be familial.
- Occasionally myelofibrosis is preceded by exposure to benzene or ionizing radiation.
- 25 percent of patients are asymptomatic at time of diagnosis.

- Fatigue, weakness, shortness of breath, palpitations, weight loss, night sweats, and bone pain are common presenting symptoms.
- Left upper quadrant fullness, pain or dragging sensation, left shoulder pain, and early satiety may result from splenic enlargement and/or infarction.
- Hepatomegaly is present in 67 percent of patients. Splenomegaly is present in 100 percent and is massive in one-third.
- Wasting, peripheral edema, or bone tenderness may occur.
- Neutrophilic dermatosis may be present.
- Portal hypertension and esophageal varices:
  - Increased splenoportal blood flow and decreased hepatic vascular compliance lead to portal hypertension, ascites, esophageal and gastric varices, intraluminal gastrointestinal bleeding, and hepatic encephalopathy.
  - Portal vein thrombosis may occur and sometimes is the initial problem.
- Immune manifestations include anti–red cell antibodies, antinuclear antibodies, anti–gamma globulins, antiphospholipid antibodies, and others.
- Osteosclerosis may develop with increased bone density evident on radiographs and marrow biopsy.
- Periostitis may lead to severe bone pain.
- Increased bone blood flow (up to 25 percent of cardiac output) may accelerate atherosclerosis or congestive heart failure.

LABORATORY FEATURES

- Normocytic-normochromic anemia is found in most patients.
- Aniso- and poikilocytosis, tear-drop red cells (dacrocytes), and nucleated red cells are consistently seen in the peripheral blood.
- Reticulocyte count is variable.
- Anemia may be worsened by an expanded plasma volume and/or splenic trapping of red cells.
- Hemolysis may be present and may be autoimmune, with a positive antiglobulin (Coombs) test.
- Occasionally, the acid hemolysis test and sucrose hemolysis test for paroxysmal nocturnal hemoglobinuria are positive.
- Acquired hemoglobin H disease with hypochromic microcytic red cells and red cell inclusions staining with brilliant cresyl blue has been described, as has erythroid aplasia.
- The total leukocyte count is usually less than 40,000/µl, but may be as high as 100,000/µl with neutrophilic granulocytosis.
- Neutropenia occurs in 15 percent.
- Myelocytes and metamyelocytes are present in the blood of all patients, along with a low proportion of blasts (1 to 5 percent).
- Neutrophil alkaline phosphatase scores are variable.

- Basophils may be slightly increased in number.
- Neutrophils may have impaired phagocytosis, decreased myeloperoxidase activity, and other functional changes.
- About one-third of patients have elevated platelet counts, and one-third have mild to moderate thrombocytopenia.
- Giant platelets, abnormal platelet granulation, and occasional circulating dwarf megakaryocytes are characteristic.
- The bleeding time may be prolonged and platelet aggregation with epinephrine may be impaired along with depletion of dense granule ADP and decreased lipoxygenase activity in platelets.
- Pancytopenia occurs in 10 percent of patients, usually secondary to ineffective hemopoiesis coupled with splenic sequestration.
- Increased numbers of circulating pluripotential, granulocytic, monocytic, and erythroid progenitor cells are found.
- Serum levels of uric acid, lactic dehydrogenase, alkaline phosphatase, and bilirubin are often elevated.
- Serum levels of albumin, cholesterol, and high-density lipoproteins are usually decreased.

MARROW

- Marrow aspiration is usually unsuccessful because of fibrosis ("dry tap").
- Biopsy is often quite cellular, with variable degrees of erythroid, granulocytic, and megakaryocytic hyperplasia.
- Collagen fibrosis can be demonstrated and can be extreme, along with osteosclerotic changes. Silver stain invariably shows increased reticulin, often extreme.
- Megakaryocytes can be prominent even in hypocellular densely fibrotic specimens, and may show giant or dwarf forms, abnormal nuclear lobulation, and naked nuclei.
- Granulocytes may show hyper- or hypolobulation, acquired Pelger-Hüet anomaly, nuclear blebs, and nuclear-cytoplasmic asynchrony.
- Dilated marrow sinusoids are common, with intrasinusoidal immature hemopoietic cells and megakaryocytes.

CYTOGENETICS

- Cytogenetic abnormalities are present in 50 percent of hemopoietic cells. Aneuploidy (mono- or trisomy) or pseudodiploidy (partial deletions and translocations) are common. Rarely the Philadelphia chromosome has been present. These cytogenetic abnormalities are not seen in fibroblasts.

DIFFERENTIAL DIAGNOSIS

- Chronic myelogenous leukemia: In CML, the white count is often greater than $100,000/\mu l$, red cell shape is usually normal, and marrow fibrosis is minimal. The Philadelphia chromosome and/or *bcr-abl* fusion gene are present.

- Myelodysplasia: Pancytopenia and maturation abnormalities may occur in both myelodysplasia and myelofibrosis. Prominent splenomegaly and marrow fibrosis may help distinguish idiopathic myelofibrosis from a myelodysplastic syndrome.
- Hairy cell leukemia may show classical findings of idiopathic myelofibrosis, but the presence of abnormal mononuclear (hairy) cells separates the two disorders.
- Disorders with reactive marrow fibrosis include metastatic carcinoma (breast, prostate), disseminated mycobacterial infection, mastocytosis, myeloma, renal osteodystrophy, angioimmunoblastic lymphadenopathy, gray platelet syndrome, systemic lupus erythematosus, polyarteritis nodosa, neuroblastoma, rickets, Langerhans cell histiocytosis, and malignant histiocytosis.
- Coincidental disorders have included lymphoma, chronic lymphocytic leukemia, hairy cell leukemia, macroglobulinemia, amyloidosis, myeloma, and monoclonal gammopathy.

TRANSITIONS BETWEEN IDIOPATHIC MYELOFIBROSIS AND OTHER MYELOPROLIFERATIVE DISORDERS

- All stem cell diseases may have increased reticulin in the bone marrow, but only idiopathic myelofibrosis has collagen fibrosis.
- Acute megakaryocytic leukemia may show intense marrow fibrosis (acute myelofibrosis), but splenomegaly is absent.
- Polycythemia vera: 10 percent of patients treated with phlebotomy or myelosuppression will develop classical idiopathic myelofibrosis, usually in a progressive pattern over a period of many years.
- Primary thrombocytosis may evolve into classical idiopathic myelofibrosis.
- Acute leukemia develops in about 5 to 10 percent of patients with *de novo* idiopathic myelofibrosis, and in about 20 percent of those with polycythemia vera who have transformed into idiopathic myelofibrosis, especially those who have been treated with myelosuppressive agents. A myelodysplastic disorder may precede the development of acute leukemia.

TREATMENT

- Many patients are asymptomatic for long periods of time and will not require therapy. There is currently no cure other than marrow transplantation, which may be difficult if fibrosis is extensive.
- Severe anemia may improve with androgen therapy in some patients (testosterone, oxymetholone, fluoxymesterone, danazol). Careful monitoring of hepatic function and periodic liver imaging with ultrasound to detect liver tumors are essential.

- Glucocorticoids may occasionally be helpful in patients with significant hemolytic anemia. High-dose glucocorticoids have been reported to ameliorate idiopathic myelofibrosis in children.
- Decreases in splenic and hepatic size, improvement in constitutional symptoms (fever, bone pain, weight loss, night sweats), and improvement in blood counts (increase in hematocrit, decrease in elevated platelet counts, and decreased marrow fibrosis) can occasionally be obtained with cautious doses of chemotherapeutic agents such as busulfan, other alkylating agents, or hydroxyurea.
- Interferon-α has been useful in treating splenic enlargement, bone pain, and thrombocytosis.
- Radiation therapy may be useful for
  - severe splenic pain or massive splenic enlargement.
  - ascites from peritoneal myeloid metaplasia
  - focal areas of bone pain (periostitis or osteolysis from granulocytic sarcoma)
  - Extramedullary tumors, especially of the epidural space
- Major indications of splenectomy
  - painful, enlarged spleen
  - excessive transfusion requirement
  - refractory hemolysis
  - severe thrombocytopenia
  - portal hypertension
- Patients with prolonged bleeding times, prothrombin times, or partial thromboplastin times are at serious risk of bleeding during and after surgery, and require meticulous preoperative evaluation and replacement therapy, surgical hemostasis, and postoperative care.
- Portal hypertension as a result of increased splenic blood flow is improved by splenectomy.
- Postsplenectomy morbidity is about 30 percent and mortality about 10 percent.

COURSE AND PROGNOSIS

- Median survival is approximately 5 years after diagnosis (range: 1 to 15 years).
- Poor prognostic signs are anemia, thrombocytopenia, hepatomegaly, unexplained fever, and prominent hemolysis.
- Major causes of death are infection, hemorrhage, postsplenectomy mortality, and transformation into acute leukemia.
- Spontaneous remissions are rare.

For a more detailed discussion, see Marshall A. Lichtman: Idiopathic myelofibrosis (agnogenic myeloid metaplasia), Chap. 30, p. 331, in *Williams Hematology*, 5/e, 1995.

11 ESSENTIAL (PRIMARY) THROMBOCYTHEMIA

Essential thrombocythemia is a clonal disorder of the multipotential stem cell with predominant phenotypic expression in the megakaryocyte-platelet lineage, but with involvement of all cell lines.

CLINICAL FEATURES

- Usually develops between ages 50 and 70. Sex distribution is equal.
- Because platelet counts are now often done as a routine, the disorder is being discovered in younger individuals and in patients who are asymptomatic.
- Rare familial cases have been reported.
- Constitutional or hypermetabolic symptoms are very uncommon.
- Mild splenomegaly is found in 40 to 50 percent of patients.
- Patients may have ecchymoses and bruising.
- Bleeding and thrombotic complications are major causes of morbidity and mortality.
- Bleeding is common and is characteristic of platelet or vascular disorders: mucosal, gastrointestinal, cutaneous, and postoperative.
- Use of aspirin may occasionally lead to serious bleeding complications.
- Thrombosis, more often arterial than venous, is commonly in cerebrovascular, peripheral vascular, and coronary vessels.
- 25 percent of all thrombotic events are lower extremity deep venous thrombosis.

Erythromelalgia and Digital Microvascular Ischemia

- Caused by vascular occlusion with platelet thrombi.
- Patients have intense burning or pain, especially in feet.
- Symptoms are exacerbated by heat, exercise, and dependency, and relieved by cold and elevation of extremity.
- Painful vascular insufficiency may lead to gangrene and necrosis with normal peripheral pulses and patent major vessels on angiography.
- These problems often respond dramatically and promptly to small doses of aspirin and/or reduction of platelet count.

Cerebrovascular Ischemia

- Symptoms may be nonspecific (headache, dizziness, decreased mental acuity) and signs may be focal (transient ischemic attacks, seizures, or retinal artery occlusion).
- Visual changes include double or blurred vision, scotomata (often scintillating), field cuts, amaurosis fugax.
- Small doses of aspirin and/or reduction in platelet count may provide relief.

Recurrent Abortions and Fetal Growth Retardation

- Multiple placental infarctions may lead to placental insufficiency with recurrent spontaneous abortions, fetal growth retardation, premature deliveries, and abruptio placentae.
- May require use of aspirin during pregnancy, but avoid at least 1 week prior to delivery to reduce risk of maternal or neonatal bleeding complications.

Hepatic and Portal Vein Thrombosis

- May lead to splenomegaly, esophageal varices, and bouts of hepatic encephalopathy.

BLOOD AND MARROW FINDINGS

- Platelet counts may range from only slightly above normal to several million platelets per microliter.
- Platelets may be large, pale blue–staining, and hypogranular. Nucleated megakaryocyte fragments having a lymphoblastoid appearance may be seen occasionally.
- Mild leukocytosis and mild anemia are common.
- The leukocyte differential count is usually normal, without nucleated red cells.
- Marrow shows increased cellularity with megakaryocytic hyperplasia and masses of platelet debris ("platelet drifts"). Megakaryocytes are frequently giant, with increased ploidy, and occur in clusters. Significant megakaryocytic dysplasia is uncommon.

CLINICAL TESTS OF HEMOSTASIS

- Abnormal tests serve as a marker for the disease but do not predict for bleeding and/or thrombosis.
- The bleeding time is prolonged in less than 20 percent of patients.
- Platelet aggregation abnormalities are variable:
  - Loss of responsiveness to epinephrine is characteristic.
  - Reduced responses to collagen, ADP, and arachidonic acid occur in less than one-third of patients.
  - May have platelet hyperaggregability or spontaneous aggregation in vitro.

DIFFERENTIAL DIAGNOSIS

- Diagnosis is made by exclusion, since there is no specific marker for the disease. The following should be demonstrated:
  - The patient is not iron deficient and has a normal to low red cell mass when iron sufficient or iron repleted.
  - The Philadelphia chromosome is absent.
  - There is no evidence for myelofibrosis.
  - There is no recognizable cause for secondary thrombocytosis (see Chap. 69).

THERAPY

Asymptomatic Patients

- The need to treat asymptomatic patients is controversial.
- No evidence exists to show that chronic cytoreductive therapy improves prognosis, but no prospective controlled trials have been done.

Symptomatic Patients

- Lowering the platelet count in patients with active bleeding and/or thrombosis is beneficial and may be life-saving.
- Prompt reduction is especially warranted in patients with microvascular digital or cerebrovascular ischemia.

Treatment Options

- Urgent platelet count reduction (hours) can be achieved by plateletpheresis, but the benefit is short-lived, often with a rebound increase in platelet count. Plateletpheresis should be followed by treatment with longer-acting agents.
- Rapid reduction (days) can be achieved with nitrogen mustard, cytosine arabinoside, or anthracycline drugs.
- Long-term reduction (weeks to months):
  - Hydroxyurea therapy is effective, using a starting dose of 15 to 30 mg/kg/day orally. The dose should be adjusted every 1 to 2 weeks according to the response.
  - Recombinant interferon-α is also effective, with a starting dose of 3 million units subcutaneously, daily.
  - Anagrelide may also be used to reduce the platelet count. The starting dose is 2 to 3 mg daily.
- Antiplatelet agents:
  - Aspirin in normal or increased doses (>900 mg/day) may cause marked prolongation of the bleeding time and serious bleeding episodes.
  - A cautious trial of low-dose aspirin (<650 mg/day) may give gratifying clinical responses.

COURSE AND PROGNOSIS

- Survival rates are similar to those of a normal age-matched population, but treatment failures and/or fatalities occur, even in younger patients.
- Rarely may transform into another myeloproliferative disorder, including frank acute leukemia.
- In view of the relatively benign nature of the disease in many patients, the use of leukemogenic agents in treatment should be minimized.

For a more detailed discussion, see Andrew I. Schafer: Essential (primary) thrombocythemia, Chap. 31, p. 340, in *Williams Hematology*, 5/e, 1995.

---

12 PURE RED CELL APLASIA

Pure red cell aplasia describes anemia caused by an isolated depletion of erythroblasts. Three types are recognized:

1. Acute red cell aplasia
2. Chronic red cell aplasia—constitutional
3. Chronic red cell aplasia—acquired

ACUTE PURE RED CELL APLASIA

- Transient erythroblastopenia occurs in both children and adults.
- Clinically apparent usually in patients with a hemolytic disorder, such as hereditary spherocytosis or sickle cell anemia, where a transient reduction in erythropoiesis causes a rapid fall in hemoglobin level—the so-called aplastic crisis.
- May also be seen in patients who are hematologically normal.
- True prevalence is unknown, and it is assumed that many cases are not detected.

Etiology

- Most patients with aplastic crises are infected with parvovirus B-19, but other viral infections may also be responsible.
- IgG inhibitors of erythroid colony formation in vitro have been found in some patients with a condition called *transient erythroblastopenia of childhood.*
- Drugs may induce aplastic crises, either by an immunological mechanism or by direct toxicity. Drugs which have been implicated are listed in Table 43-1, in *Williams Hematology,* 5/e.

Clinical Features

- Frequently the patient has had a recent, febrile illness, often with upper respiratory or gastrointestinal symptoms.
- Listlessness and increasing pallor may be present.
- Usually no significant changes are found on physical examination.
- Severe bone pain may occur during the recovery phase.

Laboratory Features

- Evidence of an underlying hematologic disorder, such as hereditary spherocytosis, may be present.
- Anemia and reticulocytopenia are characteristic.
- Granulocyte and platelet counts are usually normal, but may be decreased.
- Pyrimidine 5′-nucleotidase activity in red cells is diminished.
- Erythroid elements are depleted in the marrow early in the illness, but reappear promptly with recovery, and the erythroblastopenia may be missed.

- Reticulocytosis occurs with recovery, and nucleated red cells may appear in the blood.
- Serum iron levels are high and serum iron-binding capacity is fully saturated during the aplastic phase. Serum iron levels fall during recovery.

Differential Diagnosis

- Reduction in hemoglobin level with reticulocytopenia in a patient with known hemolytic anemia suggests this diagnosis. Reticulocyte count will be maintained or elevated if bleeding or increased hemolysis is the cause of the worsening anemia.
- Absence of involvement of leukocytes or platelets, and the erythroid aplasia in the marrow, eliminates other causes of anemia.
- Transient erythroblastopenia of childhood is differentiated from chronic forms of red cell aplasia by rapid recovery.

Therapy, Course, and Prognosis

- Discontinuation of drugs when possible, treatment of any associated illnesses, and maintenance of hemoglobin level by transfusion.
- Recovery occurs spontaneously in days or weeks.

CHRONIC PURE RED CELL APLASIA—CONSTITUTIONAL

- A form of pure red cell aplasia occurring early in childhood. Also known as the Diamond-Blackfan syndrome.
- May be familial, with possible autosomal dominant or recessive inheritance.
- Cause unknown. May be due to an inherited defect in stem cells or an abnormal hemopoietic microenvironment.

Clinical Features

- Onset with pallor, listlessness, and poor appetite. May progress to severe anemia, with cardiac failure, dyspnea, and hepatosplenomegaly.
- Signs of iron overload or glucocorticoid excess may develop after treatment.

Laboratory Features

- Normocytic, normochromic anemia with absolute reticulocytopenia in all cases.
- Leukocyte count is normal or slightly decreased.
- Platelet count is often increased.
- Marrow is cellular, with marked erythroid hypoplasia. The few erythroid cells present may have megaloblastic changes. Other marrow cells are normal.

- Serum iron levels are elevated, and transferrin saturation is increased.
- In most cases, the fetal hemoglobin level is elevated, the concentration of i antigen on the erythrocyte surface is increased, and erythrocyte adenosine deaminase activity is elevated.
- Erythropoietin levels are elevated.

Differential Diagnosis

- Reticulocytopenia and the absence of erythroblasts in an otherwise normal marrow are characteristic of this disorder.
- Acute red cell aplasia is characterized by sudden onset and prompt resolution.

Therapy, Course, and Prognosis

- Transfusions will relieve symptoms of anemia but lead to iron overload.
- Glucocorticoid therapy may be beneficial, probably by making erythroid progenitor cells more sensitive to growth factors.
- Glucocorticoid therapy should be initiated with prednisone at a daily dose of 1 to 2 mg/kg orally. Dosage is reduced to a maintenance level if a reticulocyte response occurs. Therapy should be continued for 4 to 6 weeks if no response occurs sooner. A trial of high doses of methylprednisolone may then be considered.
- Continuous glucocorticoid therapy is often required, and severe side effects frequently develop.
- Most deaths are due to complications of therapy.
- A few patients have developed acute leukemia.

CHRONIC PURE RED CELL APLASIA—ACQUIRED

- An unusual disorder of adults characterized by markedly diminished red cell production.
- May be associated with thymoma, but the true prevalence of this combination is unknown, and it appears to be less common than believed earlier.
- May also be found in association with other diseases, such as chronic lymphocytic leukemia or large granular lymphocytic leukemia.
- An immune mechanism is believed responsible in about one-half of patients.
- Persistent B-19 parvovirus infection may be responsible in some immunocompromised patients.

Clinical Features

- Pallor and other signs and symptoms of anemia are usual.
- Side effects of multiple transfusions and prolonged glucocorticoid therapy lead to additional clinical findings.

Laboratory Features

- Blood shows normochromic, normo- or macrocytic anemia with absolute reticulocytopenia, and a normal leukocyte and platelet count.
- The marrow is normocellular, with normal granulocytes and megakaryocytes, but with severe erythroid hypoplasia or aplasia.
- The serum iron level is elevated, the iron-binding capacity almost fully saturated, and the utilization of iron is low.
- The disorder is frequently associated with serum antibodies, such as antinuclear antibodies, cold and warm hemagglutinins, and heterophile antibodies.
- Thymic enlargement, if present, is usually detected as an anterior mediastinal mass on routine chest films, but more detailed examination may be required.

Differential Diagnosis

- The disorder is suggested by evidence of marked erythroid hypoplasia. In some cases nuclear abnormalities in myeloid and platelet precursors may raise the possibility of a myelodysplastic syndrome.

Therapy, Course, and Prognosis

- Red cell transfusion can be used to prevent or treat symptoms of anemia, but iron overload is a predictable complication, and acquired red cell antibodies often make it difficult to obtain compatible blood and diminish the effectiveness of transfusion.
- Erythropoietin is unlikely to be of benefit.
- Thymectomy should be done if thymic enlargement is present.
- Glucocorticoids may be effective in low doses for long-term maintenance, but often large doses are required for protracted periods, with consequent severe side effects.
- Immunosuppressive drugs, such as cyclophosphamide or 6-mercaptopurine, have been used successfully, but are potentially leukemogenic.
- Intravenous gamma globulin has also been effective and may eradicate B-19 parvovirus infection in some patients.
- Antithymic and antilymphocyte sera have also been used successfully.
- Plasmapheresis may be helpful.
- With current therapy, about 50 percent of patients enter remission.
- Median survival of patients with idiopathic disease is greater than 10 years. Common causes of death are hemosiderosis, glucocorticoid-induced hemorrhage or infection, and aplastic anemia.

For a more detailed discussion, see Allan J. Erslev: Pure red cell aplasia, Chap. 41, p. 448, in *Williams Hematology,* 5/e, 1995.

13 ANEMIA OF CHRONIC RENAL FAILURE

ETIOLOGY AND PATHOGENESIS

- Reduced production of erythropoietin appears to be the most significant factor in the development of anemia in uremia.
- The plasma volume varies widely in renal failure, with consequent variations in the hematocrit.
- A modest reduction in red cell life-span occurs in uremia, probably from mechanical disruption of metabolically impaired cells.
- Iron deficiency occurs from blood loss in the dialysis tubing, laboratory testing, or external bleeding, sometimes due to uremia-induced platelet dysfunction. Iron utilization may be impaired by aluminum absorbed from dialysis water.
- Folic acid may be lost in the dialysis bath.

CLINICAL AND LABORATORY FEATURES

- The anemia is normocytic and normochromic, with a normal or slightly reduced number of reticulocytes.
- Acanthocytes or schistocytes are seen on the blood film.
- The total and differential leukocyte count and the platelet count are usually normal.
- Platelet function is abnormal, in proportion to the degree of uremia and effectiveness of dialysis.
- The cellularity and maturation sequences in the marrow are normal. Despite the anemia there is no erythroid hyperplasia.
- Iron utilization is decreased.

THERAPY, COURSE, AND PROGNOSIS

- Replacement therapy with erythropoietin will correct the anemia in nearly all patients. Amelioration of the anemia has improved the quality of life for uremic patients and has led to a decrease in the bleeding time and to favorable endocrine changes.
- Erythropoietin has usually been given intravenously in dialysis patients, but subcutaneous administration may be equally effective.
- Usual starting dose is 50 to 100 U/kg three times weekly. Hematocrits of 32 to 38 percent can usually be achieved within 10 weeks and then maintained by adjusting the dose. Usually 50 U/kg three times a week are required.
- Patients with renal disease who do not yet require dialysis have also benefited from erythropoietin therapy, usually given subcutaneously.
- Adequate iron stores must be maintained by supplemental iron administration, usually orally.
- Folic acid supplementation is also necessary.

- Complications of erythropoietin therapy include hypertension, seizures, thrombosis of shunts, and hyperkalemia. Blood pressure should be carefully monitored throughout the treatment.
- A small number of patients do not respond to erythropoietin, most often because of iron deficiency but also because of aluminum toxicity or marrow fibrosis secondary to hyperparathyroidism.
- Red cell transfusion will compensate rapidly for acute blood loss and prior to the availability of erythropoietin was used extensively to maintain hemoglobin levels in uremic patients.
- Androgen therapy can improve the anemia of uremia, although side effects are hirsutism, virilization, skin infections, and liver toxicity.

For a more detailed discussion, see Jaime Caro, Allan J. Erslev: Anemia of chronic renal failure, Chap. 42, p. 456, in *Williams Hematology,* 5/e, 1995.

---

14 ANEMIA OF ENDOCRINE DISORDERS

ANEMIA OF PITUITARY DEFICIENCY

- Hypophyseal dysfunction or ablation is followed by development of normocytic, normochromic anemia, often associated with leukopenia.
- Replacement therapy with a combination of thyroid, adrenal, and gonadal hormones usually corrects the anemia.

ANEMIA OF THYROID DYSFUNCTION

- Some patients with myxedema have a mild-to-moderate normochromic and normocytic anemia that appears to be due to decreased red cell production.
- The plasma volume is decreased in myxedema, sometimes masking the true degree of anemia.
- The most common cause of anemia in myxedema in humans is iron deficiency. Menorrhagia occurs frequently in women with hypothyroidism and appears responsible for the iron deficiency. Myxedematous men may also be iron deficient, possibly because of poor iron absorption.
- Macrocytosis is often found in anemic patients with myxedema, usually because of accompanying folic acid deficiency. Vitamin B_{12} deficiency due to associated pernicious anemia may also occur.
- Patients with hyperthyroidism have increased red cell volume but do not appear to have polycythemia because the plasma volume is also increased.

ANEMIA OF ADRENAL DYSFUNCTION

- Humans with adrenal insufficiency have normocytic, normochromic anemia with accompanying reduction in plasma volume so that the true level of anemia is not evident from the hemoglobin level or hematocrit.
- Erythrocytosis develops in patients receiving ACTH or glucocorticoids, by a mechanism presently not understood.

ANEMIA OF GONADAL DYSFUNCTION

- Androgens stimulate erythropoiesis by increasing the production of erythropoietin (5α-H isomer), and by enhancing the effect of erythropoietin on marrow progenitor cells (5 β-H isomer)
- In normal adult males the hemoglobin level is 1 to 2 g/dl higher than in females, but with gonadal dysfunction the hemoglobin level in males is similar to that of the normal female.
- Estrogens in large doses cause moderately severe anemia by a mechanism not clearly defined.

ANEMIA OF PREGNANCY

- In humans the anemia of pregnancy is frequently caused or aggravated by iron deficiency, or, less often, folic acid deficiency.
- In normal women, anemia develops about the eighth week of pregnancy, progresses slowly until the 32d to 34th week, after which it is stable until it improves just before delivery. The hemoglobin level is usually about 10 g/dl in the last trimester.
- The total red cell volume increases about 20 percent during pregnancy, but the plasma volume increases about 30 percent, leading to dilutional anemia.

ANEMIA OF PARATHYROID DYSFUNCTION

- Primary hyperparathyroidism is occasionally accompanied by anemia, and parathyroidectomy in uremia may lead to improvement in the anemia.
- Hyperparathyroidism appears to cause anemia either by interfering with erythropoietin production or by leading to marrow sclerosis with reduction in red cell production.

ANEMIA OF PANCREATIC DYSFUNCTION

- Anemia is common in diabetes but appears to be the result of complications of the disease, rather than due to insulin deficiency.

For a more detailed discussion, see Allan J. Erslev: Anemia of endocrine disorders, Chap. 43, p. 462, in *Williams Hematology*, 5/e, 1995.

---

15 CONGENITAL DYSERYTHROPOIETIC ANEMIAS

Congenital dyserythropoietic anemias are a group of hereditary refractory anemias characterized by ineffective erythropoiesis, erythroid multinuclearity, and secondary hemosiderosis. Three types have been distinguished. In addition, a number of patients with similar, but not identical, forms of congenital dyserythropoietic anemia have been described.

CONGENITAL DYSERYTHROPOIETIC ANEMIA TYPE I

Clinical and Laboratory Features

- Presents in infancy or adolescence
- Autosomal recessive inheritance
- Moderate anemia (hematocrit 25 to 36 percent)
- Slight hyperbilirubinemia
- Splenomegaly
- Specific marrow findings summarized in Table 15-1

Differential Diagnosis

- May be confused with the thalassemia syndromes because of the similar blood findings and evidence of ineffective erythropoiesis.

TABLE 15-1 Congenital Dyserythropoietic Anemia, Types I, II, III—Marrow and Serological Features

CDA type	Marrow	Serology
I	Most erythroid cells abnormal: megaloblastoid changes; large cells with incompletely divided nuclear segments; double nuclei, internuclear chromatin bridges.	No serologic abnormalities.
II (HEMPAS)	Late polychromatophilic and orthochromic erythroblasts often contain 2 to 7 normal-appearing nuclei.	Cells possess unique HEMPAS antigen and are lysed by 30% of acidified normal sera; increased agglutination by anti-i, increased lysis by anti-I.
III	Giant erythroblasts, up to 50 μm in diameter, with up to 12 nuclei; prominent basophilic stippling.	Data inadequate; a single case showed increased agglutination by anti-i and increased lysis by anti-I, but a negative acidified serum test.

Source: Table 44-1 of *Williams Hematology*, 5/e, p. 467.

- The megaloblastoid marrow findings may suggest folic acid or vitamin B_{12} deficiency.

Treatment

- Transfusion not required.
- Phlebotomy or chelating agents may be beneficial for iron overload.

CONGENITAL DYSERYTHROPOIETIC ANEMIA TYPE II (HEMPAS)

- HEMPAS is an acronym for Hereditary Erythroblastic Multinuclearity associated with a Positive Acidified Serum test.

Clinical and Laboratory Features

- Autosomal recessive inheritance.
- Anemia varies from mild to severe.
- Reticulocyte count normal or decreased.
- Moderate-to-marked aniso- and poikilocytosis, anisochromia, and contracted spherocytes.
- Body iron stores and serum iron levels increased, and frank hemochromatosis occurs.
- Marrow and serological features are summarized in Table 15-1.

Treatment

- Partial benefit may be obtained with splenectomy.

CONGENITAL DYSERYTHROPOIETIC ANEMIA TYPE III

Clinical and Laboratory Features

- Autosomal dominant inheritance.
- Anemia may be mild or severe.
- Defect is intrinsic to progenitor cells.
- Marrow and serologic features presented in Table 15-1.

Treatment

- Transfusion-dependent patients have benefited from splenectomy.

For a more detailed discussion, see Ernest Beutler: The congenital dyserythropoietic anemias, Chap. 44, p. 467, in *Williams Hematology*, 5/e, 1995.

---

16 THE MEGALOBLASTIC ANEMIAS

DEFINITION

- Disorders caused by impaired synthesis of DNA.
- Characteristics are megaloblastic cells, typically present in the erythroid series as large cells with immature-appearing nuclei but with increasing hemoglobinization of the cytoplasm—often referred to as *nuclear-cytoplasmic asynchrony.*
- Megaloblastic granulocytic precursors are also present, and megakaryocytes may be abnormally large with nuclear abnormalities.

ETIOLOGY AND PATHOGENESIS

- Some examples of megaloblastic anemia, such as that with methotrexate toxicity, are due to deficient formation of dTTP because of the "methylfolate trap."
- In nutritional megaloblastic anemia there is evidence for impaired conversion of dUMP to dTMP. However, this finding does not provide a basis for the megaloblastic morphology, which remains poorly understood.

Clinical Features

- Anemia develops slowly, and the presenting symptoms are those of severe anemia, with weakness, palpitation, fatigue, light-headedness, and shortness of breath.
- The skin often assumes a lemon-yellow hue because of pallor combined with slight jaundice.

Laboratory Features

- Erythrocytes show marked aniso- and poikilocytosis, with many oval macrocytes and, in severe cases, basophilic stippling, Howell-Jolly bodies, and Cabot rings. Erythrocytes with megaloblastic nuclei may be present.
- Reticulocyte count is low.
- Anemia is macrocytic, with MCV of 100 to 150 fl or more, but coexisting iron deficiency, thalassemia trait, or inflammation may prevent macrocytosis.
- Leukopenia and thrombocytopenia are frequently present.
- Hypersegmented neutrophils are an early sign of megaloblastosis. Typically, the nuclei of more than 5 percent of the cells have more than five lobes.
- Platelets are smaller than usual, and vary more widely in size.
- Marrow shows erythroid hyperplasia with striking megaloblastic changes. Promegaloblasts with mitotic figures are abundant in severe

cases. The number of sideroblasts is increased, and macrophage iron content may also be increased.

- Coexisting iron deficiency may reduce the megaloblastic erythroid response, but hypersegmented neutrophils are still present in the blood, and giant metamyelocytes and bands persist in the marrow.
- Treatment of a patient with folic acid or cobalamin more than 12 h before marrow biopsy may mask the megaloblastic changes.
- Serum bilirubin, iron, and ferritin levels are somewhat elevated.
- Serum lactic dehydrogenase activity is markedly elevated, increasing with the severity of the anemia.
- Serum muramidase (lysozyme) activity is also high.

Cytokinetics

- Intramedullary destruction of red cell precursors (*ineffective erythropoiesis*) is a major feature of megaloblastic anemia. Ineffective granulopoiesis and thrombopoiesis are also present.
- Extramedullary hemolysis occurs. The red cell life span is reduced by 30 to 50 percent.
- Platelets are functionally abnormal in severe megaloblastic anemia.

FOLIC ACID DEFICIENCY

- Causes of folic acid deficiency are summarized in Table 16-1.
- An inadequate diet is the principal cause of folic acid deficiency. Folic acid reserves are small, and deficiency can develop rapidly.
- Alcohol can depress serum folate levels and accelerate the appearance of megaloblastic anemia in people with early folate deficiency.

Clinical Features

- Megaloblastic anemia with laboratory evidence of folic acid deficiency; full response to physiological doses of folic acid.

Laboratory Features

- Serum folate levels are reduced, but a low level may merely reflect reduced oral intake in the few days preceding the test.
- Red cell folic acid levels are reduced in folic acid deficiency but are also low in cobalamin deficiency; they are not low if the folate deficiency develops rapidly.

Differential Diagnosis

- Because of the possible development of neurologic complications in untreated patients with cobalamin deficiency, it is important to evaluate all patients with macrocytic anemia for both cobalamin and folic acid deficiency.

TABLE 16-1 Causes of Megaloblastic Anemias

Folate deficiency	Acute megaloblastic anemia
Decreased intake	Nitrous oxide exposure
Poor nutrition	Severe illness with:
Old age, poverty, alcoholism	Extensive transfusion
Hyperalimentation	Dialysis
Hemodialysis	Total parenteral nutrition
Premature infants	Exposure to weak folate antago-
Children on synthetic diets	nists (e.g., trimethoprim)
Goat's milk anemia	Drugs (see Table 16-2)
Impaired absorption	Inborn errors
Nontropical sprue	Cobalamin deficiency
Tropical sprue	Errors of folate metabolism
Other disease of the small	Errors of cobalamin metabolism
intestine	Others
Increased requirements	Hereditary orotic aciduria
Pregnancy	Lesch-Nyhan syndrome
Increased cell turnover	Thiamine-responsive megalo-
Chronic hemolytic anemia	blastic anemia
Exfoliative dermatitis	
Cobalamin deficiency	
Impaired absorption	
Gastric causes	
Pernicious anemia	
Gastrectomy	
Zollinger-Ellison syndrome	
Intestinal causes	
Ileal resection or disease	
Blind loop syndrome	
Fish tapeworm	
Pancreatic insufficiency	
Decreased intake	
Vegetarianism	

Source: Table 45-1 of *Williams Hematology*, 5/e, p. 471.

- Macrocytosis occurs without megaloblastic anemia in liver disease, hypothyroidism, aplastic anemia, myelodysplasia, pregnancy, and reticulocytosis, but in these settings the MCV rarely exceeds 110 fl.
- Folic acid deficiency responds to physiological doses of folic acid (200 μg/day), but cobalamin deficiency responds only to folic acid doses of 5 mg/day. Because neurologic complications may develop in patients with cobalamin deficiency treated with folic acid, a trial with folic acid is not recommended as a diagnostic test.

Therapy, Course, and Prognosis

- Folic acid is administered orally at a dose of 1 to 5 mg daily. At this dosage patients with malabsorption will still respond.
- Pregnant women should receive 1 mg of folic acid daily. Women at

risk for cobalamin deficiency, such as strict vegetarians, may also be given vitamin B_{12}, 1 mg parenterally every 3 months during the pregnancy.

COBALAMIN DEFICIENCY

- Causes of cobalamin deficiency are presented in Table 16-1.
- Cobalamin deficiency usually results from impaired absorption, most often due to pernicious anemia.

Pernicious Anemia

- Disease of later life, usually after age 40, due to failure of secretion of intrinsic factor by the gastric mucosa.
- Autoimmune disease in which there is immune destruction of the acid- and pepsin-secreting cells of the stomach.
- Some inherited predisposition exists.
- Gastric atrophy and achlorhydria occur in all patients.
- Brings with it a twofold increase in the incidence of gastric cancer.

Gastrectomy Syndromes

- Cobalamin deficiency develops within 5 to 6 years of total gastrectomy, due to loss of secretion of intrinsic factor and consequent failure to absorb cobalamins. The delay in onset of the anemia reflects the time required to exhaust cobalamin stores after absorption ceases.
- Cobalamin absorption may also be impaired after subtotal gastrectomy.

Zollinger-Ellison Syndrome

- Sufficient acid may be secreted to inactivate pancreatic proteases necessary for cobalamin absorption.

"Blind Loop" Syndrome

- Intestinal stasis from anatomical lesions or impaired motility may lead to intestinal colonization with bacteria which bind cobalamin before it can be absorbed.

Diphyllobothrium latum *Infestation*

- These parasites bind cobalamin and prevent absorption. Only about 3 percent of people infested with the parasites become anemic.

Pancreatic Disease

- Pancreatic exocrine insufficiency leads to deficiency of pancreatic proteases necessary for cobalamin absorption. Schilling tests (see below) are frequently positive with pancreatic disease but clinically significant deficiency of cobalamin is rare.

Dietary Cobalamin Deficiency

- Occurs rarely, usually in vegetarians who also avoid dairy products and eggs ("vegans").
- Breast-fed infants of vegan mothers may also develop cobalamin deficiency.

Clinical Features

- The clinical features of cobalamin deficiency are those of megaloblastic anemia generally, plus neurologic abnormalities specifically due to cobalamin deficiency.
- Neurologic abnormalities may occur in the absence of anemia and may be irreversible.
- The neurologic disorder usually begins with paresthesias of the fingers and toes and disturbances of vibration and position sense. The earliest signs are said to be loss of position sense in the second toe, and loss of vibration sense to 256 Hz but not to 128 Hz.
- If untreated, the disorder progresses to spastic ataxia because of demyelination of the posterior and lateral columns of the spinal cord, referred to as *combined system disease.*
- Cobalamin deficiency also affects the brain, and patients may develop somnolence and perversion of taste, smell, and vision, sometimes with optic atrophy.
- Dementia or frank psychosis may occur, the latter sometimes referred to as "megaloblastic madness."

Laboratory Features

- Serum cobalamin levels are low in most patients, but may be normal in cobalamin deficiency due to nitrous oxide inhalation and in some of the inherited abnormalities of cobalamin metabolism (see below).
- Serum cobalamin levels may be low with normal tissue levels in vegetarians, people taking megadoses of vitamin C, pregnancy (25 percent), transcobalamin I deficiency, or folate deficiency (30 percent).
- Serum folate levels may be high in cobalamin deficiency and may be normal in combined folate and cobalamin deficiency.
- Methylmalonic aciduria and elevated serum levels of methylmalonic acid or homocysteine are reliable indicators of cobalamin deficiency.
- Cobalamin absorption can be determined by measuring urinary radioactivity after ingestion of an oral dose of radioactive cobalamin, the Schilling test. If excretion of radioactivity is low, the test is repeated with the addition of oral intrinsic factor. Normal excretion of radioactivity indicates the original abnormality was due to deficiency of intrinsic factor.
- Some individuals are able to absorb free cobalamin but cannot release it from food and may therefore become cobalamin deficient. Such

patients will have a normal Schilling test, but the abnormality can be detected by a modification of the test which uses radioactive cobalamin in food.

- The major source of error in the Schilling test is incomplete urine collection. Renal disease may also delay excretion of the radioactive vitamin.

Differential Diagnosis

- Cobalamin deficiency leads to the general features of megaloblastic anemia with additional neurologic problems in some patients. The diagnosis is made from laboratory evidence of the deficiency. The specific diagnosis of pernicious anemia is made by demonstrating malabsorption of cobalamin, corrected by intrinsic factor.

Treatment, Course, and Prognosis

- Treatment consists of parenteral administration of cyanocobalamin (vitamin B_{12}) or hydroxycobalamin in doses sufficient to replete tissue stores and provide daily requirements.
- Toxicity is nil, but cobalamin doses larger than 100 μg saturate the transport proteins and much is lost in the urine.
- A typical treatment schedule consists of 1000 μg of vitamin B_{12} intramuscularly daily for 2 weeks, then weekly until the hematocrit is normal, and then monthly for life.
- It has been recommended that after initial therapy to return the hematocrit to normal, patients with neurologic abnormalities should receive 1000 μg every 2 weeks for 6 months.
- Infection can interfere with the response to vitamin B_{12} therapy.
- Transfusion may be required if the clinical picture requires prompt alleviation of anemia.
- Following initiation of cobalamin therapy there is often a prompt improvement in the sense of well being.
- Marrow erythropoiesis converts from megaloblastic to normoblastic beginning about 12 h after treatment is started.
- Reticulocytosis appears on day 3 to 5, and reaches a peak on day 4 to 10. The hemoglobin concentration should become normal within 1 to 2 months.
- Leukocyte and platelet counts normalize promptly, although neutrophil hypersegmentation persists for 10 to 14 days.
- Elevated serum bilirubin, serum iron, and lactic dehydrogenase levels fall rapidly.
- Severe hypokalemia may develop after cobalamin therapy, and death from hypokalemia has occurred. Potassium levels must be monitored and appropriate replacement given.
- Cobalamin therapy should be administered to all patients after total

gastrectomy. After partial gastrectomy patients should be followed carefully for the development of anemia.
- The anemia of the blind loop syndrome will respond to parenteral cobalamin therapy, but it also responds to oral antibiotic therapy or successful correction of an anatomical abnormality.
- About 1 percent of an oral dose of vitamin B_{12} is absorbed even in the absence of intrinsic factor. Therefore, patients with pernicious anemia can be successfully treated with oral vitamin B_{12} in doses of 1000 µg/day. Patients receiving such therapy should be carefully followed to ensure response.

ACUTE MEGALOBLASTIC ANEMIA

- Acute megaloblastic anemia refers to a syndrome of rapidly developing thrombocytopenia and/or leukopenia, with very little change in the hemoglobin level. The marrow is floridly megaloblastic.
- The most common cause is nitrous oxide anesthesia. Nitrous oxide destroys methylcobalamin, inducing cobalamin deficiency. The marrow becomes megaloblastic within 12 to 24 h. Hypersegmented neutrophils appear in the blood after 5 days.
- The effects of nitrous oxide disappear in a few days. Administration of folinic acid or vitamin B_{12} will accelerate recovery.
- Fatal megaloblastic anemia has occurred in patients with tetanus who were treated with nitrous oxide for weeks.
- Acute megaloblastic anemia may occur in seriously ill patients in intensive care units, patients transfused extensively, patients on dialysis or total parenteral nutrition, or patients receiving weak folic acid antagonists. The diagnosis is made from finding a megaloblastic marrow. Treatment is with parenteral folic acid (5 mg) and cobalamin (1 mg).

MEGALOBLASTIC ANEMIA CAUSED BY DRUGS

- A partial list of drugs that cause megaloblastic anemia is presented in Table 16-2.
- Methotrexate acts by inhibiting dihydrofolate reductase, the enzyme which reduces folic acid to the active, tetrahydro form. Methotrexate toxicity is treated with folinic acid, which is already fully reduced, and therefore can bypass the inhibited dihydrofolate reductase.

MEGALOBLASTIC ANEMIA IN CHILDHOOD

- Cobalamin malabsorption occurs in the presence of normal intrinsic factor in an inherited disorder of childhood (*selective malabsorption of cobalamin,* or *Imerslund-Gräsbeck disease*). There is associated albuminuria. Anemia usually develops before age 2. Treatment is with parenteral cobalamin.

TABLE 16-2 Some Drugs That Cause Megaloblastic Anemia

Agents	Comments
Antifolates	
Methotrexate Aminopterin	Very potent inhibitors of dihydrofolate reductase. Treat overdose with folinic acid.
Pyrimethamine Trimethoprim Sulfasalazine Chlorguanide (Proguanil) Triamterine	Much weaker than methotrexate and aminopterin. Treat with folinic acid or by withdrawing the drug. Can cause acute megaloblastic anemia in susceptible patients, especially those with low folate stores.
Purine analogs	
6-Mercaptopurine 6-Thioguanine Azathioprine	Megaloblastosis precedes hypoplasia. Usually mild. Responds to folinic acid but not folate.
Acyclovir	Megaloblastosis at high doses.
Pyrimidine analogs	
5-Fluorouracil Floxuridine (5-fluoro-deoxyuridine)	Mild megaloblastosis.
6-Azauridine	Blocks uridine monophosphate production by inhibiting orotidyl decarboxylase. Occasional megaloblastosis with orotic acid and orotidine in urine.
Zidovudine (AZT)	Severe megaloblastic anemia is the major side effect.
Ribonucleotide reductase inhibitor	
Hydroxyurea	Marked megaloblastosis within 1 to 2 days of starting therapy. Quickly reverse by withdrawing drug.
Cytarabine (cytosine arabinoside)	Early megaloblastosis is routine.
Anticonvulsants	
Phenytoin (diphenylhydantoin) Phenobarbital Primidone	Occasional megaloblastosis, associated with low folate levels. Responds to high dose folate (1–5 mg/day). Why anticonvulsants cause low folate is not understood.

Source: Adapted from Table 45-3 of *Williams Hematology*, 5/e, p. 482.

- *Congenital intrinsic factor deficiency* is an autosomal recessive disorder in which parietal cells fail to produce intrinsic factor. The disease presents at 6 to 24 months of age. Treatment is with parenteral cobalamin.
- *Transcobalamin II deficiency* is an autosomal recessive disorder which leads to megaloblastic anemia in early infancy. Serum cobalamin

levels are normal, but there is severe tissue cobalamin deficiency because transcobalamin II mediates transport of cobalamins into the tissues. The diagnosis is made by measuring serum transcobalamin II concentration. Treatment is with sufficiently large doses of cobalamin to override the deficient transport.

- *True juvenile pernicious anemia* is an extremely rare disorder usually presenting in adolescence. The diagnosis and treatment are as for the adult disease.

OTHER MEGALOBLASTIC ANEMIAS AND CHANGES

- Megaloblastic anemia may occur in some patients with inborn errors of cobalamin metabolism, inborn errors of folate metabolism, hereditary orotic aciduria, and the Lesch-Nyhan syndrome. A thiamine responsive megaloblastic anemia has also been reported.
- Megaloblastic changes have also been found in the congenital dyserythropoietic anemias, myelodysplastic syndromes, and erythroleukemia.

For a more detailed discussion, see Bernard M. Babior: Metabolic aspects of folic acid and cobalamin, Chap. 35, p. 380; and The megaloblastic anemias, Chap. 45, p. 471, in *Williams Hematology,* 5/e, 1995.

---

17 IRON DEFICIENCY

Iron deficiency is one of the most common chronic maladies in humans. For example, one-third to one-half of healthy females of reproductive age in the United States have absent iron stores, and 10 percent have iron deficiency anemia.

- Iron deficiency occurs in stages:
  - Iron depletion: storage iron decreased or absent.
  - Iron deficiency: storage iron decreased or absent with low serum iron concentration and transferrin saturation.
  - Iron deficiency anemia: storage iron decreased or absent, low serum iron concentration and transferrin saturation, and low hemoglobin level and reduced hematocrit.

The causes of iron deficiency are

- inadequate dietary intake of iron, primarily in infants and children
- malabsorption of iron
- chronic blood loss
- diversion of maternal iron to fetus/infant during pregnancy/lactation
- intravascular hemolysis with hemoglobinuria
- combinations of the above

DIETARY CAUSES

- Infants most often develop iron deficiency from unsupplemented milk diets.
- In children, poor diet plus intestinal parasites and/or bleeding gastrointestinal lesions are the usual causes.
- In the United States, average iron intake is 5 to 7 mg/kcal. Children and young women are in precarious iron balance and at risk for iron deficiency.

MALABSORPTION

- Iron absorption is decreased in the malabsorption syndromes.
- After subtotal gastrectomy, malabsorption of iron occurs in 50 percent of patients because of rapid gastrointestinal transit and because food bypasses the site of maximal absorption due to location of anastomosis.
- In addition, in postgastrectomy anemia there may be bleeding from anastomotic ulcer(s).
- Medicinal iron is well absorbed after partial gastrectomy.

CHRONIC BLOOD LOSS

- Chronic blood loss may occur from the respiratory, gastrointestinal, or genitourinary tracts or from phlebotomy for blood donation or laboratory testing, or it may be self-induced.
- Menorrhagia is a common cause of iron deficiency.

- The most common cause of iron deficiency in men and postmenopausal women is gastrointestinal bleeding.

PREGNANCY AND LACTATION

- The average iron loss is 900 mg. Lactation losses of iron average 30 mg/month.

PATHOGENESIS

- Lack of iron interferes with heme synthesis, which leads to reduced hemoglobin synthesis and defective erythropoiesis.
- There is decreased activity of iron-containing proteins, such as the cytochromes and succinic dehydrogenase.
- Neurologic dysfunction may occur, with impaired intellectual performance, paresthesias, etc.
- Gastric acid secretion is reduced, often irreversibly.
- Atrophy of oral and gastrointestinal mucosa may occur.

CLINICAL FEATURES

- Patients develop the general symptoms of anemia. However, there is poor correlation between hemoglobin levels and severity of symptoms. Some patients with marked iron deficiency may deny the common symptoms of fatigue, weakness, or palpitations.
- Irritability and headache occur frequently.
- Children may have poor attention span, poor response to sensory stimuli, retarded developmental and behavioral achievement, and retarded longitudinal growth.
- Paresthesias and burning of the tongue may occur, possibly due to tissue iron deficiency.
- Pica, craving to eat unusual substances such as clay or ice, is a classic manifestation.

PHYSICAL EXAMINATION

- Pallor
- Smooth red tongue, stomatitis
- Angular cheilitis
- Koilonychia (rare)
- Retinal hemorrhages/exudates (severe anemia)
- Accelerated retinopathy in diabetics
- Splenomegaly (occasionally)

LABORATORY CHANGES

Red Blood Cells

- Earliest change is anisocytosis and increased red cell distribution width (RDW).

- Mild ovalocytosis, target cells.
- Elongated hypochromic elliptocytes (pencil cells).
- Progressive hypochromia (low MCH) and microcytosis (low MCV), MCHC variable.
- Reticulocytes normal or reduced.
- The erythrocyte count, hemoglobin level, and hematocrit are all proportionately reduced.

Leukocytes

- Leukopenia (3000 to 4400/µl) is found in a small number of patients. Differential count is normal.

Platelets

- Thrombocytopenia develops in 28 percent of children and may occur in adults.
- Thrombocytosis found in
  - 35 percent of children
  - 50 to 75 percent of adults—usually secondary to chronic active blood loss

Marrow

- Marrow cellularity and M/E ratio variable.
- Decreased to absent sideroblasts.
- Decreased to absent hemosiderin by Prussian blue staining.
- Erythroblasts may be small, with narrow rim of ragged cytoplasm and poor hemoglobin formation

Serum Iron Concentration

- Usually low but may be normal.
- May be *reduced* with concomitant acute or chronic inflammation, malignancy, acute myocardial infarction, in the absence of iron deficiency.
- May be *elevated* 3 to 7 days after chemotherapy, or immediately after ingesting iron-containing medications. After receiving parenteral iron, the level may be elevated for weeks.

Total Iron Binding Capacity (TIBC)

- Usually increased in iron deficiency
- Saturation (iron/TIBC) is often 15 percent or less but this is *not* specific for iron deficiency.

Serum Ferritin

- Levels of less than 10 µg/liter are characteristic of iron deficient anemia.
- Levels of 10 to 20 µg/liter are presumptive, but not diagnostic.
- May be *elevated* with concomitant inflammatory diseases (e.g.,

rheumatoid arthritis), Gaucher disease, chronic renal disease, malignancy, hepatitis, or iron administration.
- Iron deficiency can be suspected in rheumatoid arthritis if the ferritin level is less than 60 μg/liter.

Free Erythrocyte Protoporphyrin (FEP)

- Concentration is usually increased in iron deficiency.
- Very sensitive for diagnosis of iron deficiency and suitable for large-scale screening of children, detecting both iron deficiency and lead poisoning.

DIAGNOSIS

- The physician who establishes a diagnosis of iron deficiency from blood loss has the obligation to determine the site and cause of hemorrhage.

Special Studies

- Multiple stools should be tested for occult blood.
  - Bleeding may be intermittent.
  - Tests are insensitive to <5 to 10 ml blood loss/day.
- ^{51}Cr RBC labeling may be used to quantitate blood loss.
- Angiography may be helpful if active bleeding is 0.5 ml/min or greater.
- Pertechnetate uptake studies may detect a Meckel diverticulum.
- Radiographic/endoscopic studies may detect the source of gastrointestinal bleeding.
- Exploratory laparotomy as last resort if source not apparent.
- Hemosiderin-laden macrophages in sputum if intrapulmonary bleeding suspected.

Differential Diagnosis

- Fe deficiency vs. thalassemia vs. anemia of chronic disease (see Table 17-1)

TREATMENT

Therapeutic Trial

- Should be via oral route.
- Expect
  - peak reticulocytosis at 1 to 2 weeks, although reticulocyte response may be minimal
  - significant increase in hemoglobin concentration at 3 to 4 weeks
  - one-half of hemoglobin deficit corrected at 4 to 5 weeks
  - hemoglobin level normal at 2 to 4 months
- Unless there is continued bleeding, absence of these changes indi-

TABLE 17-1 Differential Diagnosis

Laboratory test	Thalassemias	Anemia of chronic disease	Iron deficiency anemia
RBC	Majority have >5 × 10^6 RBC/μl	Usually low	Usually low
MCV	Usually 60 to 70	Low in 20 to 30 percent	Rarely as low as 60 to 70
Serum ferritin level	Normal or increased	Normal or increased	Low
Elevated Hb A$_2$, F, H, or Lepore	Usually present	Absent	Absent
Serum iron concentration	Normal to high	Low	Low
TIBC	Normal to Low	Usually low	Usually high
Transferrin saturation	Normal to high	Usually >15% but often low	Usually low but may be normal

cates that iron deficiency is not the cause of anemia. Iron treatment should be stopped and another mechanism sought (see also "Failure to respond," below).

Oral Iron Therapy

- Dietary sources may not be sufficient for treatment.
- Safest, cheapest are oral ferrous salts.
- Nonenteric coated forms are preferred.
- Avoid multiple hematinics.
- Do not give with meals or antacids or inhibitors of acid production.
- Continue for 12 months after hemoglobin level is normal to replenish iron stores.
- Daily total of 150 to 200 mg elemental iron in 3 to 4 doses, each 1 h before meals (65 mg of elemental iron is contained in 325 mg of ferrous sulfate USP, or in 200 mg dried ferrous sulfate).
- 10 to 20 percent of patients will have gastrointestinal intolerance to pills with pyrosis, constipation, diarrhea, and/or metallic taste and require
  - total daily dose reduction
  - change of oral iron preparation

Parenteral Iron Therapy

- Routine use rarely justified.
- Indications are

- malabsorption
- intolerance to oral iron preparations (colitis, enteritis)
- need in excess of amount that can be given orally
- patient uncooperative or unavailable for follow-up
- Iron dextran:
  - Only product available in United States.
  - 50 mg elemental iron per milliliter.
  - Approximately 70 percent readily available for Hb synthesis.
  - May be given IM or IV.
  - Be aware of danger of anaphylaxis or other systemic side effects.
  - See text or product information sheet for dosage calculations.

Length of Treatment

- Continue therapy for 12 months after hemoglobin level is normal, in order to replenish iron stores.
- Therapy may be needed indefinitely if bleeding continues.

Failure to Respond to Therapy

- Wrong oral preparation (enteric coated, insoluble iron, too little iron in each dose).
- Bleeding not controlled.
- Therapy not long enough to show response.
- Patient not taking medication.
- Concomitant deficiencies (vitamin B_{12}, folate, thyroid).
- Concomitant illness:
  - inflammation, infection, malignancy, hepatic disease, renal disease
- Diagnosis incorrect:
  - thalassemia, lead poisoning, etc.

For a more detailed discussion, see Virgil F. Fairbands, Ernest Beutler: Iron deficiency, Chap. 46, p. 490; and Iron metabolism, Chap. 34, p. 369, in *Williams Hematology,* 5/e, 1995.

---

18 ANEMIA DUE TO OTHER NUTRITIONAL DEFICIENCIES

VITAMIN A DEFICIENCY

- Anemia is characterized by reduced MCV, MCHC, and aniso- and poikilocytosis.
- Similar to the anemia of chronic disease with reduced serum iron concentration, normal or low serum total iron-binding capacity and increased liver and marrow iron stores, and failure to respond to treatment with medicinal iron.
- Responds to vitamin A repletion.

VITAMIN B_6 DEFICIENCY: PYRIDOXAL, PYRIDOXINE, PYRIDOXAMINE

- May lead to hypochromic microcytic anemia.
- Microcytic anemia may occur in patients taking isoniazid, which interferes with B_6 metabolism. Such anemias may be corrected with large doses of pyridoxine.
- Some patients who are not vitamin B_6 deficient may have sideroblastic anemia, which will partially respond to high doses of pyridoxine (see Chaps. 6 and 41).

RIBOFLAVIN DEFICIENCY

- Volunteers receiving a riboflavin-deficient diet plus a riboflavin antagonist (galactoflavin) developed vacuolated erythroid precursors, followed by pure red cell aplasia—all reversed by administration of riboflavin.
- Reduced erythrocyte glutathione reductase activity occurs in riboflavin deficiency, but is not associated with hemolysis or oxidant-induced injury.

VITAMIN C (ASCORBIC ACID) DEFICIENCY

- Anemia in humans with scurvy may be macrocytic, normocytic, or microcytic, and the marrow may be hypocellular, normocellular, or hypercellular. In 10 percent of patients the marrow is frankly megaloblastic.
- Macrocytic anemia may develop with vitamin C deficiency because vitamin C interacts with folic acid in the generation of tetrahydrofolic acid.
- Microcytic anemia may develop because vitamin C is important in iron metabolism, facilitating the absorption and transport of iron.
- Iron deficiency in children is often associated with dietary vitamin C deficiency.
- Normocytic normochromic anemia with a reticulocytosis of 5 to 10 percent also develops in scurvy, perhaps from compromised cellular antioxidant defense mechanisms.

- The anemia of vitamin C deficiency responds promptly to administration of vitamin C. Sufficient folic acid and iron must be present for the response to occur.

VITAMIN E (α-TOCOPHEROL) DEFICIENCY

- Vitamin E serves as an antioxidant in humans.
- The vitamin E requirement varies with polyunsaturated fatty acid content of diet and the content of peroxidizable lipids in tissues.
- Neonatal period: Low-birth-weight infants have low serum and tissue concentrations of vitamin E.
  - If they receive a diet rich in polyunsaturated fatty acids and adequate in iron but inadequate in vitamin E, they will develop hemolytic anemia by 4 to 6 weeks of age.
  - Anemia is often associated with altered red cell morphology, thrombocytosis, and edema of the dorsum of the feet and pretibial area.
  - These abnormalities are reversed promptly by treatment with vitamin E.
- Chronic fat malabsorption, such as is common in cystic fibrosis, will lead to vitamin E deficiency if daily supplements of the water-soluble form of this vitamin are not given. In such patients, the red cell life span is reduced, but anemia does not develop.

COPPER DEFICIENCY

- Copper is required for absorption and utilization of iron, perhaps functioning by maintaining iron in the ferric state for transferrin transport.
- Cooper deficiency occurs in malnourished children and in infants and adults receiving parenteral alimentation, and can also be caused by chronic ingestion of massive quantities of zinc, which impairs copper absorption.
- Copper deficiency causes a microcytic anemia with hypoferremia, neutropenia, and vacuolated erythroid precursors in marrow, which does not respond to iron therapy.
- Young children with copper deficiency may show osteoporosis, flaring of ribs, and other bony abnormalities.
- Diagnosis is established by demonstration of low serum ceruloplasmin or copper levels, or by therapeutic trial with copper at a dose of 0.2 mg/kg/day. A 10 percent solution of copper sulfate contains 25 mg of copper per ml.
- Low serum copper values may also be seen in hypoproteinemic states (exudative enteropathies, nephrosis) and Wilson disease.

ZINC DEFICIENCY

- May accompany thalassemia or sickle cell disease and may be produced by intensive desferrioxamine therapy.
- Isolated zinc deficiency does not produce anemia.

ANEMIA OF STARVATION

- Semistarvation causes mild to moderate normocytic normochromic anemia with reduced marrow erythroid precursors. The anemia appears to be dilutional.
- Complete starvation for 9 to 12 weeks leads to anemia and marrow hypocellularity, which responds to resumption of a normal diet. The anemia may be a response to a hypometabolic state with consequent decrease in oxygen requirements.

ANEMIA OF PROTEIN DEFICIENCY (KWASHIORKOR)

- In protein-calorie malnutrition, the hemoglobin level may fall to 8 g/dl, but some children may not be anemic because the reduced red cell mass is masked by a reduced plasma volume.
- Anemia is normocytic, normochromic, with significant aniso- and poikilocytosis.
- Leukocyte and platelet counts are usually normal.
- The marrow is usually normally cellular or hypocellular with reduced erythroid precursors.
- Patients respond slowly to high-protein diets.
- After 3 or 4 weeks of treatment, there may be an episode of erythroid aplasia which responds to riboflavin or prednisone.
- Occult deficiencies may become manifest during the repletion period: e.g., iron, folic acid, vitamin E, and vitamin B_{12}.

ALCOHOLISM

- Chronic alcohol ingestion is often associated with anemia, which may be due to multiple causes:
  - nutritional deficiencies
  - chronic gastrointestinal bleeding
  - hepatic dysfunction
  - hemolytic anemia
  - hypersplenism from portal hypertension
  - direct toxic effects of ethanol on erythropoiesis and on folate metabolism
- Macrocytic anemia occurs commonly in hospitalized alcoholic patients and is often associated with megaloblastic changes and sometimes with ringed sideroblasts.
  - Megaloblastic anemia in alcoholism is almost always due to folic acid deficiency.
  - Megaloblastic anemia is more common in drinkers of wine or whiskey, which have low folate content, than in drinkers of beer, which is a rich source of folate.
  - Alcoholics often have associated iron deficiency, producing a "dimorphic" blood picture (macrocytes, hypersegmented neutrophils, and hypochromic microcytes).

- Iron deficiency may be unmasked after treatment with folic acid alone by demonstration of an emerging population of microcytic red cells. Treatment with iron alone may unmask folate deficiency, by demonstration of an emerging population of macrocytes.
- Mild macrocytosis (MCV 100 to 110 fl) is found in 82 to 96 percent of chronic alcoholics.
  - Anemia is usually absent, macrocytes are typically round, and neutrophil hypersegmentation is not present.
  - The patients are not folate deficient, and the macrocytosis persists until the patient abstains from alcohol.

For a more detailed discussion, see Frank A. Oski: Anemia due to other nutritional deficiencies, Chap. 47, p. 511, in *Williams Hematology,* 5/e, 1995.

---

19 ANEMIA ASSOCIATED WITH MARROW INFILTRATION

DEFINITIONS

- Anemia or pancytopenia associated with extensive marrow infiltration is called *myelophthisic anemia*.
- *Leukoerythroblastosis* refers to anemia with schistocytes, teardrop-shaped red cells, nucleated red cells, megakaryocytic fragments, and immature myeloid cells in the blood.

ETIOLOGY AND PATHOGENESIS

- Conditions causing marrow infiltration are listed in Table 19-1.
- In most cases the infiltration is focal, with surrounding areas of normal or hyperactive marrow.
- Myelophthisic anemia is most likely caused by humoral factors or injury to the microenvironment.
- Disruption of the microenvironment by infiltration with foreign cells leads to premature release of immature blood cells from the marrow.

TABLE 19-1 Causes of Marrow Infiltration

1. Metastatic malignancy
    Most commonly from lung, breast, prostate
        Possible from almost any source

2. Hematologic malignancy
    Stem cell disorders
      Acute myelogenous leukemia
      Chronic myelogenous leukemia
      Polycythemia vera
      Agnogenic myeloid metaplasia
      Preleukemia
      Malignant histiocytosis
    Lymphocytic disorders
      Acute lymphocytic leukemia
      Chronic lymphocytic leukemia
      Hairy cell leukemia
      Plasma cell myeloma
      Lymphoma
      Hodgkin disease

3. Infections, inflammations, granulomas
      Bacterial (staphylococcus, typhoid)
      Fungal (mucormycosis, histoplasma)
      Miliary tuberculosis
      Sarcoidosis

4. Metabolic disorders
      Gaucher disease
      Other lipid storage disease

Source: Table 48-1 of *Williams Hematology*, 5/e, p. 516.

CLINICAL FEATURES

- The clinical features of marrow infiltrative disorders are usually those of the underlying disease.

LABORATORY FEATURES

- Anemia is mild to moderate.
- Leukocyte and platelet counts may be high or low.
- Blood film may show aniso- and poikilocytosis, with schistocytes, teardrop cells, nucleated red cells, immature neutrophils, and mega-karyocytic fragments.
- Leukocyte alkaline phosphatase activity is normal or increased.
- Cancer cells may occasionally be found on the blood film.
- Marrow biopsy is the most reliable diagnostic procedure. Marrow aspiration may also be of value. Aspiration or biopsy is most likely to be positive if taken from a tender area of bone.
- Sites of marrow infiltration may be detected by bone scan or by MRI.

DIFFERENTIAL DIAGNOSIS

- Leukoerythroblastosis may occur with severe blood loss, transient hypoxia, or marrow necrosis.
- Idiopathic myelofibrosis (see Chap. 10) may be confused with meta-static disease with focal fibrosis.

TREATMENT

- Splenectomy may be beneficial when there is concomitant hyper-splenism.
- Marrow infiltration may not adversely affect the response to treatment of malignant disease.
- Therapy with erythropoietin may be helpful.

For a more detailed discussion, see Allan J. Erslev: Anemia associated with marrow infiltration, Chap. 48, p. 516, in *Williams Hematology,* 5/e, 1995.

---

20 ANEMIA OF CHRONIC DISEASE

DEFINITION

- Anemia associated with chronic infection, inflammatory disease, or neoplastic disease.
- 1 to 2 months of sustained disease is required for anemia to develop.
- Anemia is moderate, with a hemoglobin level between 7 and 11 g/dl, and is rarely symptomatic.
- Common features are
  - low serum iron level
  - low serum total iron-binding capacity
  - increased marrow iron stores
  - reduced rate of red cell production

PATHOGENESIS

- Red cell life span is reduced by 20 to 30 percent.
- Impaired release of iron from macrophages leads to a low level of serum iron and consequent low saturation of transferrin. This change occurs early, for example, within 24 h of surgery.
- Production of erythropoietin (EPO) is decreased in response to anemia, and the ability of erythroid precursors to respond to EPO is impaired.

CLINICAL AND LABORATORY FEATURES

- Anemia is usually overshadowed by symptoms of the primary disease.
- Diagnosis depends on laboratory findings:
  - Initially normochromic, normocytic anemia; hypochromic, microcytic features develop as disease progresses.
  - Low serum iron level and somewhat decreased serum transferrin concentration; decreased percent saturation of transferrin.
  - Level of serum ferritin, an acute phase protein, is inappropriately elevated with respect to storage iron.
  - Bone marrow contains increased storage iron. The M/E ratio is normal, and the percentage of sideroblasts is decreased.
  - In iron deficiency anemia, low serum iron, increased transferrin, decreased storage iron, decreased serum ferritin.

DIFFERENTIAL DIAGNOSIS

- Dilution anemia, in patients with far advanced neoplastic disease.
- Drug-induced marrow suppression, or drug-induced hemolysis.
- Iron deficiency anemia.
- Anemia of chronic renal failure.
- Myelophthisic anemia, due to carcinoma or lymphoma replacing marrow.

THERAPY

- No treatment may be necessary.
- Iron (by mouth or parenterally) is contraindicated.
- Cobalt chloride and androgenic steroids may be of benefit but have unacceptable side effects.
- Packed red cell transfusions may be given, if the anemia is symptomatic.
- EPO therapy is effective.
  - Dose: 100 to 150 U/kg of rhEPO three times weekly, SC or IV.
  - The lower the baseline endogenous EPO concentration and the more severe the anemia the better the results.

For a more detailed discussion, see Allan J. Erslev: Anemia of chronic disease, Chap. 49, in *Williams Hematology,* 5/e, 1995.

---

21 IRON OVERLOAD

Iron overload denotes an excess of iron in the body. The various causes are summarized in Table 21-1.

HEREDITARY HEMOCHROMATOSIS

Etiology and Pathogenesis

- Autosomal recessive disorder. Heterozygotes do not develop the disease.
- Gene is on the short arm of chromosome 6, closely linked to the HLA locus. Patients have a high frequency of HLA-A3 and B7 alleles.
- Excessive iron absorption through the gastrointestinal mucosa leads to accumulation of ferritin and hemosiderin in most cells in the body, especially in hepatocytes, bile duct epithelium, and macrophages.
- Prevalent in populations of European origin.

Clinical Features

- Hemochromatosis usually presents in the fifth decade or later and is rare in children and young adults. The male/female ratio is 5:1, and the disease is uncommon in premenopausal women.
- Most common symptoms are weakness, lethargy, loss of libido, weight loss, and arthralgia.
- Arthralgia typically involves second and third metacarpophalangeal joints with swelling and tenderness. Hips and knees may also be involved.
- Chondrocalcinosis or calcification of periarticular ligaments is a frequent late manifestation. Synovial fluid may contain calcium pyrophosphate and apatite crystals.
- Skin becomes hyperpigmented primarily from deposition of melanin.
- Cardiac effects are common:
  - arrhythmias

TABLE 21-1 Causes of Iron Overload

Genetic	Acquired
Hereditary hemochromatosis	Chronic ingestion of medicinal iron
Thalassemia major	
Hereditary sideroblastic anemia	Transfusion iron overload
Hereditary hemolytic anemias	Acquired sideroblastic anemia
Pyruvate kinase deficiency	Porphyria cutanea tarda*
G-6-PD deficiency	African nutritional hemochromatosis*
Congenital dyserythropoietic anemia	
Neonatal hemochromatosis	Siderosis associated with splenorenal or portocaval shunts
Congenital atransferrinemia	

*Genetic component
Source: Adapted from Table 51-1 of *Williams Hematology*, 5/e, p. 529.

- cardiomegaly (may be due to restrictive or dilated cardiomyopathy)
- congestive failure
- Endocrinopathies are common:
  - pancreas (may show diffuse fibrosis and loss of islets)
  - diabetes mellitus
  - hypothyroidism (10 percent of male patients)
  - hypothalamic pituitary insufficiency, usually involving gonadotropins (about half of patients); often features
    - testicular atrophy, azoospermia, reduced libido, and impotence
    - premature menopause
- Hepatomegaly and splenomegaly are frequently present.
  - Jaundice is uncommon.
  - Esophageal varices develop late in the disease.
  - Hepatocellular carcinoma occurs in one-third of patients.
  - Patients who have hemochromatosis and also consume significant quantities of alcohol are more likely to develop hepatic fibrosis than patients who abstain from alcohol.

Laboratory Features

- Patients often have hyperglycemia and an abnormal glucose tolerance test.
- Serum iron levels exceed 180 μg/dl (32 μmol/liter) in early cases, and the transferrin saturation usually exceeds 60 percent.
- Serum total iron-binding capacity is usually normal but may be low in patients with cirrhosis.
- Serum ferritin level is greater than 500 μg/liter and commonly exceeds 1000 μg/liter.
- Serum aminotransferase activities are usually increased.
- Serum concentrations of pituitary gonadotrophins and androgens are often low.
- Serum thyroxine levels may be low and TSH concentrations increased.

Diagnosis and Screening for Disease

- Early diagnosis is imperative because complications may be irreversible and lead to death, for example, from hepatocellular carcinoma.
- Early diagnosis requires screening for iron overload. If the serum iron concentration is greater than 180 μg/dl and the transferrin saturation is above 60 percent, hemochromatosis is likely if other causes of iron overload have been ruled out.
- Serum ferritin levels are useful in screening but may be less sensitive than the serum iron level and transferrin saturation.
- Estimates of the amount of marrow iron have little or no diagnostic value.
- CT scan and MRI can demonstrate increased iron content of the liver, but high cost makes these tests inappropriate for screening.

- Liver biopsy is required in most cases to assess the degree of liver injury, to estimate the amount of iron deposition, and for direct chemical assay of iron content
  - In normal liver iron content is less than 2.8 mg/g dry weight (50 μmol/g).
  - In alcoholic liver disease, iron content is less than 5.6 mg/g (100 μmol/g).
  - In hemochromatosis, iron content exceeds 5.6 mg/g (100 μmol/g), and in hemochromatosis with cirrhosis iron content is usually greater than 11 mg/g (200 μmol/g).
- Testing for HLA antigens is of value only within the sibship. All siblings with the same HLA genotype as the patient are presumed to be at-risk homozygotes.
- Five restriction endonuclease polymorphisms are linked to the hemochromatosis gene and may prove valuable in family studies.

Treatment

- Removal of 500 ml blood by venesection once or twice a week depletes the body iron burden. Each 500 ml removes between 200 and 300 mg iron.
- The usual patient has accumulated 30 to 40 g excess iron, which will be depleted in 1 to 2 years if phlebotomy is done twice weekly.
- Adequacy of treatment may be gauged by progressive fall in hemoglobin level and the MCH.
- For chronic treatment, removal of 500 ml blood every few months is usually sufficient. Measurements of serum ferritin levels are more useful than estimates of transferrin saturation in monitoring the effects of phlebotomy.
- Alcohol and other hepatotoxins must be avoided.

Prognosis

- Life-span may be normal if treatment started during precirrhotic stage.
- Incidence of hepatocellular carcinoma is not diminished by treatment once there is hepatic fibrosis.
- Treatment may improve diabetes, cardiac function, and gonadal insufficiency.

For more detailed discussion, see Virgil F. Fairbanks, William P. Baldus: Iron overload, Chap. 51, p. 529, in *Williams Hematology,* 5/e, 1995.

22 HEREDITARY SPHEROCYTOSIS, ELLIPTOCYTOSIS, AND RELATED DISORDERS

HEREDITARY SPHEROCYTOSIS

Hereditary spherocytosis (HS) is an inherited condition with hemolysis of variable intensity, spherocytosis, and increased osmotic fragility of red blood cells. There is a favorable response to splenectomy.

Etiology

- Accelerated red cell destruction results from deficiency or abnormality of one or more of the red cell membrane proteins, resulting in release of membrane lipids, decreased surface area, and formation of poorly deformable spherocytes.
- The underlying molecular defects are heterogeneous and can be divided into four major groups:

  1. Partial deficiency of spectrin
  2. Combined partial deficiency of spectrin and ankyrin
  3. Partial deficiency of band 3 protein
  4. Deficiency of protein 4.2 and other less common defects

Partial Spectrin Deficiency

- In dominantly inherited HS only one point mutation has been found. This is located in a highly conserved region of β spectrin, which is involved in binding to protein 4.1; binding to both protein 4.1 and actin is abnormal.
- In recessively inherited HS, all known defects involve α spectrin.

Combined Spectrin/Ankyrin Deficiency

- Involves loss or reduced expression of the ankyrin gene. As ankyrin is the primary spectrin binding site on the membrane, proportional decrease in spectrin is noted.

Partial Deficiency of Band 3 Protein

- Dominantly inherited disorder that presents with "pincered" red cells. As the cells age, the band 3 deficiency worsens, suggesting that the protein is unstable.

Deficiency of Protein 4.2

- Several mutations have been identified as the cause, but the pathophysiology has not been clarified.

Pathophysiology

- With spectrin deficiency larger areas of lipid bilayer are not directly supported by the submembranous skeleton, causing loss of lipid in submicroscopic vesicles.
- The red cell membrane is more permeable to sodium, which activates the Na^+, K^+-ATPase pump and leads to K^+ loss and dehydration.
- A decrease in the surface area-to-volume ratio and an increase in internal viscosity make spherocytes less deformable and unable to penetrate the walls between splenic cords and sinuses.
- While retained in the spleen the red cells undergo a poorly understood "conditioning effect," which renders the cells more osmotically fragile and more spherical.
- Ultimately, the cells are engulfed by macrophages and destroyed.
- In almost all cases the clinical findings are limited to the red cell. However, HS may occur in association with a degenerative spinal cord disorder, cardiomyopathy, or mental retardation.

Prevalence/Inheritance

- In northern Europeans the prevalence of HS is believed to be 1 : 5000, but this may be an underestimate. The prevalence in other ethnic groups is unknown.
- The severity of the condition varies greatly among kindreds, but the typical autosomal dominant form is uniform within a family.
- Several cases of recessively inherited HS have been reported.

Clinical Features

- The condition is highly variable in presentation.
- An asymptomatic carrier state has been suggested by reports of asymptomatic parents whose children presented with typical HS.
- In some cases, anemia may be absent as increased red cell production in the marrow compensates for the red cell destruction. Changes in red cell morphology may be very subtle, and the bilirubin level and reticulocyte count may be normal to slightly elevated.
- Typically, HS presents as a mild anemia first noted in the neonate; splenomegaly and mild jaundice are characteristic features; occasionally the spleen becomes very large.
- Severe transfusion dependent anemia may be seen, improved modestly by splenectomy. Most such affected individuals appear to be homozygous for an autosomal recessive HS gene.

Complications

- Aplastic crises due to parvovirus infection result in temporary reticulocytopenia and falling hematocrit.

- Acute megaloblastic changes may result from folate deficiency, particularly in the setting of pregnancy.
- Increased hemolysis may occur during infection but it is rarely severe.
- Gallstones develop in approximately 50 percent of patients, including those with mild disease and occasionally in children.
- Recurrent lower leg ulcerations or dermatitis develop in some patients; these heal quickly after splenectomy.
- Rarely extramedullary hemopoiesis may present as a mass.
- Iron overload due to frequent transfusions may occur in severely affected individuals.

Laboratory Features

- The degree of anemia varies with severity of the disease; significant reticulocytosis is found in nearly all patients. White blood cell and platelet counts are normal initially, but increased after splenectomy.
- Few red cells are truly spherocytic; usually they are swollen, lack central concavity, and appear to contain more hemoglobin than normal. These can be missed in mild HS as loss of surface area may be small. MCHC is increased in approximately 50 percent of patients, many as high as 40 g/dl. MCH and MCV are normal but the MCV represents a mean of larger reticulocytes and smaller spherocytes. Spherocytes are less prominent after splenectomy.
- "Pincered" red cells are seen in band 3 deficient individuals.
- Because of increased red cell turnover, polychromasia and occasional nucleated red cells are noted in the peripheral smear. Indicators of red cell destruction include increased serum levels of LDH and unconjugated bilirubin, decreased haptoglobin concentration, and increased amounts of urobilinogen in the urine.
- HS cells hemolyze more quickly in hypotonic salt solutions. The abnormality is more prominent in individuals with intact spleens. The osmotic fragility of HS cells is greatly increased by incubation at 37° for 24 h. Occasionally the only abnormality on testing may be a "tail" in the osmotic fragility curve, reflecting the most fragile cells.
- Other tests for detection of HS have been described but are probably no better than the incubated osmotic fragility test.

Differential Diagnosis

- Immune-mediated hemolysis and unstable hemoglobins may lead to formation of spherocytes. Spherocytes also occasionally occur in patients with an enlarged spleen or with microangiopathic hemolytic anemia. The spherocytes in HS are relatively uniform in shape and result in increased MCHC.
- HS should be considered in individuals with incidentally noted splenomegaly, gallstones at a young age, or anemia developing during pregnancy, parvovirus infections, or infectious mononucleosis.

- Diagnosis can be obscured in obstructive jaundice as red cells may normalize in appearance and increase in survival from accumulation of cholesterol and phospholipid.
- Iron deficiency also may improve shape and osmotic fragility, but survival is still shortened.
- Gilbert syndrome may be distinguished by examining red cell shape and osmotic fragility.

Therapy, Course, and Prognosis

- Because of increased red cell turnover, folic acid supplementation is of value. Patients with aplastic crisis or severe hemolysis may require transfusion.
- Splenectomy usually corrects the anemia, but red cell survival remains shortened in some patients; spherocytosis is less prominent and osmotic fragility lessens. In severely affected individuals splenectomy may only partially improve the hemolysis.
- Splenectomy is not always indicated in patients with mild disease. Splenectomy should be performed in patients with symptomatic anemia, or if gallstones are present, in patients with mild anemia.
- Occasionally, splenectomy may not correct the anemia because of an accessory spleen or the development of splenosis as a result of splenic tissue accidently spilled into the peritoneal cavity at time of surgery. If a concomitant hemolytic disorder (such as pyruvate kinase deficiency) is present, splenectomy may not be effective. Splenectomy usually is delayed until after 6 years of age because of increased susceptibility to infection in younger children. Partial splenectomy may improve anemia and retain adequate defense against infection.

HEREDITARY ELLIPTOCYTOSIS (HE) AND RELATED DISORDERS

Definition

- Encompasses a heterogeneous group of disorders with a common feature of elliptical red cells. It is divided usually into three major groups:

  1. Common HE with discoidal elliptocytes
  2. Spherocytic or ovalocytic HE
  3. Stomatocytic HE (also called Melanesian or Southeast Asian ovalocytosis) in which cells are rounder but have a longitudinal or transverse slit

Etiology and Pathogenesis

- The most common molecular defects are mutations in α or β spectrin.
- Deficiency or dysfunction of protein 4.1 can also be elliptocytogenic.

- Glycophorin C deficiency can occur from several molecular defects; homozygous individuals will have elliptocytosis but no anemia.
- Most defects which cause elliptocytosis render the red cell membrane skeleton unstable. In severely affected individuals red cell fragmentation may occur under conditions of normal shear stress.
- Red cell precursors in common HE are round, but red cells become more elliptical as they age in vivo. It is thought that HE cells are permanently stabilized in their abnormal shape by reorganization of the skeleton with new protein contacts that prevent recovery of normal shape. The main features that affect severity of hemolysis are the spectrin content and the percentage of dimeric spectrin.

Prevalence/Inheritance

- In the United States, the prevalence of HE is approximately 3 to 5 per 10,000; it is more frequent in blacks, but prevalence data are not available. The prevalence is higher in areas where malaria is endemic (0.6 percent or more in equatorial Africa).
- In both common HE and stomatocytic HE, the inheritance pattern is autosomal dominant; occasionally HE can be inherited from an asymptomatic carrier.

Clinical Features

- Completely asymptomatic individuals may carry α-spectrin mutations. Usually these are parents or siblings of patients with hereditary pyropoikilocytosis (HPP) or occasionally HE.
- Elliptocytes may be evident in minimal or mild HE. Red cell survival may be normal in such patients.
- Transient hemolysis may be noted in individuals with mild HE if they develop viral, bacterial, or protozoal infections; renal transplant rejection; vitamin B_{12} deficiency; or if they become pregnant.
- Infants with an HE defect may have a severe hemolytic anemia during the first year of life. Destabilization of the abnormal membrane is due to increased free 2,3-bisphosphoglycerate, which binds poorly to fetal hemoglobin. As fetal hemoglobin decreases in concentration the picture changes to mild HE.
- HE may result in significant hemolysis requiring splenectomy. Such patients may be heterozygotes carrying a severely dysfunctional α-spectrin mutant or homozygotes for 4.1 deficiency or β-spectrin mutations. These individuals may have all the clinical features seen in HS: gallstones, leg ulcers, frontal bossing. In addition to elliptocytes, patients with severe disease also have large numbers of poikilocytes and small red cell fragments.
- Hereditary pyropoikilocytosis (HPP) is a severe hemolytic anemia with marked microspherocytes and micropoikilocytes (MCV as low as 50 fl) and thermal instability of red cells. It is an autosomal recessive

disorder. The patients are heterozygous for an α-spectrin mutation and a defect in spectrin synthesis. The same phenotype occurs in homozygotes or double heterozygotes for one or two α-spectrin mutations, respectively. It is chiefly seen in blacks. HPP represents a subset of HE; identical spectrin mutations have been noted but the defect is more severe in HPP where a partial spectrin deficiency is also seen. HPP is clinically indistinguishable from severe homozygous HE.

Laboratory Features

- The definition of elliptocytosis based on red cell shape and percentage of affected cells is arbitrary. Axial ratios of the red cell may vary considerably, as do the number of elliptocytes seen even in patients with a clearly defined biochemical defect. The percentage of elliptocytes in normal subjects is less than 5 percent. A positive family history is more helpful in making the diagnosis than precisely describing and quantitating elliptocytes.
- Osmotic fragility is normal in mild HE but increased in severe HE, spherocytic HE, and HPP.
- In normal individuals, spectrin denatures and red cells fragment at temperature of 49 to 50°C. Generally in HPP this occurs at temperatures of 45 to 46°C, although cases of otherwise typical HPP may have normal thermal stability. Thermal instability has also been detected in HE individuals with α-spectrin mutations.

Differential Diagnosis

- Elliptocytes and poikilocytes are commonly found in many conditions, including megaloblastic anemia, myelophthisic anemias, myelodysplastic syndromes, and pyruvate kinase deficiency. Although they may be numerous the elliptocytes rarely exceed 60 percent in these conditions.
- Differentiation from HE rests on the negative family history and presence of other clinical features associated with the above diseases.
- Biochemical analysis of the membrane skeletal proteins will establish the diagnosis.

Therapy

- Mild forms need no intervention at all. In the more severely affected, splenectomy will lessen or prevent the need for transfusions.

SPHEROCYTIC HEREDITARY ELLIPTOCYTOSIS

- Shows features of both HE and HS. Also called *HE with spherocytosis* or *hereditary hemolytic ovalocytosis*.
- On peripheral blood films elliptical red cells and spherocytes or round sphero-ovalocytes are seen. Hemolysis and increased osmotic fragility

occur despite mild abnormalities in red cell morphology. The molecular basis is unknown.

STOMATOCYTIC HEREDITARY ELLIPTOCYTOSIS

- Dominantly inherited condition, widespread in certain groups in Southeast Asia, characterized by oval red cells with one or two transverse ridges or a longitudinal slit.
- Other features include increased red cell rigidity, decreased osmotic fragility, increased thermal stability, reduced expression of certain red cell antigens.
- Resistance in vitro to invasion by several malaria parasites has been described. The mechanism of this resistance is unknown.
- Caused by an abnormality of band 3 protein.

For a more detailed discussion, see Jiri Palek, Petr Jarolim: Hereditary spherocytosis, elliptocytosis, and related disorders, Chap. 52, p. 536 in *Williams Hematology*, 5/e, 1995.

---

23 ACANTHOCYTOSIS, STOMATOCYTOSIS, AND RELATED DISORDERS

ACANTHOCYTOSIS

- Spur cells or acanthocytes are red cells with multiple, irregular projections. They have been noted in several conditions.

Severe Liver Disease

- Shape change is due to accumulation of nonesterified cholesterol in the red cell membrane, but the exact mechanism is unknown. Normal red cells will acquire the defect after transfusion into an afflicted patient.
- Rapidly progressive hemolytic anemia is noted in some individuals, usually with advanced alcoholic cirrhosis.
- Splenectomy is usually not advised because of severe liver disease.

Abetalipoproteinemia

- A rare autosomal recessive disease with slight increase in membrane cholesterol/phospholipid ratio and definite increase in membrane sphingomyelin. Shape change appears as red cells age.
- Anemia is mild. Acanthocytes constitute 50 to 90 percent of cells.
- Steatorrhea develops early in life; retinitis pigmentosa and other progressive neurologic abnormalities lead to death in the second or third decade.
- Treat with dietary restriction of triglycerides and supplementation of fat soluble vitamins.

Chorea-Acanthocytosis Syndrome

- A rare inherited, presumably autosomal recessive, choreiform syndrome. The clinical features develop in adults with variable progressive neurologic abnormalities, and acanthocytosis with normal plasma lipids.
- Patients are not anemic.

McLeod Phenotype

- An X-linked disorder that can coexist with chronic granulomatous disease, Duchenne muscular dystrophy, or retinitis pigmentosa.
- Red cells in these individuals lack the 37,000-Da Kx antigen.
- Mild hemolytic anemia with a high percentage of acanthocytes.
- Areflexia, dystonia, and choreiform movements develop after the fifth decade.

116

Other Conditions

- Acanthocytes may occur in patients with anorexia nervosa, hypothyroidism, and myelodysplasia and in the postsplenectomy state.

STOMATOCYTOSIS AND RELATED DISORDERS

- In a three-dimensional view, stomatocytes have the shape of a cup or a bowl. The slit-like appearance seen on slides is an artifact caused by folding of the cells.
- Red cell cationic permeability is often disordered, but the red cell volume is variable.
- The cells are seen in a variety of disorders.

Acquired Stomatocytosis

- Stomatocytes make up less than 5 percent of the red cells of normal subjects. About 1 in 40 hospitalized patients have more than this number, in association with a variety of medical conditions.

Hereditary Stomatocytosis

- An autosomal dominant disease with moderate to severe hemolytic anemia. From 10 to 30 percent stomatocytes are present and the osmotic fragility is markedly increased. These cells have a major inward sodium leak.

Hereditary Xerocytosis (Desiccocytosis)

- A rare autosomal dominant trait with moderately severe hemolytic anemia characterized by red cell dehydration and decreased osmotic fragility.

Intermediate Syndromes

- Sporadic cases share features of the above disorders with stomatocytes and/or target cells and normal-to-increased osmotic fragility.
- Results of splenectomy in stomatocytosis and xerocytosis are varied.

Rh Deficiency Syndrome

- Rare individuals with absent (Rh null) or markedly reduced (Rh mod) Rh antigen have hemolytic anemia with stomatocytes, occasional spherocytes, and increased osmotic fragility. Splenectomy markedly improves the anemia.

Familial Lecithin-Cholesterol Acyltransferase (LCAT) Deficiency

- A rare autosomal recessive condition with corneal opacities, premature atherosclerosis, proteinuria, and mild hemolytic anemia. Marrow shows sea blue histiocytosis.

- Target cells are numerous and have a marked increase in cholesterol and phosphatidylcholine in the red cell membrane.

Familial Deficiency of High-Density Lipoproteins

- Severe deficiency or absence of HDL results in a moderately severe hemolytic anemia with stomatocytosis and cholesterol ester accumulation in many tissues.

For a more detailed discussion, see Jiri Palek: Acanthocytosis, stomatocytosis, and related disorders, Chap. 53, p. 557, in *Williams Hematology,* 5/e, 1995.

---

24 GLUCOSE-6-PHOSPHATE DEHYDROGENASE DEFICIENCY AND OTHER ENZYME ABNORMALITIES

- Clinical manifestations of inherited red cell enzyme deficiencies may be
  - episodic hemolysis after exposure to oxidants or infection
  - chronic hemolytic anemia (hereditary nonspherocytic anemia)
  - acute hemolysis after eating fava beans (favism)
  - methemoglobinemia
  - icterus neonatorum
  - no hematologic manifestations

MECHANISM OF HEMOLYSIS IN PATIENTS WITH RED CELL ENZYME ABNORMALITIES

- Oxidant challenge leads to formation of denatured hemoglobin and Heinz bodies, which make the red cells less deformable and liable to splenic destruction.
- ATP depletion may cause hemolysis by undefined mechanism(s).
- Unstable hemoglobins reduce red cell deformability by attachment of denatured globin to the red cell membrane.

GLUCOSE-6-PHOSPHATE DEHYDROGENASE DEFICIENCY

- Sex-linked disorder.
- The normal enzyme is designated G-6-PD B.
- A mutant enzyme with normal activity [G-6-PD A(+)] is found in 16 percent of African-American males.
- G-6-PD A− is the principal deficient variant found among people of African origin and most probably arose in an individual with the G-6-PD A(+) variant. G-6-PD A− has decreased stability in vivo, and such blood shows 5 to 15 percent of normal activity.
- Prevalence of G-6-PD A− in African-American males is 11 percent.
- G-6-PD deficiency in Caucasians is most often the Mediterranean type, with barely detectable enzymatic activity and severe clinical manifestations.

Inciting Drugs (see Table 24-1)

- Individual differences in the metabolism of certain drugs as well as the specific G-6-PD defect influence the extent of RBC destruction.
- Typically drug-induced hemolysis begins 1 to 3 days after drug exposure and may be associated with abdominal or back pain. The urine may become dark, even black.
- Heinz bodies appear in circulating red cells, then disappear as

TABLE 24-1 Drugs and Chemicals That Should Be Avoided by Persons with G-6-PD Deficiency

Acetanilid	Primaquine
Furazolidone (Furoxone)	Sulfacetamide
Methylene blue	Sulfamethoxazole (Gantanol)
Nalidixic acid (NeGram)	Sulfanilamide
Naphthalene	Sulfapyridine
Niridazole (Ambilhar)	Thiazolesulfone
Isobutyl nitrite	Toluidine blue
Nitrofurantoin (Furadantin)	Trinitrotoluene (TNT)
Phenazopyride (Pyridium)	Urate oxidase
Phenylhydrazine	

Source: Table 54-5 of *Williams Hematology*, 5/e, p. 573.

they are removed by the spleen, and the hemoglobin concentration decreases rapidly.
- Hemolysis is self-limited in the G-6-PD A− type but not in the more severe Mediterranean type.

Febrile Illnesses

- Hemolysis may occur within 1 to 2 days of onset of a febrile illness, usually resulting in mild anemia.
- Hemolysis occurs especially in patients with pneumonia or typhoid fever.
- Hemolysis may be fulminating in G-6-PD deficient patients with Rocky Mountain spotted fever.
- Jaundice may be particularly severe in association with infectious hepatitis.
- Reticulocytosis is usually absent and recovery from anemia is delayed until after the active infection has cleared.

Favism

- Potentially one of the most severe consequences of G-6-PD deficiency.
- Hemolysis occurs within hours to days after ingestion of the beans.
- Urine becomes red or dark, and shock, sometimes fatal, may develop rapidly.
- More common in children and occurs usually with variants that cause severe deficiency.

Icterus Neonatorum

- May occur in some newborns with G-6-PD deficiency without maternal-fetal immunologic evidence of incompatibility.
- The jaundice may led to kernicterus and mental retardation.
- Rare in neonates with the A− variant, but is more common in Mediterranean and Chinese variants.

HEREDITARY NONSPHEROCYTIC HEMOLYTIC ANEMIA

- Anemia may range from severe (hemoglobin level 5 g/dl) to a fully compensated state with normal hemoglobin concentration.
- Chronic jaundice, splenomegaly, and gallstones are common, and some patients develop ankle ulcers.
- Nonhematologic manifestations may occur, such as cataracts in some patients with G-6-PD deficiency, or glycogen storage disease in phosphofructokinase deficiency.

Pyruvate Kinase Deficiency

- The most common cause of hereditary nonspherocytic hemolytic anemia, estimated from cord blood assays to occur in 1 percent of Caucasians and 2.4 percent of African-Americans.
- Small, densely staining echinocytic red cells are common.
- Can be fatal in early childhood.
- The gene prevalent among the Amish of Pennsylvania causes particularly severe disease.

LABORATORY FEATURES

- Erythrocytes with enzyme deficiencies have normal morphology in the absence of hemolysis.
- Heinz bodies appear in the early stages of drug-induced hemolysis in patients with G-6-PD deficiencies.
- Spherocytosis and red cell fragmentation are present in severe cases.
- Increased serum bilirubin concentration, decreased haptoglobin levels, and increased serum lactic dehydrogenase activity all may be present when hemolysis occurs.
- Leukopenia may occur in patients with splenomegaly.

Diagnosis

- Depends on demonstration of the enzyme deficiency.
- Recommended initially to screen for G-6-PD and pyruvate kinase (PK) activity and to perform an isopropanol stability test for unstable hemoglobins.
- Assays or screening tests for G-6-PD deficiency are best performed in a healthy affected (hemizygous) male.
- Diagnosis may be difficult during hemolytic episode in G-6-PD A − patients because young red cells have high levels of G-6-PD.
  - Most dense red cells (oldest, lowest activity) can be tested following differential centrifugation.
  - Family studies may be helpful.
  - May have to retest when fully recovered.
- Presence of basophilic stippling suggests lead poisoning or pyrimidine 5'-nucleotidase deficiency.

- When nucleotide substitution is known, heterozygotes are easily detected by PCR-based analysis, which is also useful for prenatal diagnosis.
- Erythrocyte enzyme assays are discussed in detail in Chap. L13 in *Williams Hematology,* 5/e.

TREATMENT

- G-6-PD-deficient individuals should avoid "oxidant" drugs (see Table 24-1).
- Transfusions should be given only in the most severe examples of G-6-PD deficiency, such as favism.
- Maintain good urine flow in patients with hemoglobinuria.
- Exchange transfusion may be necessary in infants, but G-6-PD-deficient blood must not be given.
- Splenectomy is often considered in patients with hereditary non-spherocytic hemolytic anemia.
  - Severity of disease and functional impairment are important considerations.
  - Value differs according to family defect, and family history of response to splenectomy, if available, is most useful guide.
  - If cholecystectomy is required, splenectomy may be done at the same time.
- Glucocorticoids are of no known value.
- Folic acid therapy often given, but is without proven hematologic benefit.
- Iron therapy is probably contraindicated unless iron deficient.

For a more detailed discussion, see Ernest Beutler: Glucose-6-phosphate dehydrogenase deficiency and other enzyme abnormalities, Chap. 54, p. 564, in *Williams Hematology,* 5/e, 1995.

---

25 THE THALASSEMIAS

DEFINITION

- A group of disorders, each resulting from an inherited defect in rate of synthesis of one or more globin chains.
- Resultant imbalance of globin chain production causes ineffective erythropoiesis, defective hemoglobin production, hemolysis, and anemia of variable degree.

ETIOLOGY AND PATHOGENESIS

Genetic Control and Synthesis of Hemoglobin

- Each Hb molecule consists of two separate pairs of identical globin chains.
- Adult Hb is ~96 percent Hb A ($\alpha_2\beta_2$) and ~2.5 percent Hb A_2 ($\alpha_2\delta_2$)
- Fetal life: Hb F ($\alpha_2\gamma_2$) predominates. Position 136 of some γ chains is occupied by glycine and in others by alanine. These are designated $^G\gamma$ and $^A\gamma$, respectively: At birth Hb F is a mixture of $\alpha_2{}^G\gamma_2$ and $\alpha_2{}^A\gamma_2$ in ratio of 3:1.
- Embryonic Hb: Hb Gower 1 ($\zeta_2\epsilon_2$), Hb Gower 2 ($\alpha_2\epsilon_2$), and Hb Portland ($\zeta_2\gamma_2$), before 8th week of intrauterine life.
- During fetal life, switches occur from ζ- to α- and from ϵ- to γ-chain production, followed by β- and δ-chain production after birth.

Globin Gene Clusters

- α-Gene cluster (chromosome 16) consists of one functional ζ gene and two α genes (α2 and α1).
  - Exons of the two α-globin genes have identical sequences.
  - Production of α2 mRNA exceeds that of α1, by factor of 1.5 to 3.
- β-Gene cluster (chromosome 11) consists of one functional ϵ gene, a $^G\gamma$ gene, an $^A\gamma$ gene, a δ gene, and a β gene.
- Flanking regions contain conserved sequences essential for gene expression.

Regulation of Globin Gene Clusters

- Primary transcript is large mRNA precursor, with both intron and exon sequences, which is extensively processed in the nucleus to yield the final mRNA.
- Expression of the globin genes is regulated by complex control mechanisms.
- Some forms of thalassemia appear to be due to abnormalities of these regulatory steps.

Developmental Changes in Globin Gene Expression

- β-Globin produced at low levels beginning at 8 to 10 weeks of fetal life, increases considerably at about 36 weeks gestation.

123

- γ-Globin produced at high levels early, starts to decline at ~36 weeks.
- At birth β-globin and γ-globin production are approximately equal.
- By age 1, γ-globin production is less than 1 percent of total non-α-globin production.
- Mechanism of switches not clear, but probably involves a "time clock" in hemopoietic stem cell.
- Fetal hemoglobin synthesis may be reactivated at low level in adults, in states of hemopoietic stress.

MOLECULAR BASIS OF THE THALASSEMIAS

- A large number of mutations cause thalassemia (e.g., over 100 for β thalassemia).
- The molecular basis of the thalassemias is discussed in detail in Chap. 55 of *Williams Hematology,* 5/e, p. 581.

DIFFERENT FORMS OF THALASSEMIA

- β Thalassemias are of two main varieties:
  - β^0 Thalassemia, with total absence of β-chain production.
  - β^+ Thalassemia, with partial deficiency of β-chain production.
  - Hallmark of both is elevation of Hb A_2 in heterozygotes.
- $\delta\beta$ Thalassemias are heterogeneous:
  - In some cases no δ or β chains are produced.
  - In others, the non-α chains are fusion $\delta\beta$ chains: N-terminal residue of δ chain fused to C-terminal residues of the β chain; fusion variants are called *Lepore hemoglobins.*
- δ Thalassemias:
  - Decreased Hb A_2 in heterozygotes and absent Hb A_2 in homozygotes.
  - No clinical significance.
- Hereditary persistence of fetal hemoglobin (HPFH):
  - Heterogeneous genetically (deletion and nondeletion forms).
  - Characterized by persistence of Hb F in adult life.
  - No clinical significance, but may have mild thalassemic changes.
- α Thalassemias are usually due to deletion of one or more of the four α genes (two globin genes per haploid chromosome):
  - In α^0 thalassemias, no α chains are produced from the affected chromosome.
  - In α^+ thalassemias, α chains are produced from one but not the other gene of an affected chromosome.
  - Two major clinical phenotypes: Hb Bart's hydrops fetalis, homozygosity for α^0 thalassemia, and Hb- in H disease, a compound heterozygous state for α^0 and α^+ thalassemia.

PATHOPHYSIOLOGY

Imbalanced Globin Chain Synthesis (The Major Problem)

- Homozygous β thalassemia
  - β-Globin synthesis absent or greatly reduced, resulting in hypochromic microcytic red cells.
  - Excess α chains precipitate in red cell precursors, resulting in intramedullary destruction of the abnormal erythroid cells (ineffective erythropoiesis) and hemolysis.
  - Clinical manifestations appear after neonatal switch from γ-chain to β-chain production.
- Heterozygous β thalassemia
  - Usually only mild hypochromic microcytic anemia, with elevated Hb A_2.
  - Some are more severe due to poor heme-binding properties and instability, with red cell inclusions containing precipitated β chains as well as excess α chains.
- α Thalassemias
  - Defective α-chain production: manifestations in both fetal and adult life.
  - Excess γ chains become soluble $γ_4$ homotetramers or Hb Bart's.
  - Excess β chains become soluble $β_4$ homotetramers or Hb H, which is slightly unstable and precipitates as red cells age, forming inclusion bodies.
  - Both Hb Bart's and Hb H have no heme-heme interaction and have high oxygen affinity.
  - Hb Bart's hydrops fetalis: severe intrauterine hypoxia, gross hydrops, severe erythroblastosis, enormously hypertrophied placenta.
  - Defect in hemoglobin synthesis leads to hypochromic, microcytic cells.
  - Less ineffective erythropoiesis than occurs in β thalassemia.

Persistent Fetal Homoglobin Production and Cellular Heterogeneity

- In $β^0$ thalassemias, except for small amounts of Hb A_2, Hb F is the only hemoglobin produced.
- In thalassemias, as in normal individuals, Hb F is heterogeneously distributed among the red cells.
- Because of elevated Hb F in β thalassemias, red cells have high oxygen affinity.

Consequence of Compensatory Mechanisms for the Anemia of Thalassemia

- Severe anemia and the high O_2 affinity of Hb F in homozygous β thalassemia produce severe tissue hypoxia.

- High O_2 affinity of Hb Bart's and Hb H accentuate hypoxia in severe forms of α thalassemia.
- Erythropoietin production and expansion of marrow lead to deformities of skull with frequent sinus and ear infections, porous long bones, and pathologic fractures.
- Massive erythropoiesis diverts calories, also leads to hyperuricemia, gout, and folate deficiency.

Splenomegaly; Dilutional Anemia

- Removal of precipitate globin chains leads to work hypertrophy and splenomegaly.
- Spleen may sequester red cells and expand plasma volume, exacerbating anemia.

Abnormal Iron Metabolism

- β^0 Thalassemia homozygotes have increased iron absorption due to anemia, increased iron deposition from hemolysis, and transfusional siderosis.
- Iron accumulates in endocrine glands, liver, and most importantly, myocardium.
- Consequences: diabetes, hypoparathyroidism, hypogonadism, and death from heart failure.

Disordered Red Cell Metabolism

- Inclusions of α or β chains cause shortened red cell survival.
- Oxidant damage to membrane results in abnormalities of permeability.
- Abnormalities may be enhanced by vitamin E deficiency.

Clinical Heterogeneity

- All manifestations of β thalassemia are related to excess α chains.
- Degree of globin-chain imbalance determines severity.
- Coinheritance of α thalassemia or of genes for enhanced γ-chain production may reduce the severity of β thalassemias.
- Adequate transfusion of patients with severe β thalassemia can overcome the serious consequences of excess α-chain production.

POPULATION GENETICS

- β Thalassemias: Mediterranean populations, Middle East, India and Pakistan, Southeast Asia, southern Russia, China.
  - Rare in Africa, except Liberia and parts of North Africa.
  - Sporadic in all races: Anglo-Saxon β-thalassemia major has been described.
- α Thalassemias: Widespread in Africa, Mediterranean populations, Middle East, Southeast Asia.

- α^o Thalassemias: Mediterranean and Asian populations (therefore, Hb Bart's hydrops syndrome and Hb H disease largely restricted to Southeast Asia and Mediterranean). Extremely rare in Africa and Middle East.
- Thalassemic red cells appear to protect against malarial parasites.
  - Parasitized α-thalassemia cells (or β-thalassemia cells) bind more antibody from *Plasmodium falciparum* malaria patients than do normal red cells.
  - Protection may be immune-mediated.

CLINICAL FEATURES

β Thalassemias

- β-Thalassemia major: clinically severe, requiring transfusions.
- β-Thalassemia intermedia: milder, later onset, requiring either few or no transfusions.
- β-Thalassemia minor: heterozygous carrier.

β-*Thalassemia Major*

- Homozygous or compound heterozygous state.
- Infants well at birth, anemia develops in first few months of life, becomes progressively more severe. Failure to thrive.
- Onset of symptoms after first year of life more typical of β-thalassemia intermedia.
- Inadequately transfused child:
  - Stunted growth. Expanded marrow leads to bossing of skull, expanded maxilla, widened diploë, gross skeletal deformities.
  - Grossly enlarged liver and spleen. Secondary thrombocytopenia and leukopenia.
  - Skin pigmentation. Chronic leg ulceration.
  - Hypermetabolic state: fever, wasting, hyperuricemia.
  - Frequent infections, folate deficiency, spontaneous fractures, dental problems.
  - Symptoms of iron loading by time of puberty; poor growth; endocrine problems (diabetes mellitus, adrenal insufficiency); cardiac problems, death by the third decade due to cardiac siderosis.
- Adequately transfused child grows and develops normally until effects of iron loading appear by end of first decade.

β-*Thalassemia Intermedia*

- Wide spectrum of disability:
- Severe forms: later appearing anemia than β-thalassemia major; usually requires transfusion. Retarded growth and development. Skeletal deformities. Splenomegaly.

- Milder forms: asymptomatic, transfusion-independent, Hb levels 10 to 12 g/dl.

β-*Thalassemia Minor*

- Usually no clinical disability. Discovered by blood cell examination.

α Thalassemias

- Interactions of α-thalassemia haplotypes result in four broad phenotypic categories:
  - Normal ($\alpha\alpha/\alpha\alpha$); silent carrier ($-\alpha/\alpha\alpha$).
  - α-Thalassemia trait ($-\alpha/-\alpha$) or ($--/\alpha\alpha$). Mild hematologic changes, but no clinical abnormality. Low MCV, low MCH, varying levels of Hb Bart's at birth [Hb Bart's (γ_4)].
  - Hb H disease ($--/-\alpha$). Hypochromic, hemolytic anemia [Hb H(β_4)].
  - Hb Bart's hydrops fetalis syndrome ($--/--$). Incompatible with life.

Hemoglobin Bart's Hydrops Fetalis Syndrome

- Frequent cause of stillbirth in Southeast Asia. If alive at birth, infant dies within hours.
- Pallor, massive edema, hepatosplenomegaly. Hydrops resembles that of Rh incompatibility.
- High incidence of maternal toxemia of pregnancy. Enlarged placenta.
- At autopsy: massive extramedullary hemopoiesis.

Hemoglobin H Disease

- Clinical findings vary:
  - Lifelong microcytic, hemolytic anemia with variable splenomegaly and bone changes.
  - Hb A is major hemoglobin present; Hb H varies from 5 to 30 percent, and there may be traces of Hb Bart's. In Southeast Asia, 40 percent of cases have traces of Hb Constant Spring.

α-*Thalassemia Trait*

- Asymptomatic without splenomegaly or any physical findings. Laboratory findings noted below.
- Both parents of infants with Hb Bart's hydrops fetalis have α^0-thalassemia trait.
- One parent of Hb H disease child has α^0-thalassemia trait, the other α^+-thalassemia trait.

LABORATORY FEATURES

β Thalassemias

β-*Thalassemia Major*

- Severe anemia: Hb 2 to 3 g/dl. Blood film: marked anisopoikilo-cytosis, hypochromia, target cells, basophilic stippling, large poiki-locytes. Nucleated red cells numerous. Reticulocytes moderately increased. Inclusions of Hb in hypochromic red cells (these can be supravitally stained by methyl violet). After splenectomy: more inclusions, large flat macrocytes, small deformed microcytes.
- Leukocyte and platelet counts normal or slightly elevated.
- Marrow: marked erythroid hyperplasia; abnormal erythroblasts with stippling, increased sideroblasts. Markedly increased storage iron.
- Markedly ineffective erythropoiesis. Shortened red cell survival.
- Hemoglobin: fetal hemoglobin increased, from <10 percent to >90 percent. Hb A absent in β^0 thalassemia. Hb A_2 low, normal, or high; always elevated, however, if expressed as a proportion of Hb A.

β-*Thalassemia Minor*

- Mild, if any, anemia: hemoglobin 9 to 11 g/dl.
- Microcytic hypochromic red cells: MCV 50 to 70 fl, MCH 20 to 22 pg. MCV valuable screen for thalassemia trait.
- Hemoglobin: Hb A_2 may be depressed into normal range by iron deficiency.

α Thalassemias

Hemoglobin Bart's Hydrops Fetalis Syndrome

- Blood film: severe thalassemic changes; many nucleated RBC.
- Hemoglobin: Hb Bart's predominates; Hb Portland ($\zeta_2\gamma_2$) 10 to 20 percent.

Hemoglobin H Disease

- Blood film: hypochromic microcytic RBC, increased polychro-masia.
- Mild reticulocytosis (~5 percent).
- Hb H inclusions demonstrable in almost all RBC in blood incubated with brilliant cresyl blue.

α^0-*Thalassemia and* α^+-*Thalassemia Traits*

- Similar appearance of blood film and cell counts as in β-thalassemia trait.

- α^0-Thalassemia trait:
  - 5 to 15 percent Hb Bart's at birth, disappears during maturation.
  - Rare cells with Hb H inclusions can be demonstrated in some cases.
- α^+-Thalassemia trait:
  - 1 to 2 percent Hb Bart's at birth in some but not all cases.
  - Gene mapping analysis is only certain method of diagnosing α-thalassemia carrier states.

DIFFERENTIAL DIAGNOSIS

- For an approach to the diagnosis of thalassemia syndromes see Fig. 25-1.

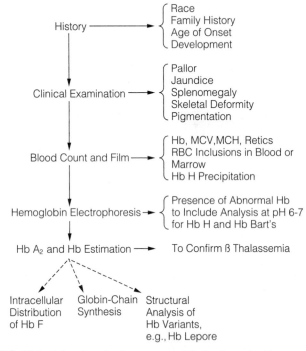

FIG. 25-1   A flowchart showing an approach to the diagnosis of the thalassemia syndromes. *(From Weatherall DJ: The thalassemias, Fig. 55-20, in Williams Hematology, 5/e, 1995, Chap. 55, p. 605.)*

- In childhood, hereditary sideroblastic anemias may resemble thalassemia, but marrow examination should permit differentiation (see Chap. 41).
- High fetal hemoglobin levels found in juvenile chronic myelomonocytic leukemia can cause confusion, but examination of the marrow should be definitive (see Chap. 8).
- Diagnosis of the rarer forms of thalassemia is discussed in Chap. 55 of *Williams Hematology,* 5/e, p. 581.

THERAPY, COURSE, AND PROGNOSIS

Transfusion

- In children, maintain Hb-10 to 14 g/dl by transfusing red cells every 6 to 8 weeks to assure normal growth and development. Use washed, filtered, or frozen cells to avoid transfusion reactions. Children maintained at high Hb level do not develop hypersplenism.

Iron Chelation

- Rationale: Every child on high-transfusion regimen will develop and die from myocardial siderosis.
- Subcutaneous infusion of deferoxamine, 12 h, overnight: determine dose to achieve maximal urinary iron excretion
- Continue nightly infusions of deferoxamine on outpatient basis, monitor by measurements of urinary iron excretion. Ascorbic acid, 50 to 100 mg/day, increases iron excretion.
- Deferoxamine requires extreme care, because of toxic effects, such as
  - local erythema and painful subcutaneous nodules
  - neurosensory toxicity in 30 percent; high-frequency hearing loss; ocular toxicity

Special Considerations

- β-Thalassemia major: high standard of pediatric care required. Early treatment of infections. Folate supplements. Careful attention to respiratory infections and dental care because of bony deformities of skull. When iron-loading is present, endocrine replacement therapy may be needed.
- Hb H disease: avoid oxidant drugs. Splenectomy may be needed if anemia and splenomegaly are severe. Caution: splenectomy may be followed by thromboembolic disease.

Bone Marrow Transplantation, for β-Thalassemia Major

- Feasible with HLA-identical sibling donors if performed early.
- In the absence of risk factors (irregular chelation, hepatomegaly,

portal fibrosis), approximately 93 percent of children have 3-year, event-free survival.
- For patients with one or two risk factors, the rejection-free survival rate is 77 percent; with all three risk factors, 53 percent.

Experimental Approaches to Treatment

- Increase γ-globin synthesis in patients with β thalassemia or sickle cell anemia using demethlyating or cytotoxic agents, or arginine butyrate.
- Somatic gene therapy is discussed in Chap. 19, Gene therapy, in *Williams Hematology,* 5/e, p. 195.

Prognosis

- Thalassemia major:
  - Sharp increase in death rate after age 15. Survival prolonged if iron loading is significantly lowered.
  - Bone marrow transplantation done early in life with HLA-identical sibling donors can lead to cure.
- Homozygous thalassemia intermedia:
  - May develop iron loading and severe bone disease in 3 to 4 decades.
  - High incidence of diabetes mellitus, due to iron loading of pancreas.

PREVENTION

- Prospective genetic counseling, warning carriers of potential risks, has been unsuccessful.
- For prenatal diagnosis screen mothers at first prenatal visit; if mother is thalassemia carrier, screen father; if both are carriers of gene for severe form of thalassemia, offer prenatal diagnostic testing and termination of pregnancy.
  - Fetal blood sampling at 18th week and globin chain synthesis analysis: fetal mortality of 3 to 4 percent, error rate of 1 to 2 percent. Using this approach, new cases of β thalassemia have been decreased significantly in Mediterranean countries.
  - Chorionic villus sampling at 9 to 10 weeks and fetal DNA analysis: appears preferable. Using Southern blotting, oligonucleotide probes, or restriction fragment length polymorphism linkage analysis, a decision whether fetus is affected or not is possible in 80 percent of cases. Newer approaches using polymerase chain reaction and oligonucleotide probes likely to improve early detection.

For a more detailed discussion, see D. J. Weatherall: The thalassemias, Chap. 55, p. 581, in *Williams Hematology,* 5/e, 1995.

26 SICKLE CELL DISEASE AND RELATED DISORDERS

The molecular biology of these hemoglobinopathies is well understood, but clinical progress has been limited. Hemoglobin variants were initially designated by letter, but after the letters of the alphabet were used up, they were named for where they were found. If they had a particular feature previously described by a letter, the location was added as a subscript (e.g., Hb M$_{saskatoon}$). In a fully characterized hemoglobin the amino acid change is described in a superscript to the appropriate globin chain (e.g., Hb S, $\alpha_2\beta_2^{6Glu-Val}$).

The term *sickle cell disorder* describes states in which sickling of red cells occurs on deoxygenation. Sickle cell diseases are disorders in which clinical manifestations are prominent.

SICKLE CELL DISEASE

Sickle cell anemia (Hb SS), hemoglobin SC, sickle cell β thalassemia, and hemoglobin SD produce significant symptoms. These diseases are marked by periods of well-being interspersed with episodes of deterioration, but the severity of clinical manifestations varies widely among patients. Generally, sickle cell anemia is the most severe, but there is considerable overlap in clinical presentations among these diseases.

Background

Biochemical Basis

- Hemoglobin S is due to substitution of valine for glutamic acid at position 6 in the β chain resulting from replacement of adenine by thymine in the DNA code (GAG→GTG).
- Molecules of deoxyhemoglobin S have a strong tendency to aggregate in a highly ordered fashion, resulting in multiple microtubules arranged in helical form. The firm gel that results causes the sickled shape of the red cell. Blood viscosity increases, vascular stasis develops, and tissue damage may occur.
- When a cell sickles and unsickles repeatedly, irreversible membrane damage occurs and the cell is destroyed.

Variability in Sickling

- Susceptibility to sickling is proportional to the concentration of hemoglobin S. Individuals with sickle cell trait have less than 50 percent hemoglobin S in their cells and are virtually without symptoms. Cellular dehydration (such as in the hyperosmolar milieu in renal papillae) will increase sickling by increasing the concentration of intracorpuscular hemoglobin.
- Some hemoglobins, such as C and D, can enhance the sickling process, whereas others, such as F, can impede. The degree of

133

protection conferred by elevated hemoglobin F levels is unclear; apparently a threshold phenomenon exists, so that there is no effect beneath a certain level of hemoglobin F.

- Deoxygenation is the most important factor in the development of sickling. The severity of the deoxygenation required depends on the percentage of hemoglobin S in the cells. The mild decrease in O_2 tension in pressurized aircraft should not cause sickling; however occasional crises in this setting have been reported.
- Since the duration of hypoxia is also important, areas of vascular stasis (such as the spleen) with lower O_2 tension are more prone to vascular occlusion and infarction.
- Low temperature slows sickling in vitro, but in patients cold weather may precipitate crisis presumably because of vasoconstriction.
- Lower pH shifts O_2 dissociation curve to the right, favoring the deoxy conformation of hemoglobin. Even when O_2 tension is adequate, sickling is greatly enhanced with acidosis; alkalosis will retard sickling but decrease tissue oxygen delivery.
- In the microvasculature, flow is affected by the rigidity of the sickled cells and adherence to the endothelium. Shear stresses in higher flow areas can break down the gel structure of hemoglobin S.
- Crises are often precipitated by infections, due to many factors including dehydration from fever and GI losses of fluids, acidosis from poor oral intake, and hypoxia from pneumonia.

Inheritance

- Patients with Hb SS are homozygous for the sickle hemoglobin gene and have inherited one gene from each parent. 7.8% of African Americans have sickle trait; 1 in 650 will have sickle cell anemia.
- The birth frequency of hemoglobin SC disease is 1 in 1120 newborns. The birth frequency of sickle β thalassemia is approximately 1 in 3200. Occurrence of sickle disease can theoretically be prevented by detection of carriers and counseling regarding the possibility of not having children. In addition to sickle cell disease, carriers for β thalassemia and hemoglobin C must also be detected. The actual effect of screening programs has not yet been ascertained.
- Although the sickle cell gene is found in a variety of areas (Middle East, Greece, India), its greatest prevalence is in tropical Africa, with heterozygote frequency as high as 40 percent. A geographical association with areas of high malaria prevalence suggests an advantage to individuals with sickle cell trait. It is theorized that the infected cell is preferentially sickled and destroyed; this results in shorter duration of infection and decreased mortality.

Clinical Features and Treatment

- In newborns, high levels of fetal hemoglobin are protective for the first 8 to 10 weeks; thereafter the manifestations of sickle cell disease are apparent. There is great variability between affected individuals, but many patients are in good health most of the time. In children, most problems are related to pain or infection. In adults, many problems are more chronic, related to organ damage.

- No effective routine treatment for sickle cell disease has been found, so care is directed toward treatment of complications. Folic acid replacement is commonly recommended to increase erythropoiesis. Transfusions are not given routinely; prophylactic transfusions will decrease the number of crises, but the risks of transfusion are significant. Pneumococcal vaccine should be given and penicillin prophylaxis administered up to the age of 6.

- Patients undergoing anesthesia are at increased risk and must be observed closely for conditions such as hypoxia or acidosis that will precipitate crisis. Simple or exchange transfusions may help to avoid complications. There is no clear advantage for exchange except in emergent settings or if iron overload is a concern.

Crises

- Vaso-occlusive crisis is the most common, occurring with a frequency from almost daily to yearly. Tissue hypoxia and infarction can occur anywhere in the body. It is important to carefully evaluate the patient to distinguish between painful crises and pain due to another process. In crisis the patient should be kept warm and given adequate hydration and pain control (see Chap. 2 in Williams Hematology, 5/e); in addition, oxygen may be beneficial. The period of crisis usually resolves in hours to days.

- Aplastic crises occur when erythropoiesis is suppressed. As red blood cell survival is greatly shortened in sickle cell disease, even temporary marrow injury is rapidly manifested with a dramatic fall in hemoglobin. Infection (most notably parvovirus B19) can cause this picture but also folic acid deficiency, which is particularly a concern during pregnancy.

- Sequestration crises occurs in children or the occasional adult with an enlarged spleen. For unclear reasons there is a sudden massive pooling of red blood cells in the spleen; this can cause hypotension and even death.

- Hemolytic crises are quite rare. Shortened red cell survival is intrinsic to the disease but a rapidly increased rate of destruction can occur.

Other Clinical Manifestations

Bone

- Young children with hemoglobin SS tend to be short. Puberty is delayed, but growth occurs in late adolescence and adults are of normal size.

- Erythroid hyperplasia in the marrow results in widening of the medullary spaces and thinning of the cortex. The vertebral bodies may show biconcavities on the upper and lower surface (codfish spine).
- Bone infarctions can be followed by periosteal reaction and areas of osteosclerosis. Dactylitis occurs in children usually up to 4 years of age, probably related to avascular necrosis. In adults avascular necrosis occurs chiefly in the femoral and humeral heads; joint replacement is occasionally required.

Genitourinary System

- The environment of the renal medulla (hyperosmolar, hypoxic) predisposes to sickling. Hyposthenuria, papillary necrosis, and hematuria are commonly present.
- Priapism is more commonly seen in hemoglobin SS disease. If not treated quickly with exchange transfusion or possible surgical decompression, permanent dysfunction can occur.

Spleen

- In hemoglobin SS disease, splenomegaly (but poor splenic function) in childhood is followed by repeated infarction and a small fibrotic spleen in the adult.
- Splenomegaly commonly persists in patients with hemoglobin SC or sickle β thalassemia.

Hepatobiliary System

- About one-third of sickle cell disease patients will manifest hepatic dysfunction of multifactorial origin. Sickle cell–induced cholestasis can be very serious and even fatal, although exchange transfusion has been reported as an effective treatment. Hepatitis may develop due to transfusions. The liver, sometimes chronically enlarged, can also enlarge transiently during a painful crisis. Gallstones are seen in 50 to 75 percent of adults; they have been seen in children as young as 6 years of age. Although there is some debate, asymptomatic cholelithiasis probably should not be operated on.

Cardiopulmonary System

- In vaso-occlusive crisis, tachycardia, flow murmurs, and an active precordium, related to pain and anemia, are commonly seen.
- Pulmonary infiltrates are commonly seen, often from infection, but also sometimes from pulmonary infarction. X-ray findings cannot delineate between the two, and close observation of the "acute chest syndrome" (fever, leukocytosis, infiltrate) is warranted. Empiric

antibiotics should be considered, but if serious clinical deterioration occurs, exchange transfusion should be instituted quickly.

Eye

- Neovascularization occurs after obstruction of retinal vessels, resulting in hemorrhage and possible blindness; laser coagulation can prevent this complication. Visual loss is more common in hemoglobin SC disease.

Central Nervous System

- Cerebral vascular accidents occur more commonly in children, usually without warning. Recurrence is common (in at least two-thirds) usually within 3 years, hence a regular transfusion program is recommended to reduce hemoglobin S levels below 50 percent.
- Other problems, including seizures, coma, headaches, and parasthesias, can occur.

Leg Ulcers

- These are uncommon in childhood but occur frequently in adults and are related to stasis. They can be very difficult to reverse; treatments include bed rest, elevation, and zinc sulfate dressings. A transfusion program or skin grafting can enhance healing.

Pregnancy

- Oral contraceptives may slightly increase the risk of thromboembolism, but this is less of a risk than pregnancy. Patients should be closely watched during pregnancy; prophylactic transfusions have appeared to help some patients, but this is not routinely accepted as necessary. Low birth weight and increased fetal loss are noted, probably related to placental vascular occlusions. Maternal mortality averages 1.6 percent.

Laboratory Features

- Hemoglobin level is usually between 5 and 11 g/dl. Anemia is normochromic and normocytic, but considerable variation in red cell size and shape is noted. Sickled cells and targets are seen; reticulocytosis is almost always present.
- Leukocytosis and thrombocytosis are common, even in patients without acute problems; these may be due to a reactive marrow along with demargination of peripheral leukocytes.
- Modest elevations in whole body iron content are common; however, hemochromatosis is rare.
- Hemoglobin electrophoresis will document presence of hemoglobin S. Hemoglobins F and A_2 are particularly increased in patients with sickle cell β thalassemia. Despite high levels of hemoglobin F at birth, electrophoresis can detect hemoglobin S in the newborn.

Experimental Management

- Marrow transplants have been performed, primarily in Europe. Encouraging results have been seen but the morbidity and mortality of graft versus host disease must be considered.
- Modalities employed in attempts to ameliorate the sickling process include induction of methemoglobinemia, inhalation of carbon monoxide, use of urea and pyridoxine, and attempts to decrease intracorpuscular hemoglobin concentration. None of these or others have been safely effective as yet.
- Several agents (hydroxyurea, erythropoietin, cytosine arabinoside, 5-azacytidine) can increase fetal hemoglobin levels and decrease sickling episodes. These are under study at present.

SICKLE CELL TRAIT

- In sickle cell trait less than half of the hemoglobin in each red blood cell is hemoglobin S. This effectively protects against sickling except in the most severe circumstances. It affects approximately 8 percent of African Americans.
- Numerous anecdotal reports suggest that sickle cell trait may be injurious, but the morbidity and mortality are extremely low and difficult to quantitate.
- In a Veterans Administration study of 65,000 adult African-American patients, a slightly higher incidence of hematuria (2.5 vs. 1.3 percent) and pulmonary embolus (2.2 vs. 1.5 percent) was found in patients with sickle cell trait. Sudden death following severe exercise occurs statistically more often in patients with sickle cell trait. The concerns about splenic infarction in commercial air flight appear unwarranted.

HEMOGLOBIN C DISEASE

- Glutamic acid in the sixth position of the beta chain is replaced by lysine in hemoglobin C disease. Red blood cells are more rigid than normal and intracellular crystals of hemoglobin C are found; target cells are numerous. The prevalence in African Americans is 2 to 3 percent.
- Splenomegaly and mild anemia are almost always present in the homozygous state. No treatment is required and the prognosis is excellent.

HEMOGLOBIN D DISEASE

- This hemoglobin variant has normal solubility but migrates like hemoglobin S on electrophoresis. The highest incidence is in northwest India (3 percent). The heterozygous state is asymptomatic; no firmly diagnosed homozygous patients have been described.

Hemoglobin SD occurs rarely and is mild. Hemoglobin D β thalassemia is also rare.

HEMOGLOBIN E DISEASE

- This is due to a β-chain mutation ($\beta^{26glu-lys}$) which results in a moderately unstable hemoglobin when exposed to oxidation. Some mRNA may be spliced improperly, giving a thalassemia-like picture.
- This is a relatively common abnormal hemoglobin, found chiefly in Southeast Asia. Only a few homozygous patients have been described; they have marked microcytosis and mild anemia. Hemoglobin E trait is asymptomatic, but mild microcytosis is seen. In association with β thalassemia a moderate anemia and splenomegaly are found; a splenectomy may be considered in this setting.

OTHER HEMOGLOBINOPATHIES

- Rare compared with those described above. Many are of no clinical significance but have helped to elucidate the structure and function of hemoglobin. Others can produce cyanosis or are unstable. These are described in other chapters.

For a more detailed discussion, see Richard B. Patt, Richard Payne: Pain management, Chap. 21, p. 203; Ernest Beutler: The sickle cell diseases and related disorders, Chap. 56, p. 616; Haewon C. Kim et al: Separation of hemoglobins, Chap. L10, p. L35; Fetal hemoglobin, Chap. L11, p. L42; Sickle hemoglobin, Chap. L12, p. L43 in *Williams Hematology*, 5/e, 1995.

---

27 HEMOGLOBINOPATHIES ASSOCIATED WITH UNSTABLE HEMOGLOBIN

- The unstable hemoglobins discussed here result from a mutation that changes the amino acid sequence of one of the globin chains, leading to precipitates that attach to the red cell membrane (Heinz bodies).
- Homotetramers of normal beta chains (hemoglobin H) or gamma chains (hemoglobin Bart's) are also unstable. These hemoglobins are found in α thalassemias (Chap. 25).

ETIOLOGY AND PATHOGENESIS

- The tetrameric hemoglobin molecule has numerous noncovalent forces that maintain the structure of each subunit and bind the subunits to each other.
- Amino acid substitutions or deletions weaken these forces allowing hemoglobin to denature and precipitate as insoluble globins, which may attach to the cell membrane (Heinz bodies).
- Heinz bodies impair erythrocyte deformability, impeding the ability to negotiate the splenic sinuses; "pitting" of Heinz bodies causes loss of membrane and ultimately destruction of red cells.

INHERITANCE

- An autosomal dominant disorder; most patients are heterozygotes.
- Rarely patients develop an unstable hemoglobin as a result of a new mutation.
- Over 80 percent have a defect in the β chain.
- Most patients have a combination of hemoglobin A and unstable hemoglobin in their red cells.

CLINICAL FEATURES

- Hemolysis is usually well compensated. A patient with an unstable hemoglobin with high O_2 affinity may have a hemoglobin level in the upper normal range.
- Infection or treatment with oxidant drugs may precipitate hemolytic episodes, making the diagnosis apparent.
- In particularly unstable variants involving β-chain mutations, chronic hemolytic anemia may become evident during the first year of life as γ chains (fetal hemoglobin) are replaced by mutant β chains.
- Physical findings include jaundice, splenomegaly, and pallor.

- Some patients have dark urine probably from the catabolism of free heme groups or Heinz bodies.

LABORATORY FEATURES

- Hemoglobin concentration may be normal or decreased. The MCV is usually decreased due to loss of hemoglobin from denaturation and pitting.
- Blood film may show hypochromia, poikilocytosis, polychromasia, anisocytosis, and basophilic stippling.
- After splenectomy Heinz bodies may be found in circulating red cells.
- Reticulocytosis is often out of proportion to the severity of the anemia, particularly when the abnormal hemoglobin has a high oxygen affinity.
- Diagnosis is confirmed by demonstration of an unstable hemoglobin. This may be done by
  - isopropanol stability test
  - heat stability test
  - staining with brilliant cresyl blue to generate Heinz bodies
- Hemoglobin electrophoresis may be useful, but a normal pattern does not rule out an unstable hemoglobin.
- Determination of the P_{50} may be helpful.
- Unstable hemoglobins can also be detected by DNA analysis.

DIFFERENTIAL DIAGNOSIS

- Consider the possibility of an unstable hemoglobin in all patients with a hereditary nonspherocytic hemolytic anemia, especially with hypochromic red cells and reticulocytosis out of proportion to the degree of anemia.
- Not all patients with a positive test for unstable hemoglobin have this disorder; a false positive isopropanol stability test may be seen in patients with sickle hemoglobin, or elevated levels of methemoglobin or hemoglobin F.
- Hemoglobin H and hemoglobin Bart's are unstable. These can be detected by electrophoresis and are found in patients with α thalassemia.

TREATMENT, COURSE, AND PROGNOSIS

- Most patients have a relatively benign course.
- Gallstones are common, often requiring cholecystectomy.
- Hemolytic episodes may be caused by infection or by oxidative drugs.
- Treatment is usually not required. Folic acid is often given, although benefit is not proven. Splenectomy is useful in some patients but may cause deleterious effects in patients with high-oxygen-affinity hemoglobins.

For a more detailed discussion, see Ernest Beutler: Hemoglobinopathies associated with unstable hemoglobin, Chap. 57, p. 650; and Heinz body staining, Chap. L5, p. L26; see also Haewon C. Kim, Elias Schwartz: Unstable hemoglobins, Chap. L9, p. L33; and Haewon C. Kim, Kazuhiko Adachi, Elias Schwartz: Separation of hemoglobins, Chap. L10, p. L35, in *Williams Hematology,* 5/e, 1995.

28 METHEMOGLOBINEMIA AND OTHER CAUSES OF CYANOSIS

Cyanosis is most frequently due to low arterial oxygen saturation because of cardiac or pulmonary disease, but rarely it may be due to increased concentrations of methemoglobin or sulfhemoglobin, or to abnormal hemoglobins with low oxygen affinity.

TOXIC METHEMOGLOBINEMIA

- Drugs or chemicals may cause methemoglobinemia either by oxidizing hemoglobin directly or by enhancing its oxidization by molecular oxygen. Common agents causing methemoglobinemia are listed in Table 28-1.
- Infants are more susceptible because of low levels of NADH diaphorase in the newborn period.
- Severe acute methemoglobinemia impairs oxygen delivery, and levels exceeding 60 to 70 percent may be fatal. Chronic methemoglobinemia is usually asymptomatic, but at levels greater than 20 percent, mild erythrocytosis is seen.
- Treatment with intravenous methylene blue (given at 1 to 2 mg/kg over 5 min) is rapidly effective (within 1 to 2 h). Excessive methylene blue, or its use in G-6-PD-deficient patients, can cause acute hemolysis.

NADH DIAPHORASE DEFICIENCY

- NADH diaphorase catalyzes the reduction of cytochrome b_5, which in turn reduces methemoglobin to hemoglobin.
- Hereditary deficiency of NADH diaphorase results in an accumulation

TABLE 28-1 Drugs That Cause Methemoglobinemia

Phenazopyridine (Pyridium)
Sulfamethoxazole
Dapsone
Aniline
Paraquat/monolinuron
Nitrate
Nitroglycerin
Amyl nitrite
Isobutyl nitrite
Sodium nitrite
Local anesthetics
  Benzocaine
  Prilocaine

Source: Table 58-1 of *Williams Hematology*, 5/e, p. 655.

of methemoglobin. In some patients, cells other than erythrocytes may be involved, and progressive encephalopathy may occur.

- Methemoglobin levels vary between 8 and 40 percent, and the NADH diaphorase level is less than 20 percent of normal.
- Treatment is with ascorbic acid (200 to 600 mg/day orally, divided into four doses).

CYTOCHROME b₅ DEFICIENCY

- Rarely the cytochrome b_5 itself is deficient, causing the same clinical picture as NADH diaphorase deficiency.

HEMOGLOBINS M

- Some amino acid substitutions in hemoglobin lead to enhanced formation or stabilization of methemoglobin. These abnormal proteins are termed hemoglobins M (see Table 58-2 in *Williams Hematology*, 5/e, p. 656).
- Cyanosis may be evident at birth in hemoglobin M disease with the α-chain mutant; in the β-chain variant this will evolve over 6 to 9 weeks as hemoglobin F is replaced by hemoglobin A.
- Hemolysis is present in certain variants and may be exacerbated by drugs.
- No effective treatment for hemoglobin M is known.

LOW OXYGEN AFFINITY HEMOGLOBINS

- Some hemoglobin variants bring about improved tissue oxygen delivery because of their decreased oxygen affinity (Table 58-2 of *Williams Hematology*, 5/e, p. 657).
- As the body perceives adequate oxygen delivery, erythropoietin is decreased and a mild anemia results.

SULFHEMOGLOBIN

- In vitro sulfhemoglobin can be produced by addition of hydrogen sulfide to hemoglobin.
- In vivo sulfhemoglobin can be induced in some individuals by ingestion of drugs, or may occur without apparent cause.
- Cyanosis is present and occasionally mild hemolysis occurs. Sulfhemoglobinemia is usually tolerated and does not affect overall health. Sulfhemoglobin cannot be changed back to normal hemoglobin.

For a more detailed discussion, see Ernest Beutler: Methemoglobinemia and other causes of cyanosis, Chap. 58, p. 654, in *Williams Hematology*, 5/e, 1995.

29 TRAUMATIC CARDIAC HEMOLYTIC ANEMIA, MARCH HEMOGLOBINURIA, AND SPORTS ANEMIA

TRAUMATIC CARDIAC HEMOLYTIC ANEMIA

Definition

- Complications of prosthetic heart valves that lead to turbulence and high shear stresses within a space enclosed by a foreign surface result in red cell fragmentation and hemolysis.
- Cardiac valve disorders, especially severe aortic or subaortic stenosis, may also cause hemolysis.

Clinical Features

- Hemolytic anemia is usually mild and compensated but may be severe.
- More important clinically is the thrombogenicity of nonendothelialized surfaces, which promote platelet thrombosis and embolization.

Laboratory Features

- Blood film: schistocytes (red cell fragments) present, including helmet cells, triangular cells, and spherocytes
- Increased reticulocyte count, increased serum lactate dehydrogenase activity, increased plasma hemoglobin concentration; urine hemosiderin present
- Decreased serum haptoglobin concentration
- Decreased platelet count may indicate platelet thrombi on valve surfaces.

Differential Diagnosis

- Based on the presence of schistocytes on the blood film and evidence of chronic hemolysis in a patient with a cardiac valve disorder or an artificial heart valve.

Treatment

- For severe anemia: replacement of the prosthesis.
  - Transfusion may be necessary preoperatively and may diminish the hemolysis.
- For milder anemia: ensure maximal erythropoiesis.
  - Replace urinary iron loss with ferrous sulfate, 300 mg/day orally.
  - Give folic acid, 1 mg/day orally.
- For severe anemia ineligible for reoperation:

145

- Propranolol, to decrease shearing force between foreign material and red cells.
- Recombinant human erythropoietin treatment may eliminate transfusion requirements.

MARCH HEMOGLOBINURIA AND SPORTS ANEMIA

Definition

- Mild anemia occurs in individuals involved in sustained, strenuous physical activity.
- Pathogenesis is complex and appears to involve the following:
  - Hemoglobinuria may occur from trauma sustained by intravascular red cells in the feet of long distance runners or in the hands of karate practitioners or persons playing the congo drums.
  - Gastrointestinal bleeding occurs in about 20 percent of long distance runners but is usually not enough to cause anemia.
  - Decreased serum ferritin concentration is found in most athletes during intense training, presumably from iron loss in sweat, but this is insufficient to cause iron deficiency anemia.
  - Increased plasma volume and red cell mass develops in athletes, with gain in plasma volume exceeding gain in red cell mass.
  - Increased extraction of O_2 by muscles leads to increased production of 2,3-BPG by red cells with shift of oxygen dissociation curve to the right, improving O_2 delivery to tissues, decreasing erythropoietin production.

Clinical and Laboratory Features

- Concentration of hemoglobin and hematocrit are at lower limits of normal; red cells tend to be macrocytic.
- Reticulocyte count may be increased, especially in active runners.
- Serum iron, ferritin, and haptoglobin concentrations are usually moderately decreased.
- Hemoglobinuria may be noted for 6 to 12 h in runners after a race.

Differential Diagnosis

- Hemoglobinuria follows exercise rather than chilling of the body [as in paroxysmal cold hemoglobinuria (PCH)] or sleep [paroxysmal nocturnal hemoglobinuria (PNH)]. If doubt arises, the Donath-Landsteiner test for PCH and/or the sucrose lysis test for PNH should be performed.
- Myoglobinuria can be distinguished from hemoglobinuria by chemical tests of urine (see Chap. L16D of *Williams Hematology*, 5/e).
- Athletes with occult blood in stools should be tested for underlying gastrointestinal tract abnormality, despite the frequency of subclinical gastrointestinal bleeding after strenuous exercise.

Therapy

- For march hemoglobinuria: reassure the patient; add cushioned insoles to the shoes; and suggest that changing the gait may ameliorate the condition.
- For sports anemia, no treatment is indicated; the condition may be a beneficial adaptation to tissue demands for oxygen.

For a more detailed discussion, see Allan J. Erslev: Traumatic cardiac hemolytic anemia, Chap. 59, p. 663; and March hemoglobinuria and sports anemia, Chap. 61, p. 669, in *Williams Hematology,* 5/e, 1995.

---

30 MICROANGIOPATHIC HEMOLYTIC ANEMIA

DEFINITION

- Intravascular hemolysis due to fragmentation of normal red cells passing through abnormal arterioles.
- Deposition of platelets and fibrin is most common cause of microvascular lesions.

ETIOLOGY AND PATHOGENESIS

- Intravascular coagulation, with deposition of platelets and fibrin in small arterioles, is the common antecedent.
- Red cells stick to fibrin and are fragmented by force of blood flow, resulting in both intravascular and extravascular hemolysis.
- Underlying disorders:
  - Invasive carcinoma, especially mucin-producing adenocarcinomas.
  - Complications of pregnancy: preeclampsia, eclampsia, abruptio placentae.
  - Malignant hypertension.
  - Thrombotic thrombocytopenic purpura (TTP), hemolytic uremic syndrome (HUS)
  - Drugs, especially antineoplastic agents: most often mitomycin, but also bleomycin, daunorubicin in combination with cytosine arabinoside, cisplatin. The HUS may occur weeks or months after discontinuing mitomycin therapy.
  - Posttransplantation of kidney or liver.
  - Postallogeneic or autologous marrow transplantation.
  - Generalized vasculitis associated with immune disorders, e.g., systemic lupus erythematosus, polyarteritis nodosa, Wegener's granulomatosus, scleroderma.
  - Localized vascular abnormalities: cutaneous cavernous hemangiomas, hemangioendothelioma of the liver.

CLINICAL FEATURES

- Symptoms and signs are related to the primary process and the organs affected by the intravascular deposition of platelets and fibrin.
- Severe anemia and kidney failure may contribute to the constitutional symptoms.

LABORATORY FINDINGS

- Blood film: schistocytes prominent, including helmet cells, triangular cells, spherocytes.
- Elevation of reticulocyte count, and increased concentrations of plasma hemoglobin, urine hemoglobin, and hemosiderin. Serum lac-

tate dehydrogenase activity is increased, and the level correlates with disease activity.
- Decreased serum haptoglobin level.
- Coagulation abnormalities due to consumption coagulopathy:
  - Overt: decreased levels of factors V, VIII, antithrombin III, fibrinogen; elevated fibrin(ogen) degradation products.
  - Subtle: increased plasma concentration of fibrinopeptide A, fibrin D dimer.
- If deposition of platelets predominates there is minimal or no evidence of intravascular coagulation.

DIFFERENTIAL DIAGNOSIS

- Other types of intravascular hemolysis: paroxysmal nocturnal hemoglobinuria, paroxysmal cold hemoglobinuria, some cases of autoimmune hemolytic anemia.
- Distinguishing features: schistocytes on the blood film, thrombocytopenia, negative direct antiglobulin test, evidence of intravascular coagulation, identification of the primary process.

TREATMENT

- Directed toward management of primary process underlying the microangiopathy.
- Red cell transfusions to maintain adequate level of hemoglobin.
- Platelet transfusions for bleeding due to thrombocytopenia.
- Heparin use is controversial.
- If the hemolytic uremic syndrome is associated with mitomycin C, immunoadsorption of the patient's plasma by staphylococcal protein A may be beneficial.

For a more detailed discussion, see Jose Martinez: Microangiopathic hemolytic anemia, Chap. 60, p. 665, in *Williams Hematology,* 5/e, 1995.

31 HEMOLYTIC ANEMIA DUE TO CHEMICAL AND PHYSICAL AGENTS

HEMOLYSIS INDUCED BY DRUGS OR CHEMICALS

- Certain drugs can induce hemolysis in individuals with abnormalities of erythrocytic enzymes, such as glucose-6-phosphate dehydrogenase, or with an unstable hemoglobin (see Chaps. 24 and 27). Such drugs can also cause hemolysis in normal individuals if given in sufficiently large doses.
- Other drugs induce hemolytic anemia through an immunological mechanism (see Chap. 35).
- The drugs and chemicals discussed here cause hemolysis by other mechanisms.

ARSENIC HYDRIDE (ARSINE, AsH₃)

- Arsine gas is formed in many industrial processes.
- Inhalation of arsine gas can lead to severe anemia, hemoglobinuria, and jaundice.

LEAD

- Lead poisoning in adults usually is the result of industrial exposure. In children it usually is due to ingestion of lead paint flakes or chewing lead-painted objects.
- Lead intoxication leads to anemia. There is a modest decrease in red cell life-span, but the anemia is more the result of inhibition of heme synthesis.
- Lead also inhibits pyrimidine 5'-nucleotidase, and this may be responsible for the basophilic stippling of red cells found in lead poisoning.
- The anemia is usually mild in adults but may be severe in children. Red cells are normocytic and slightly hypochromic.
- Basophilic stippling may be fine or coarse and is most likely found in polychromatophilic cells.
- Ringed sideroblasts are frequently found in the marrow.

COPPER

- Hemolytic anemia may be induced by high levels of copper in patients hemodialyzed with fluid contaminated by copper tubing, or in patients with Wilson disease.
- The hemolysis is probably due to inhibition of erythrocytic enzymes by copper.

CHLORATES

- Ingestion of sodium or potassium chlorate, or contamination of dialysis fluid with chloramines, can cause oxidative damage with formation of Heinz bodies and methemoglobin and with development of hemolytic anemia.

MISCELLANEOUS DRUGS AND CHEMICALS

- Other drugs and chemicals that may cause hemolytic anemia are listed in Table 62-1 of *Williams Hematology,* 5/e.

WATER

- Water administered intravenously, inhaled in near drowning, or gaining access to the circulation during irrigation procedures can cause hemolysis.

OXYGEN

- Hemolytic anemia has developed in patients receiving hyperbaric oxygenation and in astronauts exposed to 100% oxygen.

INSECT AND ARACHNID VENOMS

- Severe hemolysis may occur in some patients following bites by bees, wasps, spiders, or scorpions.
- Snake bites are not often a cause of hemolysis.

HEAT

- Patients with extensive burns may develop severe hemolytic anemia apparently due to direct damage to the red cells by heat.
- Blood films of many burned patients show spherocytes and fragmentation, and the osmotic fragility may be increased.

For a more detailed discussion, see Ernest Beutler: Hemolytic anemia due to chemical and physical agents, Chap. 62, p. 670, in *Williams Hematology,* 5/e, 1995.

---

32 HEMOLYTIC ANEMIA DUE TO INFECTIONS WITH MICROORGANISMS

- Hemolysis represents a prominent part of the overall clinical picture in many infections.
  - Hemolysis may be caused by direct invasion by infecting organisms (malaria), elaboration of hemolytic toxins *(Clostridium perfringens),* or development of autoantibodies against red blood cell antigens (viral infections).

MALARIA

Etiology and Pathogenesis

- The world's most common cause of hemolytic anemia.
- Transmitted by bite of an infected female *Anopheles* mosquito.
- Parasites grow intracellularly and parasitized cells are destroyed in the spleen.
- Uninvaded cells are apparently destroyed also, possibly by oxidative damage to red blood cell lipids.
- Genetic polymorphisms that interfere with invasion of red blood cells by parasites have developed in endemic areas (G-6-PD deficiency, thalassemias, and hemoglobinopathies).

Clinical Features

- Febrile paroxysms are characteristically cyclic—*P. vivax* every 48 h, *P. malariae* every 72 h, and *P. falciparum* daily.
- Splenomegaly is typically present in chronic infection.
- Falciparum malaria is occasionally associated with very severe hemolysis and dark, almost black urine (blackwater fever).

Laboratory Features

- Diagnosis depends on demonstration of the parasites on the blood film or the appropriate DNA sequences in the blood.

Treatment/Prognosis

- The blood form of malaria is treated with quinine, chloroquine, or sulfones/sulfonamides together with pyrimethamine.
- Tissue stages of vivax malaria are effectively treated with primaquine. Primaquine, as well as certain sulfones, may produce severe hemolysis in patients with G-6-PD deficiency.
- For blackwater fever, transfusions may be necessary, and if renal failure occurs, dialysis may be required.
- With early treatment, prognosis is excellent. When therapy is delayed

or the strain is resistant, malaria (particularly falciparum) may be fatal.

BARTONELLOSIS

- *Bartonella bacilliformis* is transmitted by the sand fly.
- The organism adheres to the exterior surface of red blood cells, which are rapidly removed from the circulation by the spleen and liver.

Clinical Features

- Disease develops in two stages:
  1. acute hemolytic anemia (Oroya fever)
  2. chronic granulomatous disorder (verruca peruviana)
- Most patients manifest no clinical symptoms during the Oroya fever phase, but may develop severe anemia accompanied by anorexia, thirst, sweating, and generalized lymphadenopathy.
- Verruca peruviana is a nonhematologic disorder characterized by a bleeding warty eruption over the face and extremities.

Laboratory Features

- Severe anemia develops rapidly.
- Large numbers of nucleated red cells appear in the blood and the reticulocyte count is high.
- Diagnosis is established by demonstrating the organisms on red blood cells on a Giemsa-stained smear (red-violet rods 1 to 3 μm in length).

Treatment/Prognosis

- Mortality for untreated patients is very high. Those who survive experience sudden clinical improvement with increase in red cell count and change of the organisms from an elongated to a coccoid form.
- The acute phase responds well to treatment with penicillin, streptomycin, chloramphenicol, and the tetracyclines.

CLOSTRIDIUM PERFRINGENS (WELCHII)

- Most commonly seen in patients with septic abortion and occasionally following acute cholecystitis.
- In *C. welchii* septicemia, the toxin (a lecithinase) reacts with red blood cells surfaces, leading to severe, often fatal hemolysis with striking hemoglobinemia and hemoglobinuria; serum may be a brilliant red and the urine a dark-brown mahogany color.
- Acute renal and hepatic failure usually develop.
- The blood film shows microspherocytosis, leukocytosis with a left shift and thrombocytopenia.

- Treatment is with high-dose penicillin and surgical debridement.
- Mortality is greater than 50 percent, even with appropriate therapy.

BABESIOSIS

- Intraerythrocytic protozoa transmitted by ticks infect many species of wild and domestic animals (rodents and cattle).
- Humans are rarely infected, usually via ticks but transmission by transfusion has been reported.
- Most common in the U.S. northeastern coastal region, but also encountered in the midwest.
- Gradual onset with malaise, anorexia, fatigue, followed by fever, sweats, myalgias, and arthralgias.
- May be more severe in splenectomized patients.
- Parasites seen in the red blood cells on Giemsa-stained blood films.
- Treatment with clindamycin and quinine.
- Whole-blood exchange has been used with marked improvement.

OTHER INFECTIONS

- Viral agents may be associated with autoimmune hemolysis (see Chap. 33). The mechanisms include absorption of immune complexes, cross-reacting antibodies, and loss of tolerance.
- Evidence for CMV infection is found in a high percentage of children with lymphadenopathy and hemolytic anemia.
- High cold agglutinin titer may develop with *Mycoplasma pneumoniae* infection and occasionally results in hemolytic anemia or compensated hemolysis.
- *Microangiopathic hemolytic anemia* (see Chap. 30) may be triggered by a variety of infections, including *Shigella, Campylobacter,* and *Aspergillus.*

For a more detailed discussion, see Ernest Beutler: Hemolytic anemia due to infections with microorganisms, Chap. 63, p. 674; and Lucio Luzzatto, Allan J. Erslev: Examination of blood for malaria and other parasites, Chap. L8, p. L29, in *Williams Hematology,* 5/e, 1995.

---

33 ACQUIRED HEMOLYTIC ANEMIA DUE TO WARM-REACTING AUTOANTIBODIES

- In autoimmune hemolytic anemia (AHA), shortened red blood cell (RBC) survival is the result of host antibodies that react with autologous RBC.
- AHA may be classified by whether an underlying disease is present (secondary) or not (primary or idiopathic)(Table 33-1).
- AHA may also be classified by the nature of the antibody (Table 33-1).
  - "Warm-reacting" antibodies have optimal activity at 37°C.
  - "Cold-reacting" antibodies show affinity at lower temperatures (see Chap. 34).
  - Occasionally, mixed disorders occur with both warm and cold antibodies.
  - Warm antibody autoimmune hemolytic anemia (AHA) is the most common type.

ETIOLOGY AND PATHOGENESIS

- AHA occurs in all ages, but the incidence rises with age, in part probably because the frequency of lymphoproliferative malignancies increases with age.

TABLE 33-1 Classification of Autoimmune Hemolytic Anemia

I. On basis of serologic characteristics of involved autoimmune process:
  - A. Warm autoantibody type—autoantibody maximally active at body temperature 37°C
  - B. Cold autoantibody type—autoantibody active at temperatures below 37°C
  - C. Mixed cold and warm autoantibodies

II. On basis of presence or absence of underlying or significantly associated disorder:
  - A. Primary or idiopathic AHA
  - B. Secondary AHA:
    1. Associated with lymphoproliferative disorders
    2. Associated with the rheumatic disorders, particularly systemic lupus erythematosus
    3. Associated with certain infections
    4. Associated with certain nonlymphoid neoplasms, e.g., ovarian tumors
    5. Associated with certain chronic inflammatory diseases, e.g., ulcerative colitis
    6. Associated with ingestion of certain drugs, e.g., α-methyldopa

Source: Table 64-1 of *Williams Hematology*, 5/e, p. 677.

- In primary AHA, the autoantibody often is specific for a single RBC membrane protein, suggesting that an aberrant immune response has occurred to an autoantigen or a similar immunogen; a generalized defect in immune regulation is not seen.
- In secondary AHA, the autoantibody most likely develops from an immunoregulatory defect.
- Certain drugs (e.g., α-methyldopa) can induce specific antibodies in otherwise normal individuals by some unknown mechanism. These subside spontaneously when the drug is stopped.
- The red cells of some apparently normal individuals may be found coated with warm-reacting autoantibodies similar to those of patients with AHA. Such antibodies are noted in otherwise normal blood donors at a frequency of 1 in 10,000. A few such individuals have gone on to develop AHA.
- RBC autoantibodies are pathogenic.
  - RBC that lack the targeted antigen have a normal survival.
  - Transplacental passage of autoantibodies to a fetus can cause hemolytic anemia.
  - Antibody-coated RBC are trapped by macrophages primarily in the spleen, where they are ingested and destroyed or partially phagocytosed and a spherocyte with smaller surface area is released.
  - Macrophages have cell surface receptors for the Fc portion of IgG and for fragments of C3 and C4b. These immunoglobulin and complement proteins on the RBC surface can act cooperatively as opsonins and enhance trapping of RBC.
- Large quantities of IgG or the addition of C3b will increase trapping by macrophages in the liver.
- Direct RBC lysis by complement is unusual in warm antibody AHA, probably due to interference with complement activity by several mechanisms.
- RBC may be destroyed by monocytes or lymphocytes by direct cytotoxic activity, without phagocytosis. The extent of hemolysis due to this mechanism is unknown.

CLINICAL FEATURES

- Generally, symptoms of anemia draw attention to the disease, although jaundice may also be a presenting complaint.
- Symptoms are usually slow in onset, but rapidly developing anemia can occur.
- Physical examination may be normal if the anemia is mild. Splenomegaly is common but not always observed. Jaundice and physical findings related to more pronounced anemia may be noticed.
- AHA may be aggravated or first noticed during pregnancy. Both mother and fetus generally fare well if the condition is treated early.

LABORATORY FEATURES

General

- Anemia can range from mild to life threatening.
- Blood film reveals polychromasia (indicating reticulocytosis) and spherocytes.
- With severe cases, nucleated RBC, RBC fragments, and occasionally erythrophagocytosis by monocytes may be seen.
- Reticulocytosis is usually present if the marrow has not been injured by some other condition, although early in the course, a brief reticulocytopenia occurs in a third of the cases.
- Most patients have mild neutrophilia and normal platelet count, but occasionally neutropenia and thrombocytopenia occur.
- Evans syndrome is a rare condition in which both immune-mediated RBC and platelet destruction occur.
- Bone marrow examination usually reveals erythroid hyperplasia; occasionally an underlying lymphoproliferative disease may be uncovered.
- Unconjugated hyperbilirubinemia is often present, but usually the total bilirubin level does not exceed 5 mg/dl, with less than 15 percent conjugated.
- Haptoglobin levels are usually low, and LDH activity is elevated.
- Urinary urobilinogen is routinely increased, but hemoglobinuria is very uncommon.

Serologic Features

- The diagnosis of AHA requires demonstration of immunoglobulin and/or complement bound to the RBC.
  - This is usually achieved by the direct antiglobulin test (DAT) in which rabbit antiserum to human IgG or complement is added to suspensions of washed RBC. Agglutination of the RBC signifies the presence of surface IgG or complement.
  - The DAT is first performed with broad spectrum reagents including antibodies against both complement and immunoglobulin. If this is positive, further testing is done to define the offending antibody or complement component.
  - RBC may be coated with
    - IgG alone
    - IgG and complement
    - complement only
  - Rarely anti-IgA and anti-IgM reactions are encountered.
- Autoantibody exists in a dynamic equilibrium between RBC and plasma.
  - Free autoantibody may be detected by the indirect antiglobulin test in which the patient's plasma is incubated with normal donor RBC

which are then tested for agglutination by the addition of antiglobulin serum.

- Binding affinity for antibodies varies, but in general, plasma autoantibody is detectable in those with heavily coated RBC.
- A positive indirect test with a negative direct test probably does not indicate autoimmune disease but an alloantibody generated by a prior transfusion or pregnancy.

- Occasional patients exhibit all the features of AHA but have a negative DAT. The amount of their RBC-bound autoantibody is too low for detection by DAT but can often be demonstrated by more sensitive methods such as enzyme-linked immunoassay or radioimmunoassay.
- The relationship between the amount of bound antibody and degree of hemolysis is variable.
  - Subclasses IgG1 and IgG3 are generally more effective in causing hemolysis than IgG2 and IgG4, apparently because of greater affinity of macrophage Fc receptors for these subclasses as well as increased complement fixation abilities.
- Autoantibodies from AHA patients usually bind to all the types of RBC used for laboratory screening and therefore appear to be "nonspecific."
  - However, the autoantibodies from individual patients usually react with antigens which are present on nearly all RBC types, the so-called "public" antigens, and only appear to lack specificity.
  - Nearly half have specificity for epitopes on Rh proteins (Rh related) and hence will not react with cells of the rare Rh null type.
  - The remaining autoantibodies have a variety of specificities, but many are not defined.

DIFFERENTIAL DIAGNOSIS

- Other conditions may have spherocytosis, including hereditary spherocytosis, Zieve syndrome, and clostridial sepsis. DAT is negative in these conditions.
- Paroxysmal nocturnal hemoglobinuria and microangiopathic hemolytic anemia must also be considered, but minimal or no spherocytosis is seen and the DAT is negative.
- If the DAT is positive, further serologic characterizations are warranted to distinguish cold- from warm-reacting autoantibodies.
- In recently transfused patients, alloantibody against donor RBC may be detected by a positive DAT.
- Organ transplant recipients may develop a picture of AHA usually when an organ from a blood group O donor is transplanted into a group A recipient, probably because B lymphocytes persist in the transplanted organ and form alloantibodies against host RBC.
  - Marrow transplant patients of blood group O who receive blood group A or B marrow may develop a briefly positive DAT, and

RBC synthesized by the engrafted marrow may be hemolyzed until previously made anti-A or anti-B disappears.

- Mixed chimera also occur so that the immunocompetent host B lymphocyte continues to generate alloantibodies.

THERAPY

- Occasional patients have a positive DAT but minimal hemolysis and stable hematocrit. These patients need no treatment but should be observed for possible progression of the disease.

Transfusion

- Generally, anemia develops slowly so that RBC transfusion is not required; however, for rapid hemolysis or patients otherwise compromised (i.e., cardiac disease), transfusion may be life saving.
- Transfused RBC are destroyed as fast or faster than host RBC but may tide the patient through a dangerous time.
- Glucocorticoids quickly slow or stop hemolysis in two-thirds of the patients.
  - 20 percent of patients will achieve a complete remission.
  - 10 percent will show little or no response.
  - Best results are seen in patients with primary AHA or AHA secondary to lupus erythematosus.
- Initial treatment should be with oral prednisone at 60 to 100 mg/day.
- For the gravely ill, intravenous methylprednisolone at 300 mg daily can be given.
- When the hematocrit stabilizes, prednisone may be tapered to 15 to 20 mg/day and continued for 2 to 3 months before tapering off the drug entirely.
- Relapses are common and the patient should be closely followed.
- The mechanism(s) of action of glucocorticoids in AHA has not been clearly established.

Splenectomy

- In patients who cannot be tapered off prednisone (approximately one-third), splenectomy is the next modality of therapy to use. If response is slow and the anemia is severe, splenectomy should be considered sooner.
- Splenectomy removes the main site of RBC destruction. Hemolysis can continue, but much higher levels of RBC-bound antibody are necessary to cause the same rate of destruction. Sometimes the amount of cell-bound antibody will decrease after splenectomy, but often no change is noted.
- Approximately two-thirds of patients have complete or partial remission after splenectomy, but relapses frequently occur. If gluco-

cortocoids are still necessary, it is often possible to use a lower dosage.

- Splenectomy slightly increases the risk of pneumococcal sepsis (children more than adults), and pneumococcal vaccine should be given prior to surgery. In addition, prophylactic oral penicillin is often given to children after splenectomy.

Immunosuppressive Drugs

- For patients who fail to respond to glucocorticoids and splenectomy, cytotoxic drugs can be considered. This approach, while not universally accepted, has been beneficial in otherwise refractory patients.
- Either cyclophosphamide (60 mg/m^2) or azathioprine (80 mg/m^2) given daily can be used. Close attention to blood counts is crucial as erythropoiesis can be suppressed, temporarily worsening the anemia. Treatment can be continued for up to 6 months awaiting a response, then tapered after the desired response is attained.

Other Treatments

- Plasmapheresis has been used with some success reported, but it is controversial.
- Variable success has been achieved with high-dose intravenous immunoglobulin (400 mg/kg daily for 5 days), danazol, 2-chloro-deoxyadenosine, thymectomy in children, and administration of vinblastine-loaded RBC.

COURSE AND PROGNOSIS

- Idiopathic warm-antibody AHA runs an unpredictable course characterized by remissions and relapses.
  - Survival at 10 years is approximately 70 percent.
  - In addition to anemia, deep venous thrombosis, pulmonary emboli, splenic infarcts, and other cardiovascular events occur during active disease.
- In secondary warm-antibody AHA, prognosis is related to the underlying disease.
- Overall mortality rate in children is lower than in adults, ranging from 10 to 30 percent.
  - AHA related to infection is self-limited and responds well to glucocorticoids.
  - Children who develop chronic AHA tend to be older.

For a more detailed discussion, see Charles H. Packman, John P. Leddy: Acquired hemolytic anemia due to warm-reacting autoantibodies, Chap. 64, p. 677, in *Williams Hematology,* 5/e, 1995.

---

34 CRYOPATHIC HEMOLYTIC SYNDROMES

- Caused by autoantibodies that bind red cells best at temperatures below 37°C, usually below 31°C.
- Mediated through two major types of "cold antibody"; cold agglutinins and Donath-Landsteiner antibodies.
- Clinical features vary considerably, but in both types the complement system plays a major role in red cell destruction.

COLD AGGLUTININ–MEDIATED AUTOIMMUNE HEMOLYTIC ANEMIA

- Cold agglutinins are IgM autoantibodies that agglutinate red cells optimally between 0 to 5°C. Complement fixation occurs at higher temperatures.
- Classified as either primary (chronic cold agglutinin disease) or secondary (generally due to mycoplasma or infectious mononucleosis).
- Peak incidence for the primary (chronic) syndrome is over age 50.
- This disorder characteristically has monoclonal IgM cold agglutinins and may be considered a monoclonal gammopathy.
- Some patients develop a B-cell lymphoproliferative disorder (Waldenström macroglobulinemia).

Pathogenesis

- The specificity of cold agglutinins is usually against I/i antigens. I is expressed heavily in adult red cells, weakly on neonatal red cells. The reverse is true of the i antigen.
- Naturally occurring cold agglutinins are present in low titer (less than 1 to 32) in normal subjects, but transient hyperproduction of less clonally restricted antibodies occurs in the recovery phase of infections, such as EBV, mycoplasma, and CMV.
- I/i antigens serve as mycoplasma receptors, which may lead to altered antigen presentation and subsequent autoantibody production.
- In B-cell lymphomas, cold agglutinins may be produced by the malignant cells.
- The highest temperature at which antibodies can cause agglutination is termed the thermal amplitude. The higher the thermal amplitude, the greater the risk for clinically significant hemolysis, depending on ambient temperature.
- Cold agglutinins bind red cells in the superficial vessels impeding capillary flow, producing acrocyanosis.
- Pathogenicity is dependent on the antibody's ability to fix complement; concurrent agglutination is not required for this process.
- Red cell injury then occurs either by direct lysis or enhanced phagocytosis by macrophages.
  - Direct lysis results from propagation of the full complement sequence, but severe intravascular hemolysis from this cause is rare.

- Commonly, fragments C3b and C4b are deposited on the red cell surface, providing a stimulus for phagocytosis. The affected red cell may be engulfed and destroyed or released back into circulation as a spherocyte because of loss of some plasma membrane.
- Red cells are released with a coating of C3dg, an inactive fragment which protects the red cells from further complement fixation and agglutination but causes a positive direct antiglobulin test.

Clinical Features

- Cold-agglutinin–mediated hemolysis accounts for 10 to 20 percent of all cases of autoimmune hemolytic anemia.
- Hemolysis is generally chronic, although episodes of acute hemolysis can occur upon chilling.
- Acrocyanosis is frequently observed, but skin ulceration and necrosis are distinctly uncommon.
- Splenomegaly may occasionally be seen in the idiopathic form.
- The hemolysis due to mycoplasma infection develops as the patient recovers from the infection and is self-limited, lasting 1 to 3 weeks.
- In patients with mycoplasma infections, clinically significant hemolysis is rare.

Laboratory Features

- Anemia is usually mild to moderate. On the blood film the red cells show autoagglutination, polychromasia, and spherocytosis.
- In the chronic syndrome, serum titers of cold agglutinins (generally IgM) can be greater than 1 to 100,000. The direct antiglobulin test is positive with anticomplement reagents. The cold agglutinin itself readily dissociates from the red cell.
- Anti-I specificity is seen with idiopathic disease, mycoplasma pneumonia, and some lymphoma cases. Anti-i occurs with infectious mononucleosis and lymphomas. Rarely the antibodies will have other specificities, including Pr, M, or P antigens.

Differential Diagnosis

- When peripheral vaso-occlusive symptoms occur, Raynaud phenomenon or cryoglobulinemia should be considered.
- In drug-induced immune hemolytic anemia, the direct antiglobulin test may be positive only for complement, but the cold agglutinin titer is low.
- Mixed type autoimmune hemolysis can occur with a direct antiglobulin test positive for both IgG and complement, along with elevated cold agglutinin titers.
- Episodic hemolysis can result from paroxysmal cold hemoglobinuria, paroxysmal nocturnal hemoglobinuria, and march hemoglobinuria.

Therapy, Course, and Prognosis

- Keeping the patient warm is important and may be the only treatment needed for mild conditions.
- Chlorambucil and cyclophosphamide are useful for more severe chronic cases; α-interferon appears promising in preliminary reports.
- Splenectomy and glucocorticoids generally are not helpful, although very high dose glucocortocoids may be useful in the severely ill.
- In critically ill patients, plasmapheresis may provide temporary relief.
- Generally patients with the chronic syndrome have a stable condition and long-term survival.
- Postinfectious syndromes are self-limited, resolving in a few weeks.

PAROXYSMAL COLD HEMOGLOBINURIA

- A very rare form of hemolytic anemia characterized by recurrent massive hemolysis following exposure to cold. Formerly, this condition was more common, due to its association with syphilis. A self-limited form occurs in children following several types of viral infections.

Pathogenesis

- In the extremities, the cold reactive autoantibody (Donath-Landsteiner antibody) and early complement proteins bind to the red cells at low temperatures. Upon return to the 37°C environment, lysis occurs due to propagation of the classical complement sequence.

Clinical Features

- 2 to 5 percent of all autoimmune hemolytic anemias, but may exceed 30 percent in the pediatric population.
- Paroxysms of hemolysis occur with associated systemic symptoms—rigors, fever, diffuse myalgias, headache. These symptoms and hemoglobinuria usually last several hours. Cold induced urticaria may also occur.

Laboratory Features

- Hemoglobinuria with a rapid fall in hemoglobin level is usual and is associated with depressed complement levels. Spherocytes and erythrophagocytosis may be seen on the blood film.
- The direct antiglobulin test is positive for complement during and immediately after an attack; the Donath-Landsteiner antibody readily dissociates from the red cells.
- Antibody is detected by the biphasic Donath-Landsteiner test. Red cells are incubated with the patient's serum at 4°C, then warmed to 37°C, at which point intense hemolysis occurs.

- Classically, the antibody (IgG type) has specificity for P blood group antigens, although other specificities have been noted.

Differential Diagnosis

- Patients with paroxysmal cold hemoglobinuria lack high titers of cold agglutinins. The Donath-Landsteiner antibody is a far more potent hemolysin than most cold agglutinins.

Therapy, Course, and Prognosis

- Attacks can be prevented by avoiding cold exposure.
- Splenectomy and glucocortocoids are not of value.
- Urticaria may be treated with antihistamines.
- If related to syphilis, the hemolysis will resolve with proper treatment of the infection.
- Postinfectious paroxysmal cold hemoglobinuria may resolve spontaneously in days to weeks, although the antibody may be detectable for years.
- In the idiopathic chronic form, long-term survival is common.

For a more detailed discussion, see Charles H. Packman, John P. Leddy: Cryopathic hemolytic syndromes, Chap. 65, p. 688, in *Williams Hematology,* 5/e, 1995.

35 DRUG-RELATED IMMUNE HEMOLYTIC ANEMIA

ETIOLOGY AND PATHOGENESIS

- Drugs implicated in the production of a positive direct antiglobulin test and accelerated red cell destruction are listed in Table 35-1.
- Three mechanisms of drug-related immunologic injury to red cells are recognized:
  1. hapten/drug adsorption involving drug-dependent antibodies
  2. ternary complex formation involving drug-dependent antibodies.
  3. induction of autoantibodies that react with red cells in the absence of the inciting drug

TABLE 35-1 Association Between Drugs and Positive Direct Antiglobulin Tests

Hapten or drug adsorption mechanism	
Penicillins	Carbromal
Cephalosporins	Tolbutamide
Tetracycline	Cianidanol
Ternary complex mechanism	
Quinidine	Cephalosporins
Stibophen	Probenecid
Quinine	Nomifensine
Chlorpropamide	Diethylstilbestrol
Rifampin	Amphotericin B
Antazoline	Doxepin
Thiopental	Diclofenac
Tolmetin	
Autoantibody mechanism	
Alpha-methyldopa	Procainamide
Cephalosporins	Mefenamic acid
Cianidanol	Teniposide
Tolmetin	Latamoxef
Nomifensine	Flafenine
L-Dopa	Diclofenac
Nonimmunologic protein adsorption	
Cephalosporins	Cisplatin
Uncertain mechanism of immune injury	
Phenacetin	Steptomycin
Insecticides	Ibuprofen
Chlorpromazine	Triamterene
Melphalan	Erythromycin
Isoniazid	5-Fluorouracil
p-Aminosalicylic acid	Nalidixic acid
Acetaminophen	Sulindac
Thiazides	Omeprazol

Source: Adapted from Table 66-1 of *Williams Hematology,* 5/e, p. 69.

165

- Drug-related nonimmunologic protein adsorption may also result in a positive direct antiglobulin test without red cell injury.

HAPTEN OR DRUG ADSORPTION MECHANISM

- Occurs with drugs that bind firmly to red cell membrane proteins. Penicillin is the classical example.
- In patients receiving high-dose penicillin red cells have a substantial coating of the drug. In a small proportion of patients, an antipenicillin antibody (usually IgG) develops and binds to the penicillin on the red cell. The direct antiglobulin test then becomes positive and hemolytic anemia may ensue.
- Hemolytic anemia due to penicillin typically occurs after 7 to 10 days of treatment and ceases a few days to 2 weeks once the drug is stopped.
- Other manifestations of penicillin allergy are usually not present.
- Antibody-coated ("opsonized") red cells are destroyed mainly in the spleen.
- Antibodies eluted from red cells, or present in sera, react only against penicillin-coated red cells. This specificity distinguishes drug-dependent antibodies from true autoantibodies.
- Hemolytic anemia similar to that seen with penicillin has also been ascribed to other drugs (see Table 35-1).

TERNARY COMPLEX MECHANISM: DRUG-ANTIBODY-TARGET CELL COMPLEX

- The mechanism of red cell injury is not clearly defined, but it appears to be mediated by a cooperative interaction to generate a *ternary complex* involving the drug or drug-metabolite, a drug-binding membrane site on the target cell, and antibody, with consequent activation of complement.
- The antibody attaches to a neoantigen consisting of loosely bound drug and red cell antigen; binding of drug to the target cell is weak until stabilized by the attachment of the antibody to both drug and cell membrane.
- Some of these antibodies have specificity for blood group antigens such as Rh, Kell, Kidd, or I/i and are nonreactive with red cells lacking the alloantigen even in the presence of drug.
- The direct antiglobulin test is usually positive with anticomplement reagents.
- Intravascular hemolysis may occur after activation of complement, with hemoglobinemia and hemoglobinuria, and C3b-coated red cells may be destroyed by the spleen and liver.

AUTOANTIBODY MECHANISM

- Many drugs induce the formation of autoantibodies to autologous red cells, most importantly alpha-methyldopa (Table 35-1). The mechanism by which a drug can induce formation of an autoantibody is unknown.

- Positive direct antiglobulin tests are seen in 8 to 36 percent of those taking alpha-methyldopa. The positive test develops 3 to 6 months after the start of therapy. In contrast, less than 1 percent develop hemolytic anemia.
- Antibodies in the serum or eluted from red cells react optimally at 37°C with autologous or homologous red cells in the absence of drug.
- As in autoimmune hemolytic anemia, these antibodies frequently react with the Rh complex.
- Destruction of red cells occurs chiefly by splenic sequestration of IgG-coated red cells.

NONIMMUNOLOGIC PROTEIN ADSORPTION

- Patients receiving cephalosporins occasionally develop positive direct antiglobulin tests due to nonspecific adsorption of immunoglobulins, complement, albumin, fibrinogen, and other plasma proteins to red cell membranes.
- Hemolytic anemia has not been reported.
- The clinical importance is the potential to complicate cross-matching.

CLINICAL FEATURES

- A careful drug history should be obtained in all patients with hemolytic anemia and/or positive direct antiglobulin test.
- The severity of symptoms is dependent upon the rate of hemolysis, and the clinical picture is quite variable.
- Patients with hapten/drug adsorption (e.g., penicillin) and autoimmune (e.g., alpha-methyldopa) mechanisms generally exhibit mild to moderate red cell destruction with insidious onset of symptoms over days to weeks.
- If the ternary complex mechanism is operative (e.g., cephalosporins or quinidine), there may be sudden onset of severe hemolysis with hemoglobinuria and acute renal failure.
- Hemolysis can occur after only one dose of the drug if the patient has been previously exposed.

LABORATORY FEATURES

- Findings are similar to those of autoimmune hemolytic anemia, with anemia, reticulocytosis, and high MCV.
- Leukopenia, thrombocytopenia, hemoglobinemia, or hemoglobinuria may be observed in cases of ternary complex–mediated hemolysis.
- The serologic features are included under "Differential Diagnosis," below.

DIFFERENTIAL DIAGNOSIS

- Immune hemolysis due to drugs should be distinguished from autoimmune hemolytic anemia (warm or cold antibodies), congenital hemolytic anemias (e.g., hereditary spherocytosis), and drug-mediated hemolysis due to disorders of red cell metabolism (e.g., G-6-PD deficiency).
- In drug-related hemolytic anemia, the direct antiglobulin test is positive.
- In the hapten/drug mechanism, the key difference from autoimmune hemolytic anemia is that serum antibodies react only with drug-coated red cells. This serologic distinction plus a history of drug exposure should be decisive.
- In the ternary complex mechanism, the direct antiglobulin test is positive with anti-complement serum, similar to cold autoimmune hemolytic anemia. However, the cold agglutinin titer and Donath-Landsteiner test are normal and the indirect antiglobulin test is positive only in the presence of drug. The direct antiglobulin test becomes negative shortly after stopping the drug.
- In hemolytic anemia due to alpha-methyldopa, the direct antiglobulin reaction is strongly positive for IgG (rarely for complement) and the indirect antiglobulin reaction is positive with unmodified red cells, often showing Rh specificity. There is no specific serologic test to differentiate this disorder from warm-autoimmune hemolytic anemia with Rh complex specificities. The diagnosis is supported by recovery from anemia and disappearance of antibodies with discontinuing the drug.
- With a clinical picture of drug-immune hemolysis, it is reasonable to stop any drug while serologic studies are performed and to monitor for increase in hematocrit, decrease in reticulocytosis, and disappearance of positive antiglobulin test.
- Rechallenge with the suspected drug may confirm the diagnosis but should be tried only for compelling reasons.

THERAPY, COURSE, AND PROGNOSIS

- Discontinuation of the offending drug is often the only treatment needed, and may be life-saving in severe hemolysis mediated by the ternary complex mechanism.
- Transfuse only for severe, life-threatening anemia.
- Glucocorticoids are generally unnecessary and are of questionable efficacy.
- If high-dose penicillin is the treatment of choice in life-threatening infection, therapy need not be changed due to a positive direct antiglobulin test, unless there is overt hemolytic anemia.
- A positive direct antiglobulin test alone is not necessarily an indication

for stopping alpha-methyldopa, although it may be prudent to consider alternative antihypertensive therapy.
- Hemolysis associated with alpha-methyldopa ceases promptly after stopping the drug. The positive direct antiglobulin test gradually diminishes over weeks or months.
- Problems with cross-matching may occur in patients with a strongly positive indirect antiglobulin test (for example, alpha-methyldopa).
- Immune hemolysis due to drugs is usually mild, but occasional episodes of severe hemolysis with renal failure or death have been seen, usually due to the ternary complex mechanism.

For a more detailed discussion, see Charles H. Packman, John C. Leddy: Drug-related immune hemolytic anemia, Chap. 66, p. 691, in *Williams Hematology,* 5/e, 1995.

---

36 ALLOIMMUNE HEMOLYTIC DISEASE OF THE NEWBORN

- The life-span of fetal or newborn red cells is shortened by maternal antibodies.
- Manifestations include anemia, jaundice, and hepatosplenomegaly; in more severe cases, anasarca and kernicterus also occur.

PATHOGENESIS

- Transplacental passage of fetal red cells occurs in 75 percent of pregnancies.
- If there is blood group incompatibility between mother and fetus, the chance of maternal immunization increases with the volume of any transplacental hemorrhage.
- Larger volume transplacental hemorrhages are more likely to occur at delivery or during invasive obstetrical procedures.
- Prior blood transfusions can also immunize the mother.
- D antigen of the Rh blood group systems is involved in most serious cases.
  - Without prophylaxis, sensitization occurs in 7 to 8 percent of those at risk with an ABO-compatible fetus, and 2 percent of ABO-incompatible.
  - 2 percent of those at risk are sensitized early in the pregnancy.
  - Anti-D IgG readily crosses the placenta and leads to extravascular hemolysis in the infant.
- Anti-A and anti-B occasionally cause mild and rarely severe hemolysis. Numerous other causative antibodies have been described but are much more rare.

CLINICAL FEATURES

- With severe hemolysis, profound anemia leads to hydrops fetalis (anasarca due to cardiac failure), and most such fetuses will die in utero.
- With milder cases, hemolysis will persist until incompatible red cells or the offending IgG are cleared. (Half-life of IgG is 3 weeks.)
- Most affected infants are not jaundiced at birth because of transplacental transport of bilirubin.
  - Generally with mild disease, the bilirubin peaks at day 4 or 5 and declines slowly thereafter.
  - Premature infants may have higher levels of bilirubin because of decreased glucuronyl transferase activity.
  - With marked elevation, kernicterus may develop from deposition of bilirubin in the basal ganglia and cerebellum. Severe involvement can be fatal or lead to long-lasting neurologic defects.
- Hepatosplenomegaly is usually present.
- Occasionally severe thrombocytopenia or hypoglycemia also occur and are bad prognostic signs.

LABORATORY FEATURES

- All pregnant patients should have ABO and Rh(D) typing and testing for unusual serum antibodies early in the pregnancy.
  - If Rh negative, they should be tested again in 28 weeks before Rh immunoglobulin is given.
  - After delivery, blood should be drawn to evaluate the degree of fetal-maternal hemorrhage, so that appropriate dose of anti Rh IgG can be given.
- If alloimmunized, the mother's titer should be determined and followed in 3- or 4-week intervals after 20 weeks. If the titer becomes greater than 16, amniocentesis is often performed to test for the bilirubin level, which predicts disease severity.
- Ultrasonography allows further description of disease severity by detecting organomegaly, ascites, or edema. More specific information can be obtained by percutaneous umbilical blood sampling (mortality less than 1 percent) or chorionic villus sampling.
- After delivery, cord blood should be sampled for hemoglobin and bilirubin concentrations, the ABO-Rh type, and the direct antiglobulin test. The peripheral blood film may show nucleated red blood cells, spherocytes, and polychromatophilia.
- Hemopoiesis may be suppressed, but marrow recovery is usually complete by 2 months.
- Other diseases can cause hydrops but are distinguished from alloimmune hemolysis by the absence of maternal antibodies.

THERAPY, COURSE, AND PROGNOSIS

Fetus

- Percutaneous umbilical cord blood sampling is performed if there is a history of a prior affected infant, maternal anti-D serology, or another antibody of concern, or if there is hepatosplenomegaly or evidence of fetal distress on ultrasonography.
- Red cells may be transfused to the severely affected fetus, based on level of anemia, development of ascites, or a rising bilirubin concentration. Either the intraperitoneal or intravascular route may be used—the former is difficult in hydropic cases with ascites, as peritoneal absorption is impaired.
- For a woman with a previous alloimmunized pregnancy, transfusions should begin 10 weeks before the time of the earliest prior fetal death or transfusion, but not before 18 weeks unless hydrops is present. Transfusions are given to keep the hematocrit of the fetus in the 20 to 25 percent range and to prevent hydrops.
- O-negative, antigen-negative for any other identified antibody, CMV-negative, irradiated packed cells are used, cross-matched against the mother's blood.

- The decision as to when to deliver the fetus is complex; if possible, transfusions are given up to 34 weeks with delivery at 36 weeks.
- Other treatments, such as intravenous immunoglobulin with or without plasmapheresis, glucocorticoids, or promethazine have been used with variable success.

Neonatal

- The aim of treatment is to prevent bilirubin neurotoxicity. The risk is higher for newborns with hemolytic disease than others with a similar bilirubin level.
- Phototherapy is used prophylactically in any patient with hemolysis.
- Transfusion is indicated if the cord blood hemoglobin level is less than 13 g/dl and bilirubin level greater than 4 mg/dl. If the infant is premature or unstable parameters are present, less stringent criteria are used. After the first exchange, the rate of rise of bilirubin is used to guide subsequent transfusions.
- Double volume exchanges will remove greater than 50 percent of intravascular bilirubin. In some centers, prior to exchange, intravenous albumin is given to mobilize tissue bilirubin stores.
- ABO-compatible, Rh-negative irradiated blood is used, cross-matched against the mother.
- Erythropoietin has been used to enhance recovery in those with suppressed marrow.

PREVENTION

- Rh immunoprophylaxis is standard practice for an Rh-negative mother.
  - Intramuscular doses of 100 to 300 μg of Rh immune globulin within 72 h of delivery have decreased Rh immunization by greater than 90 percent.
  - Antenatal Rh immunoglobulin at 28 weeks is given but is under debate. Rarely sensitization may occur before the 28th week.
- Although immunoprophylaxis has greatly reduced the incidence, 10.6 per 10,000 births still occur in the United States.
- Since the only adequate prophylaxis is for the D-antigen, other rare antibodies will continue to cause hemolytic disease.

For a more detailed discussion, see Louis DePalma, Naomi C. Luban: Alloimmune hemolytic disease of the newborn, Chap. 67, p. 697, in *Williams Hematology*, 5/e, 1995.

---

37 ACUTE BLOOD LOSS ANEMIA

MAJOR EFFECTS OF RAPID HEMORRHAGE

1. Sudden depletion of blood volume may cause cardiovascular collapse, irreversible shock, and death.
2. The circulating red cell mass is depleted and oxygen transport to the tissues is impaired.

CLINICAL MANIFESTATIONS OF ACUTE BLOOD LOSS

- In acute hemorrhage, the hematocrit does not indicate the extent of blood loss. Rather, the hematocrit falls slowly over 2 or 3 days, as plasma volume is replaced from endogenous sources.
- Clinical signs and symptoms of blood loss depend on the magnitude of the hemorrhage, as outlined in Table 37-1.
- Replacement of volume loss may be accomplished with crystalloid solutions or blood components, the choice of solution depending on the clinical setting.

CLINICAL MANIFESTATIONS OF RED CELL LOSS

- Loss of red cell mass becomes a problem after volume loss has been replaced or if the hemorrhage is relatively slow.

TABLE 37-1 Reaction to Acute Blood Loss of Increasing Severity

Volume lost up to % TVB*	Volume, ml†	Clinical signs
10	500	None. Rarely see vasovagal syncope in blood bank donors.
20	1000	With the patient at rest it is still impossible to detect volume loss. Tachycardia is usual with exercise, and a slight postural drop in blood pressure may be evident.
30	1500	Neck veins are flat when supine. Postural hypotension and exercise tachycardia are generally present, but the resting, supine blood pressure and pulse still can be normal.
40	2000	Central venous pressure, cardiac output, and arterial blood pressure are below normal even when the patient is supine and at rest. The patient usually demonstrates air hunger; a rapid, thready pulse; and cold, clammy skin.
50	2500	Severe shock, death.

*TVB, total blood volume.
†For a normal 70-kg person with a 5000-ml total blood volume.
Source: Table 68-1 of *Williams Hematology*, 5/e, p. 704.

- Oxygen supply to tissues is maintained acutely by vasoconstriction in oxygen-insensitive areas and vasodilatation in essential areas.
- Plasma erythropoietin (EPO) levels increase within hours of the development of anemia after hemorrhage.
- 2,3-Bisphosphoglycerate concentration in the red cell increases, facilitating release of oxygen to the tissues.
- After acute hemorrhage the leukocyte count increases and may reach 10,000 to 30,000/μl within a few hours.
- The platelet count also increases and may reach levels approaching 1,000,000/μl.
- Metamyelocytes, myelocytes, and nucleated red cells may appear in the blood after severe hemorrhage.

ERYTHROPOIETIC RESPONSE

- EPO initiates proliferation and maturation of early erythroblasts. Erythroid hyperplasia begins promptly in the marrow and can be readily recognized in marrow specimens obtained at 5 days.
- EPO also causes premature release of reticulocytes to the circulation. An increase in the number of reticulocytes can be detected 6 to 12 h after a hemorrhage, and further increases occur over the next several days.
- Daily production of red cells can be estimated from the absolute reticulocyte count, corrected for the premature release of reticulocytes by dividing the absolute reticulocyte count by 2.
- A more vigorous marrow response is seen with a more severe hemorrhage.
- Any intrinsic marrow disease, such as tumor invasion or myelofibrosis, can severely limit the marrow response.
- An adequate supply of utilizable iron is also necessary.
- Normal marrow iron stores can be mobilized at a rate which will permit erythropoiesis to expand up to three times normal.
- If iron is also available from oral or parenteral supplements, or from some other source such as an absorbing hematoma, red cell production may increase up to four to five times normal.
- In hemolytic anemias, the red cell iron is reutilized at even greater rates, and red cell production rates of greater than five times normal can be achieved.
- Transfusion of packed red blood cells is given for immediate replacement in instances of severe anemia.
- EPO therapy has been used to speed recovery from postoperative anemia and to facilitate donations for autologous blood transfusions.

For a more detailed discussion, see Robert S. Hillman: Acute blood loss anemia, Chap. 68, p. 704, in *Williams Hematology*, 5/e, 1995.

38 HYPERSPLENISM AND HYPOSPLENISM

THE SPLEEN

- The white pulp (lymphoid tissue) functions in antigen processing and antibody production.
- The red pulp (monocyte-macrophage system) serves as a filter, retaining defective blood cells and foreign particles.

HYPERSPLENISM (increased splenic function)

- Hypersplenism is considered "appropriate" if it is an exaggeration of normal function, as in hereditary spherocytosis or idiopathic thrombocytopenic purpura, or "inappropriate" if the hyperfunction is due to vascular congestion or infiltrative disease.
- Usually associated with splenomegaly.
- Causes cytopenias with associated compensatory bone marrow hyperplasia.
- Most often corrected by splenectomy.
- Causes of hypersplenism are listed in Table 38-1, and causes of massive splenomegaly are listed in Table 38-2.

TABLE 38-1 Classification and the Most Common Causes of Splenomegaly and Hypersplenism

Splenomegaly with appropriate hypersplenism	Splenomegaly with inappropriate hypersplenism
Hereditary hemolytic anemias	Congestion (Banti syndrome)
Hereditary spherocytosis	Cirrhosis of the liver
Hereditary elliptocytosis	Portal vein thrombosis
Thalassemia	Splenic vein obstruction
Sickle cell anemia (infants)	Budd-Chiari syndrome
Autoimmune cytopenias	Congestive heart failure
Idiopathic thrombocytopenia	Infiltrative diseases
Essential neutropenia	Leukemias, chronic and acute
Acquired hemolytic anemia	Lymphomas
Infections and inflammations	Polycythemia vera
Infectious mononucleosis	Agnogenic myeloid metaplasia
Subacute bacterial endocarditis	Gaucher disease
Miliary tuberculosis	Niemann-Pick disease
Rheumatoid arthritis (Felty syndrome)	Glycogen storage disease
Lupus erythematosus	Amyloidosis
Sarcoidosis	Tumors and cysts
Brucellosis	Idiopathic
Leishmaniasis	
Schistosomiasis	
Malaria	

Source: Table 69-1 of *Williams Hematology,* 5/e, p. 709.

TABLE 38-2 Causes of Massive Splenomegaly*

Chronic myeloid leukemia
Idiopathic and secondary myelofibrosis
Malignant lymphoma
Hairy cell leukemia
Gaucher disease
Thalassemia major
Leishmaniasis (kala-azar)
Malaria

*The spleen extends into one or both lower quadrants of the abdomen.
Source: Table 69-2 of *Williams Hematology*, 5/e, p. 710, 1995.

Pathophysiology

- The normal spleen carries out appropriate filtration and elimination of aged and defective blood cells.
- This same process also removes red cells with hereditary abnormalities of RBC membrane and antibody-coated blood cells.
- The spleen may enlarge because of work hypertrophy, and the enlarged spleen may sequester and destroy normal blood cells, leading to symptomatic cytopenias.
- An expanded splenic (systemic) plasma pool may cause further anemia by dilution.
- Increased blood flow may cause portal hypertension, further splenomegaly, and associated varices.

Effect on Platelets

- Normally about one-third of platelets are sequestered in the spleen.
- Up to 90 percent of platelets may be sequestered temporarily by an enlarged spleen.
- Platelets survive almost normally in the spleen and are available, albeit slowly, when needed.

Effect on Neutrophils

- Large fraction of circulating neutrophil pool may be marginated in an enlarged spleen.
- Neutrophils survive almost normally in the spleen and like platelets slowly become available on demand.

Effect on Red Blood Cells

- Red blood cells are metabolically less sufficient than leukocytes or platelets and may be destroyed prematurely in red pulp.
- Spherocytes may be formed during prolonged metabolic conditioning in the red pulp.

Symptoms (Splenomegaly)

- Splenomegaly may be asymptomatic.
- Greatly enlarged spleens may cause abdominal discomfort, trouble sleeping on side, and early satiety.
- Splenic infarction may cause pleuritic-like left upper quadrant pain, with or without a friction rub.
- In patients with hereditary hemolytic anemias, the spleen may become acutely enlarged and painful, often following infection, with sudden aggravation of anemia (sequestration crisis).

Estimation of Splenic Size

- A normal size spleen may be palpable in young and thin patients with low diaphragms. Otherwise, a palpable spleen should be considered to be enlarged.
- Splenic size is best assessed with abdominal ultrasound examination.
- Cysts, tumors, or infarcts of the spleen may be identified by radionuclide scanning (colloid), abdominal computerized tomography, or magnetic resonance imaging.

Laboratory Features

- The number of one or all of erythrocytes, leukocytes, or platelets is reduced in the blood, with corresponding hyperplasia in the marrow.
- Cellular morphology is usually normal, but spherocytes may be present.

Splenectomy

- Splenectomy may lead to dramatic restoration of blood counts to normal in patients with hypersplenism.
- Splenectomy may alleviate portal hypertension.
- After splenectomy there may be a rapid, but temporary, rise in the platelet count, which can lead to thromboembolic complications especially in the elderly or bedridden patients.
- Chronic changes in the blood after splenectomy are listed below under "Hyposplenism, Laboratory Findings."
- Splenectomy removes a protective filter bed and renders the patient vulnerable to bacteremia.
- It also may diminish resistance to preexisting parasitic disease (malaria, bartonellosis, babesiosis) and transform dormant infestation into active disease.
- The number of disorders for which splenectomy may be recommended has decreased in recent years because of improved alternative therapies. Splenectomy is still recommended for some disorders, as discussed in specific chapters (e.g., Chap. 22, Hereditary Spherocytosis; Chap. 33, Warm Antibody Hemolytic Anemia; and Chap. 67, Throm-

TABLE 38-3 Hyposplenism

Normal infants	Gastrointestinal disorders
Congenital asplenia	Celiac disease
Old age	Regional enteritis
Repeated sequestration crises	Ulcerative colitis
Sickle hemoglobinopathies	Dermatitis herpetiformis
Essential thrombocytosis	Tumors and cysts
Malaria	Amyloidosis
Thrombosis of splenic artery or vein	Splenic irradiation
Autoimmune disorders	Postsplenectomy
Glomerulonephritis	
Systemic lupus erythematosus	
Rheumatoid arthritis	
Graft-vs.-host disease	
Sarcoidosis	

Source: Table 69-3 of *Williams Hematology*, 5/e, p. 712.

bocytopenia Due to Enhanced Platelet Destruction by Immunologic Mechanisms).

HYPOSPLENISM (decreased splenic function)

- Splenic function may be reduced by disease or surgical removal.
- Hyposplenism may or may not be associated with reduced splenic size.
- Impaired filtering causes mild thrombocytosis and increased risk of severe bloodstream infections.
- Causes of hyposplenism are listed in Table 38-3.

Infectious Complications

- Overwhelming sepsis is often fatal.
- Usually due to encapsulated bacteria, such as pneumococcus or *Hemophilus influenzae*.
- Risk greatest in very young.
- Splenectomy usually contraindicated before age 4.
- Healthy adults with splenectomy because of accidental rupture of normal spleen are still at some increased risk.

Laboratory Findings

- Slight to moderate increase in leukocyte and platelet counts.
- Target cells, deformed erythrocytes.
- Howell-Jolly bodies usually in 1 red cell in 100 to 1000.
- Pitted erythrocytes (wet preparation, using direct interference-contrast microscopy).
- Increased numbers of Heinz bodies.

- Increased numbers of nucleated red cells in patients splenectomized for various hemolytic disorders.
- 99^mTc sulfur colloid uptake is a reliable measure of the capacity of the spleen to clear particulates from the blood.

Treatment of the Hyposplenic Patient

- Immunize with polyvalent pneumococcal vaccine presplenectomy.
- Vaccinate children against *Hemophilus influenzae.*
- Prophylactic penicillin is routinely given to asplenic children.
- All febrile infections should be considered serious. Administer penicillin immediately upon onset of symptoms.
- Cover all dental work (especially extractions) with antibiotics.

For a more detailed discussion, see Leon Weiss: Structure of the spleen, Chap. 5, p. 38; and Allan J. Erslev: Hypersplenism and hyposplenism, Chap. 69, p. 709, in *Williams Hematology,* 5/e, 1995.

---

39 SECONDARY POLYCYTHEMIA (ERYTHROCYTOSIS)

APPARENT POLYCYTHEMIA (RELATIVE POLYCYTHEMIA)

- Characterized by an increased hematocrit, normal red cell mass, and low plasma volume.
- Also referred to as Gaisbock syndrome, or stress, spurious, pseudo-, and smokers' polycythemia.
- Associated with obesity, hypertension, use of diuretics and smoking.
- Differential diagnosis includes dehydration.
- Treatment should be directed toward any underlying condition, if present, such as obesity (weight reduction) or cigarette smoking (cessation of smoking).
- If phlebotomy is done, temporary hypovolemia should be avoided by infusion of albumin or other colloid.

SECONDARY POLYCYTHEMIA

- A group of disorders with increased red cell mass (absolute polycythemia) due to stimulation of erythrocyte production, through increased erythropoietin (EPO) production. The polycythemia is considered
  - appropriate if there is tissue hypoxia and the increased red cell mass minimizes the hypoxia.
  - inappropriate if tissue hypoxia is absent and the polycythemia serves no useful purpose.

High Altitude Acclimatization (Appropriate)

- Acute mountain sickness
  - Due to cerebral hypoxia and may be life-threatening. Polycythemia does not occur.
  - Subjects may have headaches, insomnia, palpitations, weakness, nausea, vomiting, and mental dullness and may develop pulmonary and cerebral edema.
  - Treatment is with acetazolamide, dexamethasone, calcium channel blockers, and/or rapid return to lower altitude.
- Chronic mountain sickness
  - Occurs after prolonged exposure to high altitudes.
  - Characterized by marked cyanosis, plethora, emotional deterioration, clubbing of the fingers, and signs of right heart failure.
  - Cure develops slowly with return to sea level. Venesection provides temporary relief.

Pulmonary Disease (Appropriate)

- Associated with cyanosis, clubbing, and arterial desaturation.
- In chronic obstructive pulmonary disease, chronic infection and inflammation may blunt erythropoietin and red cell production.

- Cautious venesection to maintain the hematocrit at less than 55 percent improves oxygen transport, exercise tolerance, and quality of life.

Alveolar Hypoventilation (Appropriate)

- Central: May be due to a cerebral vascular accident, parkinsonism, encephalitis, or barbiturate intoxication.
- Peripheral: May be due to myotonic dystrophy, poliomyelitis, spondylitis, extreme obesity.

Cardiovascular Disease (Appropriate)

- In patients with congenital right to left intracardiac shunts, hematocrit may reach 75 to 85 percent.
- Reduction of the hematocrit by phlebotomy may not be beneficial, and such therapy is controversial.
- Treatment with phlebotomy is indicated for cerebral symptoms.
- Dehydration must be avoided to prevent further increase in hematocrit.
- Other right-to-left shunts may be seen in hepatic cirrhosis (pulmonary arteriovenous or portopulmonary venous shunts), hereditary hemorrhagic telangiectasia, and idiopathic pulmonary arteriovenous aneurysms.

Hereditary High-Affinity Hemoglobins (Appropriate) (See Table 70-1, Williams Hematology, 5/e)

- Autosomal dominant inheritance.
- Fifty percent of the abnormal hemoglobins are demonstrable by starch gel electrophoresis.
- All show decreased P_{50}.

Acquired High-Affinity Hemoglobinopathy (Appropriate)

- May be due to carboxyhemoglobin (smoking) or to methemoglobin (congenital or drug-induced).

Tissue Hypoxia (Histotoxic Anoxia) (Appropriate)

- Cobalt chloride treatment inhibits oxidative metabolism and leads to an increased hematocrit.

Renal Vascular Impairment (Inappropriate)

- About 10 percent of patients develop erythrocytosis after renal transplantation.
- Erythrocytosis is mild, usually self-limited, and may be due to excessive diuretic therapy.
- Recipient's native kidneys may be the source of increased erythropoietin production which can be treated with surgical removal or

selective embolism. The offending kidneys usually autoinfarct with time.
- EPO production may be attenuated with captopril or theophylline treatment.
- Atherosclerotic obstruction of renal artery is an uncommon cause.

Renal Cysts and Hydronephrosis (Inappropriate)

- EPO can be demonstrated in cyst fluid.

Renal Tumors (Inappropriate)

- 1 to 3 percent of patients with hypernephroma have erythrocytosis, probably due to excess EPO formed by the tumor.
- Remission of polycythemia occurs after tumor removal.
- Reappearance of polycythemia heralds recurrence.
- Occasionally erythrocytosis is seen in Wilms tumor.

Other Tumors (Inappropriate)

- Uterine myoma, usually huge. Removal of the myoma routinely followed by hematologic cure.

Cerebellar Hemangiomas (Inappropriate)

- About 15 percent of patients have erythrocytosis, and EPO can be demonstrated in cyst fluid and stromal cells.
- Hepatoma causes erythrocytosis, probably due to erythropoietic production by the neoplastic cells.

Endocrine Disorders (Inappropriate)

- Pheochromocytoma, aldosterone-producing adenomas, Bartter syndrome, or dermoid cyst of ovary may be associated with increased EPO levels and erythrocytosis, which respond to removal of the tumor.
- Cushing syndrome: Hydrocortisone and other glucocorticoids may cause general marrow stimulation and mild polycythemia.
- Androgen usage:
  - Androgens of the 5α-H configuration stimulate EPO production and resultant erythrocytosis.
  - Androgens of the 5β-H configuration enhance differentiation of stem cells.

Neonatal Erythrocytosis (Inappropriate)

- Normal physiologic response to intrauterine hypoxia and high oxygen affinity fetal hemoglobin.
- May be excessive in infants of diabetic mothers.
- Late cord clamping may be contributory.
- Partial exchange transfusion sometimes performed if the hematocrit is above 65 percent at birth.

Pure (Essential) Erythrocytosis

- Usually patients are asymptomatic.
- Often there is a strong family history, suggesting either dominant or recessive inheritance.
- EPO levels may be zero, low, or elevated.
- Some patients have defects in the EPO receptor.
- Autonomous erythroid colony formation has been demonstrated in some patients.

Autotransfusion (Blood Doping)

- Autotransfusion of stored red cells prior to competition improves performance in cross-country skiers and long-distance runners but at the risk of life-threatening hyperviscosity when associated with fluid losses from strenuous activity.
- Should be suspected when an elevated hematocrit is associated with very low level of EPO in an athlete.
- Injection of commercial EPO preparations will achieve the same effect as autotransfusion.

For a more detailed discussion, see Allan J. Erslev: Secondary polycythemia (erythrocytosis), Chap. 70, p. 714, in *Williams Hematology,* 5/e, 1995.

---

40 THE PORPHYRIAS

The porphyrias are genetic deficiencies in the activity of enzymes in the heme biosynthetic pathway (Fig. 40-1). Metabolic intermediates are produced in excess, accumulate in tissues, and result in neurologic and/or photocutaneous symptoms.

CLASSIFICATION (see Table 40-1)

Hepatic (Principal Site of Enzyme Defect Is Liver)

Acute (Acute Neurovisceral Attacks)

- ADP (δ-aminolevulinic acid dehydratase porphyria)
- AIP (acute intermittent porphyria)
- HCP (hereditary coproporphyria)
- VP (variegate porphyria)

Chronic (No Acute Attacks)

- PCT (porphyria cutanea tarda)
- HEP (hepatoerythropoietic porphyria)

Erythropoietic (Principal Site of Defect Is Marrow)

- CEP (congenital erythropoietic porphyria)
- HEP (hepatoerythropoietic porphyria)
- EPP (erythropoietic protoporphyria)

SPECIFIC DISORDERS

- There are eight enzymes involved in heme synthesis, and with the exception of δ-aminolevulinic acid (ALA) synthase, the first step, each enzymatic defect is associated with a specific form(s) of porphyria.

ALA Dehydratase Porphyria (ADP)

- Autosomal recessive disorder due to an almost complete deficiency of ALA dehydratase.
- The rarest form of porphyria (4 cases reported).
- Patients have neurovisceral symptoms similar to those of AIP (see below).
- Clinical exacerbations follow stress, decreased caloric intake, ethanol consumption.
- Urine ALA excretion is increased; porphobilinogen (PBG) excretion is normal.
- Red cell ALA dehydratase activity is less than 2 percent of normal.
- Must distinguish from lead poisoning and hereditary tyrosinemia I.
- Treatment has been that given for AIP, but the response has been variable.

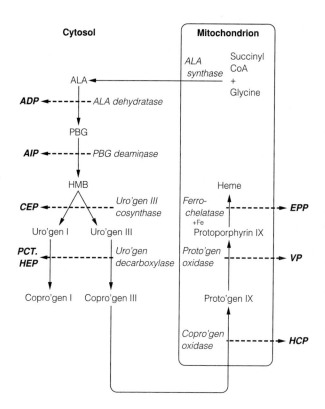

FIG. 40-1 Enzymatic defects in the porphyrias. The enzymatic defect in each porphyria is shown by a broken line. In patients, the substrate for the defective enzymatic step accumulates in the tissue, e.g., erythrocytes and plasma, and is excreted in large excess into urine and/or stool. In addition, the excretion of porphyrin precursors, i.e., δ-aminolevulinic acid (ALA) and porphobilinogen (PBG), may be increased in patients with acute hepatic porphyrias as a result of de-repression of ALA synthase activity in the liver. Abbreviations: HMB, hydroxymethylbilane; Uro'gen, uroporphyrinogen; Copro'gen, coproporphyrinogen; Proto'gen, protoporphyrinogen. Abbreviations for the names of the porphyrias are identified in the text. (From Chap. 71, Fig. 71-1 of *Williams Hematology*, 5/e.)

TABLE 40-1 Basic Outline of the Porphyrias

Names of disorders	Clinical symptoms	Prominent laboratory findings	Treatment(s)
ADP	N	↑ urine ALA	1
AIP	N	↑ urine ALA, PBG	1
CEP	PA	↑ urine URO I	2, 3
PCT	P	↑ fecal ISOCOPRO	2, 4, 5
HEP	PA	↑ fecal ISOCOPRO	2
HCP	N(P)	↑ urine/fecal COPRO	1, (2)
VP	N(P)	↑ fecal PROTO	1, 2
EPP	P(A)	↑ RBC, fecal PROTO	2, (3)

Key: N, neurologic symptoms; P, photosensitivity; A, anemia. ( ) Denotes mild symptoms.

1, Maintain good caloric intake, avoid estrogens/progestins, avoid phenobarbital and P_{450} inducers. Prompt treatment of infections, high carbohydrate intake, IV hematin.
2, Avoid sun exposure, β-carotene analogs used.
3, Hypertransfuse to shut down red cell production, splenectomy.
4, Reduce iron stores with repeated phlebotomy, chloroquine.
5, Avoid alcohol, estrogens, iron, polychlorinated hydrocarbons.

AIP, acute intermittent porphyria; ADP, ALA dehydratase deficiency; ALA, δ-aminolevulinic acid; CEP, congenital erythropoietic porphyria; COPRO, coproporphyrin; EPP, erythropoietic protoporphyria; HEP, hepatoerythropoietic porphyria; HCP, hereditary coproporphyria; ISOCOPRO, isocoproporphyrin; PBG, porphobilinogen; PCT, porphyria cutanea tarda; PROTO, protoporphyrin; URO, uroporphyrin; VP, variegate porphyria.
Source: Table 71-2 of *Williams Hematology*, 5/e, p. 728.

Acute Intermittent Porphyria (AIP)

- An autosomal dominant disorder due to partial deficiency of PBG deaminase.
- Abdominal pain occurs in almost all patients, often as the initial symptom.
  - May be severe and mimic an acute surgical abdomen.
  - Nausea, vomiting, constipation or diarrhea, abdominal distension, ileus, urinary retention are frequently present.
- Neuropathy may be motor or sensory and lead to bulbar paralysis; respiratory impairment; seizures; mental symptoms; muscle weakness; and limb, head, neck, or chest pain.
- Other clinical features may be hypertension, tachycardia, fever, and inappropriate ADH secretion.
- Attacks may last from a few days to several months.
- Up to 90 percent of individuals with documented PBG deaminase activity remain asymptomatic.
- Attacks may be precipitated by
  - drugs inducing cytochrome P_{450} (e.g., phenobarbital)

- estrogens, progesterone, puberty, menses
- reduced caloric intake, especially carbohydrates
- intercurrent illnesses, infection, alcohol, surgery
- Diagnosis:
  - Watson-Schwartz test for urinary PBG is widely used for screening.
  - Demonstration of increased ALA and PBG concentration in urine,
  - Demonstration of decreased PBG deaminase activity ($\sim$50 percent of normal). Activity is reduced in all tissues, including erythrocytes, in about 85 percent of patients. The remainder have normal red cell PBG deaminase activity but reduced activity in other cells, such as fibroblasts or lymphocytes.
- Treatment of AIP is also applied to ADP, HCP, and VP
  - Ensure adequate nutrition and caloric intake.
  - Avoid precipitating drugs (see above).
  - Initiate prompt treatment of fasting, intercurrent disease, or infection.
  - Unresponsive cases:
    - Admit to hospital.
    - Give at least 300 g/day of glucose intravenously.
    - Intravenous hematin, now considered the treatment of choice, is given intravenously, over 30 min or more, in doses up to 4 mg/kg/day. In severe cases, the dose may be repeated after 12 h. Hematin solutions are very unstable and administration frequently causes phlebitis.
  - LHRH inhibitors may be beneficial by inhibiting ovulation.

Congenital Erythropoietic Porphyria (CEP)

- Rare (200 cases reported) autosomal recessive disorder, due to an almost complete deficiency of uroporphyrinogen III cosynthase activity.
- Cutaneous photosensitivity appears early in life and is exacerbated by exposure to sunlight. Subepidermal bullous lesions develop and progress to crusted erosions which heal with scarring, pigmentary changes, hypertrichosis, and alopecia.
- Red teeth with red fluorescence under UV light are pathognomonic.
- Hemolytic anemia may be present, with splenomegaly and porphyrin-rich gallstones, and compensatory marrow expansion which results in pathologic fractures and short stature.
- Diagnosis:
  - In utero: dark brown porphyrin-rich amniotic fluid is characteristic.
  - The diagnosis may be made in the newborn from pink-dark brown staining of diapers.
  - Urinary porphyrin excretion (predominantly uroporphyrin) is increased 20- to 60-fold above normal. Fecal porphyrin is also increased.

- Treatment:
  - Avoid sunlight, skin trauma, use topical sunscreens, oral β-carotene.
  - Suppression of marrow with hypertransfusion may be beneficial.
  - Splenectomy often has been of only short-term benefit.
  - Treatment with oral charcoal may bind porphyrins.

Porphyria Cutanea Tarda (PCT)

- PCT is the most common of all porphyrias.
- Due to partial deficiency of uroporphyrinogen (URO) decarboxylase.
- Type I is sporadic, mostly presenting in adults, with normal URO decarboxylase in red cells but reduced levels in liver.
- Type II is an autosomal dominant disorder which may appear in children or in adults. Enzyme activity is reduced in both red cells and liver.
- Type III is a familial disorder with reduced URO decarboxylase activity in liver and normal levels in red cells. Type III may appear in children or adults.
- Patients have increased skin fragility; minor trauma leads to erosions.
- Sun exposure produces vesicles and bullae which heal slowly, with scarring. Hyperpigmentation, facial hypertrichosis, and alopecia may develop.
- Liver biopsy frequently shows hemosiderosis, and serum iron and ferritin concentrations are increased. Patients usually develop cirrhosis and may develop hepatoma.
- Sporadic PCT may be triggered by exposure to alcohol, estrogens, medicinal iron, polychlorinated hydrocarbons, or by pregnancy.
- Diagnosis:
  - Urinary porphyrin excretion is increased.
  - Isocoproporphyrin is often the dominant porphyrin in feces and is important in diagnosis.
- Treatment:
  - Identification and avoidance of precipitating factors, especially alcohol.
  - Phlebotomy program to reduce the patient's iron stores may be very beneficial.
  - Chloroquine therapy may be effective.

Hepatoerythropoietic Porphyria (HEP)

- A rare disorder due to homozygous deficiency in URO decarboxylase activity.
- HEP is clinically indistinguishable from CEP, with childhood onset with pink urine, severe photosensitivity, and skin fragility.

- Diagnosis:
  - Elevated urinary porphyrin excretion; isocoproporphyrin in feces; and zinc-protoporphyrin in erythrocytes.
  - Red cell URO decarboxylase activity is 2 to 10 percent of normal.
- Treatment
  - Avoid sun exposure and use topical sunscreen.
  - No response to repeated phlebotomies.

Hereditary Coproporphyria (HCP)

- An autosomal dominant disorder due to partial deficiency of coproporphyrinogen oxidase.
- 30 percent of patients show photosensitivity.
- Neurologic dysfunction indistinguishable from ADP, AIP, VP.
- Attacks precipitated by menses, pregnancy, contraceptive steroids, and drugs (phenobarbital).
- Laboratory:
  - Excessive urinary and fecal excretion of coproporphyrin III.
  - Excessive excretion of ALA, PBG, and uroporphyrin in the urine during attacks.
- Treatment:
  - Avoid precipitating factors.
  - Treat acute attacks as in AIP.

Variegate Porphyria (VP)

- VP is an autosomal dominant disorder due to partial deficiency of protoporphyrinogen oxidase.
- Neurovisceral symptoms as in ADP, AIP, HCP.
- Photosensitivity common with chronic skin changes.
- Precipitated by same factors as in ADP, AIP, HCP.
- Laboratory:
  - Increased fecal porphyrin excretion, especially protoporphyrin IX.
  - Urinary excretion of coproporphyrin, ALA, and PBG increased during attacks.
  - Plasma has porphyrin with fluorescence max at 626 nm, specific for VP.
- Treatment:
  - Neurovisceral attacks treated as for AIP.
  - Measures to reduce exposure to light, including protective clothing.

Erythropoietic Protoporphyria (EPP)

- EPP is an autosomal dominant disorder due to partial deficiency of ferrochelatase activity.

- Childhood onset of cutaneous photosensitivity, worse on face and hands and in the spring and summer but milder than in CEP, PCT, HEP, or VP.
- Gallstones are common and may present at an unusually early age.
- No neurovisceral symptoms.
- May have mild microcytic anemia.
- May develop severe cirrhosis, liver failure.
- No known precipitating factors other than light exposure.
- Laboratory:
  - Excess concentrations of protoporphyrin in red cells, plasma, bile, and feces.
- Treatment:
  - Avoidance of sun exposure, use of topical sunscreens, oral β-carotene, cholestyramine.
  - Hypertransfusion to suppress erythropoiesis may be helpful.

For a more detailed discussion, see Shigeru Sassa: The porphyrias, Chap. 71, p. 726, in *Williams Hematology,* 5/e, 1995.

---

41 HEREDITARY AND ACQUIRED SIDEROBLASTIC ANEMIAS

SIDEROBLASTIC ANEMIAS

- They may be acquired or hereditary and are characterized by:
  - ineffective erythropoiesis
  - many ringed sideroblasts and increased storage iron in the marrow
  - varying proportions of hypochromic erythrocytes in the blood
- A sideroblast is an erythroblast that contains one or more aggregates of nonheme iron appearing as Prussian blue–stainable granules
  - In normal subjects, 30 to 50 percent of late erythroblasts contain one or two such granules.
  - In sideroblastic anemias, the pathologic sideroblasts contain multiple granules distributed perinuclearly, in a ring.
  - The granules in ringed sideroblasts are in fact iron-laden mitochondria.
- Several types of intramitochondrial defects in heme synthesis occur in sideroblastic anemias.
  - These may result in either a decreased or increased level of free erythrocyte protoporphyrin (FEP).
  - Deficiency of ALA synthase of marrow erythroblasts has been documented in both the congenital disorder and the acquired disease.
  - Deficiencies in other enzymes in the heme synthetic pathway have been identified in other cases.
  - Drugs that reduce the formation of pyridoxal 5′-phosphate from pyridoxine cause decreased heme synthesis and sideroblastic anemia.
- The main factor responsible for the anemia is ineffective erythropoiesis, with increased plasma iron turnover, normal to decreased red cell survival, and increased excretion of fecal stercobilin.

Primary Acquired Sideroblastic Anemia

This is discussed in Chap. 6, Myelodysplatic Disorders.

Secondary Acquired Sideroblastic Anemia

- Most commonly associated with isonicotinic acid hydrazide (INH), pyrazinamide, and cycloserine.
- Ethanol ingestion is also a cause.
- May occur in patients with neoplastic or chronic inflammatory diseases.
- Anemia may be severe.
- Characterized by dimorphic red cells on the blood film, hypochromic and normochromic.

- If drugs are responsible, the anemia responds promptly to withdrawal of the offending agent.

Hereditary Sideroblastic Anemia

- A rare disease, usually inherited as an X-linked trait.
- Anemia appears in the first few weeks or months of life.
  - Characteristically microcytic and hypochromic
  - Prominent red cell dimorphism, with striking aniso- and poikilocytosis
  - Splenomegaly is usually present.
  - Hemochromatosis regularly develops in these patients.
  - Treatment
    - Patients with hereditary sideroblastic anemia may respond to pyridoxine in oral doses of 50 to 200 mg daily.
    - Folic acid administered concomitantly may increase the response.
    - Full normalization of the hemoglobin level is not achieved, and relapse occurs if pyridoxine therapy is stopped.
    - Efforts should be made to reduce iron overloading by phlebotomy, if possible, or by use of desferrioxamine.

For a more detailed discussion, see Ernest Beutler: Hereditary and acquired sideroblastic anemias, Chap. 72, p. 747, in *Williams Hematology,* 5/e, 1995.

---

42 NEUTROPENIA

INTRODUCTION

- *Leukopenia* refers to a reduced total leukocyte count.
- *Granulocytopenia* refers to a reduced granulocyte (neutrophils, eosinophils, and basophils) count.
- *Neutropenia* refers to a reduced neutrophil count.
- Neutropenia is a neutrophil count of less than $1500/\mu l$ from age 1 month to 10 years and less than $1800/\mu l$ over age 10 years.
- African Americans have lower mean neutrophil counts than Caucasians.
- The risk of infections is inversely related to the severity of the neutropenia: patients with counts of 1.0 to $1.8 \times 10^3/\mu l$ are at low risk, 0.5 to $1.0 \times 10^3/\mu l$ moderate risk, and less than $0.5 \times 10^3/\mu l$ high risk.
- Neutropenia due to disorders of early hematopoietic precursor cells (e.g., chemotherapy), generally results in a greater susceptibility to infections.
- The risk of infection is greater when the count is falling or when there is associated monocytopenia, lymphocytopenia, or hypogammaglobulinemia.
- Integrity of the skin and mucous membranes, blood supply to tissues, and nutritional status are also important.
- Neutropenia can be classified as: (1) disorders of production; (2) disorders of distribution and turnover; (3) drug-induced neutropenia; and (4) neutropenia with infectious diseases.

DISORDERS OF PRODUCTION

Acquired Disorders

- Cytotoxic drugs cause neutropenia by decreasing cell production, and are probably the most frequent cause in the United States.
- Neutropenia due to impaired production is a common feature of diseases affecting hemopoietic stem cells, such as leukemia, aplastic anemia, and myelodysplastic syndromes.

Congenital Neutropenia Syndromes

- *Kostmann syndrome* is an autosomal recessive disease; otitis, gingivitis, pneumonia, enteritis, peritonitis, and bacteremia usually occur in the first month of life.
  - Neutrophil count is often less than $200/\mu l$. Eosinophilia, monocytosis, and mild splenomegaly may be present.
  - Marrow usually shows some early neutrophil precursors but few myelocytes or mature neutrophils.
  - Immunoglobulin levels are usually normal or increased and chromosome analyses are normal.

- Treatment with granulocyte colony stimulating factor (G-CSF) is usually effective, and marrow transplantation may be curative.
- *Rectiular dysgenesis* consists of thymic aplasia and inability to produce neutrophils or thymus- or marrow-derived lymphocytes. Patients have extreme susceptibility to bacterial and viral infections and often die at an early age. Marrow transplantation should be considered.
- *Neutropenia associated with agammaglobulinemia* is a primary immunodeficiency disorder which is fatal unless marrow transplantation can be done.
- *Transcobalamin II deficiency* causes neutropenia because of vitamin B_{12} deficiency and megaloblastic hematopoiesis. It is corrected by vitamin B_{12} treatment.
- *Neutropenia with dysgranulopoiesis* is notable for ineffective granulopoiesis. Neutrophil precursors show abnormal granulation, vacuolization, autophagocytosis, and nuclear abnormalities.
- *Myelokathexis* is a rare disorder associated with neutrophil counts of less than 500/μl. The marrow contains abundant myeloid precursors and mature neutrophils. Marrow neutrophils show hypersegmentation, cytoplasmic vacuoles, and abnormal nuclei. Neutrophil count does not rise with infection, suggesting that the primary disorder is neutrophil release from the marrow.
- *Lazy leukocyte syndrome:* Ample marrow precursors are present, but few circulating cells. The neutrophils have a defect in intrinsic motility and do not migrate out of the marrow efficiently.
- *Glycogen storage disease Ib* is characterized by hypoglycemia, hepatosplenomegaly, seizures, and failure to thrive in infants. Neutropenia gradually develops despite normal-appearing marrow. The neutrophils have a reduced metabolic burst and chemotaxis.
- *Cartilage-hair hypoplasia syndrome* consists of short-limbed dwarfism with hyper-extensible digits, fine hair, neutropenia, lymphopenia, and frequent infections. The marrow shows granulocytic hypoplasia. There is also a defect in cellular immunity.
- The *Schwachman-Diamond syndrome* is characterized by short stature, pancreatic exocrine deficiency, and neutropenia (often less than 200/μl) beginning in the neonatal period.
- *Chediak-Higashi syndrome* is a rare autosomal recessive disorder with oculocutaneous albinism, neutropenia, recurrent infections, and giant granules in granulocytes, monocytes, and lymphocytes.

Cyclic Neutropenia

- Characterized by recurring episodes (every 21 days) of severe neutropenia lasting 3 to 6 days, with malaise, fever, mucous membrane ulcers, and lymphadenopathy.
- Onset is usually in childhood. One-third of patients have an autosomal dominant pattern of inheritance.

- Appears to be due to a defect in the regulation of hemopoietic stem cells.
- Diagnosis can be made only by serial differential counts, at least three times per week for a minimum of 6 weeks.
- Most patients survive to adulthood, and symptoms are often milder after puberty.
- Fatal clostridial bacteremia has been reported. Careful observation is warranted with each neutropenic period.
- Treatment with G-CSF is effective. It does not abolish cycling but shortens the neutropenic periods sufficiently to avoid symptoms and infections.

Chronic Idiopathic Neutropenia

- Includes familial severe or benign neutropenia, chronic benign neutropenia of childhood, and chronic idiopathic neutropenia in adults. Severe cases can resemble the Kostmann syndrome. Some patients with chronic neutropenia may have large granular lymphocyte leukemia (see Chap. 57).
- Patients have selective neutropenia and normal or near-normal red cell, reticulocyte, lymphocyte, monocyte, and platelet counts and immunoglobulin levels. The spleen is normal or minimally enlarged.
- Marrow examination shows normal cellularity or selective neutrophilic hypoplasia; the ratio of immature to mature cells is increased, suggesting ineffective granulocytopoiesis.
- Clinical course can usually be predicted based on the degree of neutropenia, marrow examination, and prior history of fever and infections. Treatment with G-CSF will increase neutrophils in most patients.

Neutropenia Due to Nutritional Deficiencies

- Neutropenia is a consistent feature of megaloblastic anemias due to vitamin B_{12} or folate deficiency.
- Copper deficiency can cause neutropenia in patients on total parenteral nutrition with inadequate supplies of trace metals.
- Mild neutropenia may occur in patients with anorexia nervosa.

DISORDERS OF NEUTROPHIL DISTRIBUTION AND TURNOVER

Alloimmune (Isoimmune) Neonatal Neutropenia

- Neutropenia due to the transplacental passage of maternal IgG antibodies to neutrophil-specific antigens inherited from the father. The disorder occurs in about 1 in 2000 neonates and usually lasts 2 to 4 months.

- Often not recognized until bacterial infections occur in an otherwise healthy infant and may be confused with neonatal sepsis.
- Hematologic picture usually consists of isolated severe neutropenia and marrow with normal cellularity but reduced numbers of mature neutrophils. Diagnosis is usually made with agglutination or immunofluorescence tests.
- Antibiotic treatment used only when necessary, and glucocorticoids should be avoided. Exchange transfusions to decrease antibody titers may be useful.

Autoimmune Neutropenia

- Neutrophil autoantibodies may accelerate neutrophil turnover and impair production.
- Patients usually have selective neutropenia and one or more positive tests for antineutrophil antibodies. It is often difficult to distinguish cases of autoimmune neutropenia from chronic idiopathic neutropenia.
- Spontaneous remissions sometimes occur; intravenous immunoglobulin is effective for some pediatric patients; response to glucocorticoids is unpredictable.
- *Systemic lupus erythematosus:* Neutropenia occurs in 50 percent of patients, anemia in 75 percent (Coombs positive in one-third), thrombocytopenia in 20 percent, and splenomegaly in 15 percent. There is increased IgG on the surface of neutrophils, and marrow cellularity and maturation are normal. The neutropenia usually does not increase susceptibility to infections, in the absence of treatment with glucocorticoids or cytotoxic drugs.
- *Rheumatoid arthritis:* Less than 3 percent of patients with classical rheumatoid arthritis have leukopenia.
- Sjögren syndrome: About 30 percent of patients have leukocyte counts of 2000 to 5000/μl, with a normal differential count. Severe neutropenia with recurrent infections is rare.
- *Felty syndrome* (rheumatoid arthritis, splenomegaly, leukopenia): Prominent neutropenia is a constant feature and troublesome infections are common in patients with absolute neutrophil counts below 200/μl.
- In Felty syndrome, no clear relationship exists between spleen size and neutrophil count. Three-quarters of patients respond to splenectomy with an increase in neutrophil count, but one-third of these relapse later. Splenectomy should be reserved for patients with severe, recurrent, or intractable infections. Improvement has been reported with gold, testosterone, methotrexate, and lithium. Treatment with colony stimulating factors is still investigational.
- Patients with Felty syndrome have lymphopenia and a very high rheumatoid factor titer. A subset of patients has large granular lymphocyte leukemia (see Chap. 57).

- Autoimmune neutropenia has been sporadically reported in *Hodgkin disease, chronic autoimmune hepatitis,* and *Crohn disease.*
- *Pure white cell aplasia* has been used to describe severe neutropenia, in association with thymoma and hypogammaglobulinemia, analogous to pure red cell aplasia.

Other Neutropenias Associated with Splenomegaly

- A variety of diseases may cause this type of neutropenia including sarcoidosis, lymphoma, tuberculosis, malaria, kala-azar, and Gaucher disease, usually in association with thrombocytopenia and anemia.
- Neutropenia associated with splenomegaly may be due to immune mechanisms or sluggish blood flow through the spleen with trapping of neutrophils. The neutropenia is usually not of clinical importance and splenectomy is rarely indicated.

DRUG-INDUCED NEUTROPENIA

- Drugs may cause neutropenia because of dose-related toxic effects or by immune mechanisms. Table 42-1 lists some of the frequently implicated drugs. A more complete list is in Table 81-1 of *Williams Hematology,* 5/e, p. 821. Information about new drugs can be obtained from the manufacturer, a drug information center, or a poison center.
- Dose-related toxicity refers to nonselective interference of the drug with protein synthesis or cell replication. Phenothiazines, antithyroid drugs, and chloramphenicol cause neutropenia by this mechanism. Dose-related toxicity is more likely to occur with multiple drugs, high plasma concentrations, slow metabolism, or renal impairment.
- The immunologic mechanism is poorly understood but appears to be similar to drug-induced hemolytic anemia. Neutropenia tends to occur relatively early in the course of treatment with drugs to which the patient has been previously exposed.
- Patients usually present with fever, myalgia, sore throat, and severe neutropenia. A high level of suspicion and careful clinical history are critical to identifying the offending drug. Differential diagnosis includes acute viral infections and acute bacterial sepsis. If other hematologic abnormalities are also present, leukemia and aplastic anemia should be considered.
- Once the offending drug is stopped, patients with sparse marrow neutrophils but normal-appearing precursor cells will have neutrophil recovery in 4 to 7 days. When early precursor cells are severely depleted, recovery may take considerably longer.

NEUTROPENIA WITH INFECTIOUS DISEASES

- Occurs with acute or chronic bacterial, viral, parasitic, or rickettsial diseases.

TABLE 42-1 Drugs Frequently Associated with Idiosyncratic Neutropenia

Analgesics and antiinflammatory agents
  Indomethacin
  Para-aminophenol derivatives
    Acetaminophen
    Phenacetin
  Pyrazolon derivatives
    Aminopyrine
    Dipyrone
    Oxyphenbutazone
    Phenylbutazone
Antimicrobials
  Chloramphenicol
  Penicillins/semisynthetic penicillins
  Sulfonamides
Antithyroid drugs
  Carbimazole
  Methimazole
  Propylthiouracil
Phenothiazines
  Chlorpromazine
  Others

Source: Adapted from Table 81-1 of *Williams Hematology,* 5/e, p. 821.

- Some agents such as those causing infectious mononucleosis, infectious hepatitis, Kawasaki disease, and HIV infection may cause neutropenia and pancytopenia by infecting hemopoietic progenitor cells.
- In severe gram-negative bacterial infections, neutropenia is probably due to increased adherence to the endothelium as well as increased utilization at the site of infection.
- Chronic infections causing splenomegaly, such as tuberculosis, brucellosis, typhoid fever, and malaria, probably cause neutropenia by splenic sequestration and marrow suppression.

CLINICAL APPROACH TO THE PATIENT PRESENTING WITH NEUTROPENIA

- Patients with the acute onset of severe neutropenia present with fever, sore throat, and inflammation in the skin or mucous membranes. This is an urgent clinical situation requiring prompt cultures, intravenous fluids, and antibiotics.
- In the absence of recent hospitalization and antibiotic exposure, infections are usually caused by organisms found on the skin, nasopharynx, and intestinal flora and are sensitive to numerous agents. Immediate evaluation should include a careful history with particular attention to drug use and physical examination with attention to skin, mucous membranes, lymph nodes, and spleen.

- Chronic neutropenia is usually found by chance or during evaluation of recurrent fevers or infections. It is useful to determine whether the neutropenia is chronic or cyclic, and the average neutrophil count when the patient is well.
- The absolute monocyte, lymphocyte, eosinophil, and platelet counts, as well as hemoglobin and immunoglobulin levels, should be determined, and the blood film should be studied carefully for atypical lymphocytes and abnormal cells.
- Marrow examination is useful to rule out leukemia and myelodysplastic disorders and may show fibrosis, hypoplasia, or atypical cells.
- It may be useful to measure antinuclear antibodies (ANA), rheumatoid factor, or obtain other serologic tests for collagen vascular diseases.
- Examination of the blood and marrow may identify the abnormal cells of myelokathexis or the Chediak-Hagashi syndrome, or identify increased numbers of large granular lymphocytes.
- Infectious and nutritional causes for chronic neutropenia are rare and seldom difficult to recognize.
- Measurements of antineutrophil antibodies, in vitro marrow colony forming activity, and studies of drug-induced neutropenia require laboratory techniques available only in research centers.
- In adults, the most difficult differentiation may be between chronic idiopathic neutropenia and the myelodysplastic syndromes.

For a more detailed discussion, see Bernard M. Babior, David M. Golde: Production, distribution, and fate of neutrophils, Chap. 76, p. 773; and David C. Dale: Neutropenia, Chap. 81, p. 815, in *Williams Hematology,* 5/e, 1995.

---

43 NEUTROPHILIA

- Neutrophilia is an increase in the absolute neutrophil count (bands and mature neutrophils) to greater than $7.5 \times 10^3/\mu l$.
- For infants less than 1 month of age, the normal range is as high as $26 \times 10^3/\mu l$.
- Extreme neutrophilia is often referred to as a *leukemoid reaction* because the height of the leukocyte count may suggest leukemia.
- Neutrophilia may occur because of
  - an increase in cell production
  - accelerated release of cells from the marrow into the blood
  - shift from the marginal to circulating pool (demargination)
  - reduced egress of neutrophils from the blood to tissues
  - a combination of these mechanisms
- The time required to develop neutrophilia may be
  - minutes (demargination)
  - hours (accelerated release of cells from marrow)
  - days (increase in cell production)

ACUTE NEUTROPHILIA

- The causes are listed in Table 43-1.
- *Pseudoneutrophilia* is caused by a shift from the marginal to circulating pool (demargination) induced by vigorous exercise, acute physical and emotional stress, or by the infusion of epinephrine.
- Marrow storage pool shifts involve the release of segmented neutrophils and bands from the marrow reserve in response to inflammation, infections, or colony stimulating factors (CSFs).

CHRONIC NEUTROPHILIA

- The causes are listed in Table 43-1.
- The neutrophil production rate increases up to threefold with chronic infections and even more in myeloproliferative disorders and in response to CSFs. The maximum response requires at least a week to develop.
- Neutrophilia due to decreased egress from the vascular compartment occurs with glucocorticoids, leukocyte adhesion deficiency (CD11/CD18 deficiency) (see Chap. 44), and recovery from infection.

DISORDERS ASSOCIATED WITH NEUTROPHILIA (Table 43-1)

- Perhaps the most frequent are conditions with elevations of endogenous epinephrine and cortisol, such as exercise or emotional stress.
- The average neutrophil count of people who smoke two packs of cigarettes daily is twice normal.
- Gram-negative infections, particularly those resulting in bacteremia or septic shock, may cause extreme neutrophilia or neutropenia.

TABLE 43-1 Major Causes of Neutrophilia

Acute neutrophilia	Chronic neutrophilia
Physical stimuli Anesthesia, cold, convulsions, exercise, heat, labor, pain, surgery	Infections Persistence of many infections that cause acute neutrophilia
Emotional stimuli Panic, rage, severe stress	Inflammation Continuation of most acute inflammatory reactions, such as chronic vasculitis, colitis, dermatitis, drug reactions, gout, myositis, nephritis, pancreatitis, periodontitis, rheumatic fever, rheumatoid arthritis, Sweet syndrome, thyroiditis
Infections Many localized and systemic acute bacterial, mycotic, rickettsial, spirochetal, and certain viral infections	Tumors Carcinomas of the breast, kidney, liver, lung, pancreas, stomach, uterus. Rarely, brain tumors, Hodgkin disease, lymphoma, melanoma, multiple myeloma
Inflammation or tissue necrosis Antigen-antibody complexes, burns, complement activation, electric shock, gout, infarction, trauma, vasculitis	Drugs, hormones, and toxins Cigarette smoking, continued exposure to many substances that produce acute neutrophilia; lithium; rarely as a reaction to other drugs
Drugs, hormones, and toxins Colony stimulating factors, endoxin, epinephrine, etiocholanolone, glucocorticoids, vaccines, venoms	Metabolic and endocrinologic disorders Eclampsia, overproduction of ACTH or glucocorticoids, thyroid storm
	Hematologic disorders Asplenia, benign idiopathic leukocytosis, chronic hemolysis, chronic hemorrhage, hereditary thrombocytopenia, myeloproliferative disorders, rebound from agranulocytosis or therapy of megaloblastic anemia
	Hereditary and congenital disorders Down syndrome

Source: Adapted from Table 82-1 of Williams Hematology, 5/e, p. 826.

- Some infections characteristically do not cause neutrophilia (e.g., typhoid fever, brucellosis, many viral infections).
- Neutrophilia in association with cancer may be due to tumor cell secretion of colony stimulating factors (paraneoplastic) or due to tumor necrosis and infection.
- In patients with cancer, subarachnoid hemorrhage, or coronary artery disease, neutrophilia portends a less favorable prognosis.
- In addition to the myeloproliferative syndromes, several unusual hematologic conditions may be associated with neutrophilia:
  - Hereditary disorders associated with thrombocytopenia may also be accompanied by leukemoid reactions (e.g., thrombocytopenia with absent radii, see Chap. 65).
  - Benign idiopathic neutrophilic leukocytosis may be acquired or may occur as an autosomal dominant trait.
- In Down syndrome, neonatal leukemoid reactions may resemble chronic myelogenous leukemia.
- Neutrophilia and drugs:
  - As noted above, catecholamines and glucocorticoids are common causes of neutrophilia.
  - Lithium causes neutrophilia, presumably due to CSF release.
  - Rarely other drugs will cause neutrophilia (e.g., ranitidine or quinidine).

EVALUATION

- In most instances, the finding of neutrophilia, with an increase in bands and with toxic granules in the mature cells can be related to an ongoing infection or inflammatory condition.
- The history should make note of smoking, drug usage, chronic anxiety, or symptoms of occult malignancy.
- If the neutrophilia is accompanied by myelocytes, promyelocytes, increased basophils, and splenomegaly, a myeloproliferative disorder should be considered.
- Measurement of the leukocyte alkaline phosphatase (LAP) can be useful in certain cases. LAP score is generally elevated in inflammatory conditions and low in chronic myelogenous leukemia and paroxysmal nocturnal hemoglobinuria.

THERAPY

- Except in extreme instances in the myeloproliferative syndromes (see Chaps. 7 and 8, under "Hyperleukocytosis"), there is no known direct adverse effect of an elevated neutrophil count.
- In some inflammatory diseases, glucocorticoids and immunosuppressive therapies are used to reduce inflammation in part by reducing distribution and production of neutrophils.

- Specific therapy, if indicated, is generally directed at the underlying cause of neutrophilia.

For a more detailed discussion, see Bernard M. Babior, David W. Golde: Production, distribution, and fate of neutrophils, Chap. 76, p. 773; David C. Dale: Neutrophilia, Chap. 82, p. 824; and Ernest Beutler: Leukocyte alkaline phosphatase, Chap. L24, p. L66, in *Williams Hematology*, 5/e, 1995.

---

44 NEUTROPHIL DISORDERS: QUALITATIVE ABNORMALITIES OF THE NEUTROPHIL

- Neutrophil dysfunction may be due to
  - antibody/complement defects
  - abnormalities of cytoplasmic movement
  - abnormal microbicidal activity

ANTIBODY/COMPLEMENT DEFECTS

- Interaction between antibodies and complement generates opsonins and stimulates chemotactic factor development.
- C3 deficiency (autosomal recessive inheritance) results in the most severe disorder.
  - Homozygotes have no detectable C3 and suffer severe bacterial infections.
  - Deficiency of other less centrally active complement proteins results in a milder condition.
- Functional deficiency of C3 also occurs due to deficiency of C3b inactivator or properdin.
- Affected individuals usually suffer from infections due to encapsulated organisms.

ABNORMALITIES OF CYTOPLASMIC MOVEMENT

Degranulation Abnormalities

Chédiak-Higashi Syndrome

- A rare autosomal recessive disorder with generalized cell dysfunction, resulting in defects in chemotaxis, degranulation, and microbicidal activity.
- Increased membrane fluidity in Chédiak-Higashi neutrophils.
- Spontaneous fusion of granules results in huge lysosomes with diluted hydrolytic enzymes.
- Phagocytosis and the respiratory burst are normal, but killing of organisms is slow.
- Neutropenia occurs due to early destruction in the marrow.

Clinical manifestations

- Because of abnormal association of melanosomes, decreased pigment is noted in skin, hair, and ocular fundi.
- Infections are common, primarily involving mucous membranes, skin, and the respiratory tract; a variety of bacteria and fungi are involved, but *Staphylococcus aureus* is the most common.

- Peripheral neuropathies (sensory and motor) occur, as well as ataxia.
- Platelet and natural killer cell dysfunction are observed.
- An accelerated phase of unclear etiology may occur at any age, characterized by rapid lymphocytic proliferation (not neoplastic) involving liver, spleen, bone marrow, and lymph nodes. Fevers (often without infection), pancytopenia, and an even higher susceptibility to infection usually lead to death.

Treatment

- High-dose ascorbic acid (200 mg/day in infants, 2 g/day in adults) is usually prescribed but is not clearly beneficial.
- Infections are treated as they arise.
- The only curative treatment is allogeneic marrow transplantation.
- In the accelerated phase, vincristine and glucocorticoids have been used but are not clearly efficacious.

Specific granule deficiency

- Exceedingly rare, autosomal recessive disorder, characterized by recurrent skin and pulmonary infections.
- "Empty" specific granules are seen on electron microscopy.
- Chemotaxis is abnormal (due to lack of adhesion molecules) and microbicidal activity is mildly impaired (due to a lack of defensins and lactoferrin).
- Treatment is supportive.

Adhesion Abnormalities

Leukocyte Adhesion Deficiency

- A rare, autosomal recessive disease, with delayed wound healing, frequent severe periodontal or soft-tissue infection, and markedly decreased pus formation despite blood neutrophilia that may exceed 100,000/μl.
- Underlying defect is decreased or absent expression of the β-2 integrin family of leukocyte adhesion proteins (CD11/CD18 complex). These integral membrane glycoproteins (including LFA-1, Mac-1, and p150,95) have noncovalently bonded α and β subunits. Several mutations in the gene encoding the β subunit have been found, resulting in profoundly impaired chemotaxis or phagocytosis; degranulation and the respiratory burst are diminished.
- Prophylactic trimethoprim-sulfamethoxazole lowers the risk of infection.
- Treatment of choice for the severely affected is marrow transplant.

Neutrophil Actin Dysfunction

- Abnormal chemotaxis and phagocytosis are expressed as recurrent severe bacterial infections.

- Defective actin polymerization occurs; an intracellular inhibitor of polymerization has been isolated.

Other Disorders of Neutrophil Motility

- Neonatal neutrophils have impaired integrin function with abnormal transendothelial movement.
- Direct inhibitors of mobility include ethanol and glucocorticoids.
- Circulating immune complexes also inhibit by binding to neutrophil Fc receptors.

Hyperimmunoglobulin E Syndrome

- Patients have markedly elevated serum IgE levels, chronic dermatitis, and recurrent bacterial infections. They may also have coarse facial features, growth retardation, and osteoporosis.
- Chemotaxis is impaired but the molecular mechanism is unknown.
- Serum IgE levels exceed 2500 IU/ml, but, as opposed to atopic patients, most of this antibody is directed against *S. aureus*.
- Marked eosinophilia and poor antibody responses to neoantigens are also seen.
- Prophylactic trimethoprim-sulfamethoxazole is used.
- Topical steroids may reduce symptoms from the dermatitis.
- Interferon-γ decreases IgE production and holds promise.

DEFECTS IN MICROBICIDAL ACTIVITY

Chronic Granulomatous Disease (CGD)

- Neutrophils have impaired production of superoxide, with markedly reduced microbicidal activity. NADPH oxidase is an electron transport chain that catalyzes the formation of superoxide. Mutations in any of the involved genes will cause CGD.
- In the resting state, the oxidase components are in two locations. The membrane bound portion, cytochrome b_{558}, is composed of two subunits—gp91-*phox* and p22-*phox*. The heavy chain has binding sites for heme, FAD, and NADPH. Three other proteins reside in the cytosol, but upon stimulation, move to the membrane and interact with gp91-*phox*. These are p47-*phox*, p67-*phox*, and a GTP-binding protein. Severity of CGD depends upon which of these components is affected. The most frequent form is due to mutation of gp91-*phox* gene on chromosome Xp21.1. Other mutations also cause CGD, but occur less frequently.

Pathogenesis

- Normally neutrophils form hydrogen peroxide, which acts as substrate for myeloperoxidase in oxidizing halide to hypochlorous acid and chloramines. These accumulate in the phagosome and kill the microbe.

- Oxidase activation acutely affects an alkaline phase in the phagosome which is important for function of neutral hydrolases. In CGD cells this alkaline phase does not occur, impairing the enzymes which digest bacteria.

Clinical Features

- The X-linked form can be evident in the first months of life, whereas autosomal forms may not be diagnosed until adulthood.
- Skin abscesses, lymphadenitis, dermatitis, pneumonias, osteomyelitis, and hepatic abscesses are all common.
- Organisms commonly involved are *S. aureus, Aspergillus* spp., and *Candida albicans.*
- Granulomata are common and cause chronic lymphadenopathy.

Laboratory Features

- For diagnosis, superoxide or hydrogen peroxide generation is measured in response to certain stimuli.
- In addition, the nitroblue tetrazolium (NBT) test can be used. In normal neutrophils, NBT is reduced to purple formazan, but with most forms of CGD no reduction occurs.
- The NBT test can also detect the X-linked carrier state, as a varied percentage of cells will be NBT negative.
- More sophisticated procdures can define the molecular defect.
- Rare severe forms of glucose-6-phosphate dehydrogenase deficiency can mimic CGD; NADPH is inadequate for normal superoxide generation.

Therapy and Prognosis

- Treatment consists of long term trimethoprim-sulfamethoxazole prophylaxis, appropriate antibiotics for particular infections, and surgical management of abscesses.
- Interferon-γ (50 μg/m^2 3 times/week) has been found to decrease the number of serious infections.
- The only known cure is marrow transplantation.

Myeloperoxidase Deficiency (MPO)

- A common autosomal recessive disorder, with a prevalence 1:2000.
- MPO catalyzes formation of hypochlorous acid; the MPO-deficient neutrophil is slower to kill ingested organisms, but after 1 h, microbicidal activity is similar to normal.
- The disorder usually does not lead to increased susceptibility to infection.
- In a few patients with diabetes mellitus and MPO deficiency severe infection with *Candida* has occurred.
- Acquired MPO deficiency can be seen in lead intoxication, myelodysplastic syndrome, myeloid leukemias, and ceroid lipofuscinosis.

EVALUATION OF SUSPECTED NEUTROPHIL DYSFUNCTION

- Frequent bacterial infections should alert the clinician to the possibility of a neutrophil defect. Many of the tests used to evaluate neutrophils are bioassays, so are subject to great variability—they must be interpreted with caution, always in light of the patient's clinical condition. These tests are reviewed in Table 83-5 in *Williams Hematology, 5/e,* p. 840.

For a more detailed discussion, see Lawrence A. Boxer: Neutrophil disorders: qualitative abnormalities of the neutrophil, Chap. 83, p. 828, in *Williams Hematology,* 5/e, 1995.

---

45 EOSINOPHILIA
AND EOSINOPENIA

- The normal absolute eosinophil count in adults is less than 400 cells/μl.
- The eosinophil count is higher in neonates.
- Eosinophils are primarily tissue dwelling, with 100 to 500 cells in the tissues for every blood eosinophil.

CAUSES OF EOSINOPHILIA (Table 45-1)

- The degree of eosinophilia can be described as
  - mild (400 to 1500 cells/μl)
  - moderate (1500 to 5000)
  - marked (>5000)
- The most common causes of eosinophilia
  - worldwide are infections with helminthic parasites
  - in industrialized countries are asthma and other allergic diseases (drugs, rhinitis, atopic dermatitis)
- Allergic diseases generally result in only mild eosinophilia.

EOSINOPHILS AND DISEASE

- Eosinophils appear to have a role in both ameliorating inflammatory responses and producing tissue damage.
- They may be important in wound healing and may act as accessory cells in T-cell–mediated reactions.
- Because eosinophils can kill parasites, it has been hypothesized that their principal role is to counter parasitic infection.
- Eosinophils can also cause severe tissue damage under certain circumstances.

ASTHMA

- Inhaled antigen produces:
  - An *early response,* with fall in forced expiratory volume due to release of mediators from mast cells.
  - A *late response* with influx of large numbers of eosinophils, activated T cells, and monocytes to the airways.
- There is a general correlation between the numbers of airway eosinophils and the severity of asthma.
- Basic proteins secreted by eosinophils are toxic for airway epithelium and may be a better guide to the degree of inflammation than eosinophil numbers.

PARASITIC DISEASE

- The mechanism of eosinophilia in parasitic disease is similar to allergic disease.

TABLE 45-1 Causes of Eosinophilia

Disease	Frequency	Degree
Infections		
Parasitic disease	Common worldwide	Moderate to high
Others	Rare	Moderate to high
Allergic diseases		
Allergic rhinitis	Common worldwide	Mild
Atopic dermatitis	Common esp. children	Mild
Urticaria/angioedema	Common	Variable
Asthma	Common	Mild
Drug reactions		
Many drugs	Uncommon	Mild to high
Neoplasms		
Eosinophilic leukemia	Rare	High
Chronic myelogenous leukemia	Uncommon	Moderate to high
Lymphoma (esp. Hodgkin)	Uncommon	Moderate
Langerhans cell histiocytosis	Rare	Mild
Solid tumors	Uncommon	Mild to high
Musculoskeletal		
Rheumatoid arthritis	Rare	Mild to high
Fasciitis	Rare	High
Gastrointestinal		
Eosinophilic gastroenteritis	Rare	Mild to moderate
Celiac disease	Uncommon	Normal
Inflammatory bowel disease	Rare	Mild to high
Allergic gastroenteritis	Rare	Mild to high
Respiratory tract		
Asthma (see Allergic diseases)		
Churg-Strauss syndrome	Rare	Moderate to high
Pulmonary eosinophilia	Uncommon	Mild to high
Bronchiectasis/cystic fibrosis	Uncommon	Mild
Skin disease		
Atopic dermatitis (see Allergic diseases)		
Bullous pemphigoid	Uncommon	Moderate
Miscellaneous causes		
IL-2 Therapy	Rare	Moderate to high
Hypereosinophilic syndrome	Rare	High
Endomyocardial fibrosis	Rare	High
Hyper-IgE syndrome	Rare	High
Eosinophilia/myalgia	Rare	Moderate to high
Toxic oil syndrome	Rare	High
Adrenocortical deficiency	Rare	Moderate

Source: Adapted from Table 84-1 of Williams Hematology, 5/e, p. 845.

- The more pronounced eosinophilia in parasitic disease is presumably due to the systemic nature of the disease compared to the more localized nature of allergic disease.
- Eosinophils can kill a number of opsonized parasite larvae but not adult worms.

IDIOPATHIC HYPEREOSINOPHILIC SYNDROME

- The sporadic occurrence of striking eosinophilia and cardiac and neurologic injury due to the noxious effects of eosinophil granule contents. Considered an inflammatory rather than a neoplastic process.

Clinical Features

- Onset with anorexia, weight loss, fatigue, nausea, abdominal pain, diarrhea, nonproductive cough, pruritic rash, fever, night sweats, and venous thrombosis.
- Most patients have cardiac involvement with congestive heart failure, new murmurs, conduction defects, and arrhythmias.
- Hepatosplenomegaly, interstitial pulmonary infiltrates, and pleural effusions may occur.
- Nervous system dysfunction may be profound, including confusion, delirium, dementia, and coma.

Laboratory Features

- Anemia occurs in most patients.
- Thrombocytopenia is seen occasionally.
- All patients have leukocytosis with a striking eosinophilia, usually greater than 1500 eosinophils/μl, and counts of 50,000/μl or more are found in over half the patients.
- The eosinophilia may be progressive.
- The marrow shows only eosinophilia.

Therapy, Course, and Prognosis

- The disease is sometimes indolent, but more often progressive and rapidly fatal.
- Symptoms may remit and relapse, but organ damage is usually progressive.
  - Cardiac failure results from endomyocardial fibrosis.
  - Central nervous system dysfunction leads to encephalopathy, polyneuropathy, or stroke.
- Episodes of venous thrombosis may complicate the course.
- In one series, over 75 percent of patients died after 3 years despite therapy with glucocorticoids or cytotoxic agents.
- Glucocorticoids and hydroxyurea have been the mainstays of treatment.
- Other therapies include etoposide, interferon and surgical replacement of severely damaged heart valves.

- Occasionally patients may evolve to overt malignancy, either hemo-poietic or lymphocytic.

EOSINOPHILIA-MYALGIA SYNDROME

- First described in 1989 with over 1500 cases reported and 30 deaths in the next 2 years.
- Caused by the ingestion of L-tryptophan containing a contaminant.
- Pathological features mimic eosinophilic fasciitis.
- Constant features are severe myalgia and eosinophil count greater than 1000/μl.
- Common findings are arthralgias, cough, dyspnea, edema, hair loss, peripheral neuropathy, and scleroderma-like skin changes.
- Glucocorticoids or NSAIDs may improve symptoms.

TOXIC OIL SYNDROME

- In 1981 in Spain, more than 20,000 people developed a syndrome of fever, cough, dyspnea, neutrophilia, and eosinophilia with over 300 deaths.
- Thought to be due to ingestion of aniline-denatured rapeseed oil.
- Pulmonary infiltrates, pleural effusion, and hypoxemia were common findings.
- One-half the patients developed a chronic illness that mimicked the eosinophilia-myalgia syndrome, with myalgias, eosinophilia, periph-eral neuritis, scleroderma-like skin lesions, hair loss, and sicca syn-drome.
- Glucocorticoids may have improved the pulmonary symptoms.

REACTIVE HYPEROSINOPHILIA AND NEOPLASMS

- Marked eosinophilia has been reported in association with a variety of lymphoid and solid tumors, believed to be due to IL-5 and other cytokines elaborated by tumor cells.
- Eosinophilia may precede the diagnosis but usually occurs concomi-tantly.
- Successful treatment of the malignancy may be associated with ame-lioration of eosinophilia.
- Eosinophilic leukemia is a subtype of acute myelogenous leukemia (see Chap. 7).

EOSINOPHILIA, ANGIITIS, AND ASTHMA

- Polyarteritis nodosa and allergic granulomatosis (Churg-Strauss angi-itis) are associated with prominent eosinophilia.
- In patients with asthma and eosinophilia, the development of multi-organ signs (skin, nervous system, kidney, joints, lung, heart, gastro-intestinal tract) should lead to consideration of these disorders.

EOSINOPHILIC FASCIITIS

- Characterized by stiffness, pain, and swelling of the arms, forearms, thighs, legs, hands, and feet in descending order of frequency.
  - Malaise, fever, weakness, and weight loss also occur.
  - Absolute eosinophil counts of greater than $1000/\mu l$ are found in most patients.
  - Biopsy is usually required for diagnosis and shows inflammation, edema, thickening, and fibrosis of the fascia and synovium.
  - Aplastic anemia, cytopenias, pernicious anemia, and leukemia have been associated.

EOSINOPHILS IN URINE AND CEREBROSPINAL FLUID

- Excretion of eosinophils in the urine is seen most often in urinary tract infection or acute interstitial nephritis.
- Cerebrospinal fluid eosinophilia may occur with infection, shunts, allergic reactions involving the meninges, and Hodgkin disease.

EOSINOPENIA

- The eosinophil count in hospitalized patients is less than $10/\mu l$ in only 0.1 percent of patients.
- Acute infections, glucocorticoids, and epinephrine all decrease the eosinophil count.

For a more detailed discussion, see A. J. Wardlaw, A. B. Kay: Eosinophils: production, biochemistry, and function, Chap. 78, p. 798; and Eosinopenia and eosinophilia, Chap. 84, p. 844, in *Williams Hematology,* 5/e, 1995.

---

46 BASOPHILIA, BASOPHILOPENIA, AND MASTOCYTOSIS

BASOPHILIA

- Normal basophil count is 20 to 80/μl.
- The causes of basophilia are listed in Table 46-1.
- An increase in the absolute basophil count may be a useful early sign of a myeloproliferative disease.
- In chronic myelogenous leukemia (CML), an increased basophil count occurs in virtually all patients.
- Acute basophilic leukemia can occur *de novo;* and basophilia may be associated with acute myelogenous or acute promyelocytic leukemia.
- Basophils in myeloproliferative diseases are derived from the malig-

TABLE 46-1 Causes of Basophilia and Basophilopenia

Basophilia
  Allergy or inflammation
    Drug, food, inhalant hypersensitivity
    Erythroderma, urticaria
    Rheumatoid arthritis
    Radiation
    Ulcerative colitis
  Endocrinopathy
    Diabetes mellitus
    Estrogen administration
    Hypothyroidism (myxedema)
  Infection
    Chickenpox
    Influenza
    Small pox
    Tuberculosis
  Iron deficiency
  Neoplasia
    Myeloproliferative diseases (CML, polycythemia vera, myelofibrosis, primary thrombocytosis)
    Carcinoma
    Basophilic leukemia

Basophilopenia
  Hereditary absence of basophils
  Glucocorticoid therapy
  Hypersensitivity reaction
    Urticaria
    Anaphylaxis
    Drug-induced reactions
  Hyperthyroidism

Source: Adapted from Table 85-1 of *Williams Hematology,* 5/e, p. 854.

nant clone and may cause symptoms of histamine release (flushing, pruritus, hypotension).

BASOPHILOPENIA

- The causes of basophilopenia are listed in Table 46-1.

MAST CELLS

- Mast cells are produced in the marrow and cannot be identified in the blood of healthy individuals by standard techniques.
- Mast cells produce mediators which may be preformed in granules, e.g., histamine, heparin, and chemotactic factors, or newly formed, e.g., arachidonic acid metabolites (e.g., prostaglandin D2) and leukotrienes.

REACTIVE MASTOCYTOSIS

- An increased number of mast cells may be seen in any tissue involved in a hypersensitivity reaction.
- An increased number may be seen in the lymph nodes and marrow in a variety of benign and malignant tumors.

BENIGN MAST CELL DISEASES

- *Cutaneous mastocytosis* may be expressed as a solitary lesion in infants or as multiple nodules in older children.
- *Urticaria pigmentosa* occurs before age 2 in 50 percent of cases and is characterized by dermal accumulations of mast cells resulting in brown papules symmetrically distributed, especially over the trunk.
- Intense pruritus and urticaria may occur from mild friction of the skin (*Darier sign*).
- Demonstration of mast cell infiltrates on skin biopsy is diagnostic.
- Urticaria pigmentosa usually subsides at puberty but can continue into adulthood, and patients may develop systemic mastocytosis.

SYSTEMIC MASTOCYTOSIS

Clinical Features

- Affects men and women equally; half are over 60 at the time of diagnosis.
- Malaise, weight loss, and fever are frequent.
- Symptoms of mediator release include urticaria, pruritus, dermatographism, abdominal cramps, diarrhea, nausea, vomiting, flushing, headaches, dizziness, palpitations, dyspnea, hypotension, syncope, and shock.
- Hyperpigmented skin lesions may be present. Lymphadenopathy, hepatomegaly, splenomegaly, and bone pain are frequently present.

- Osteoporosis complicated by fractures occurs in half the patients.

Laboratory Features

- Anemia is present in about half the cases. Mast cells in the blood indicate a transformation to leukemia.
- Marrow biopsy usually shows an increase in mast cells and skin biopsy shows mast cell accumulations.
- Osteoporosis, osteoblastic, or osteolytic lesions are common on bone x-rays.
- Measurement of plasma histamine levels and urinary excretion of the histamine metabolite 1-methyl-4-imidazoleacetic acid may be useful diagnostic tests.

Course and Prognosis

- Symptoms range from absent to progressive and disabling.
- About one-third of patients have associated hematologic malignancies.
- Overall 3-year survival is about 50 percent.

Mast Cell Leukemia

- Patients may have fever, constitutional symptoms, and severe clinical manifestations of mediator release (see above).
- Hepatomegaly, splenomegaly, and lymphadenopathy are common.
- Anemia and thrombocytopenia are nearly always present; white count varies from 10,000 to 150,000/μl, and mast cells make up 5 to 90 percent of the leukocytes.
- Marrow shows a striking increase in mast cells, sometimes up to 90 percent of cells.

Mast Cell Sarcoma

- A rare tumor, characterized by nodules at various cutaneous and mucosal sites; subsequently almost every organ becomes involved by extensive mast cell infiltration; terminally, the blood cells are nearly all immature mast cells with a monocytoid appearance.

Management

- Local lesions may be excised.
- Histamine-2 (H_2) receptor antagonists (e.g., cimetidine) can decrease gastric hyperacidity; histamine-1 (H_1) receptor antagonists (e.g., diphenhydramine, chlorpheniramine, tricyclic antidepressants) can decrease flushing, vasodilation, and headache; disodium cromoglycate, psoralen and ultraviolet light (PUVA), and glucocor-

ticoids have been reported to alleviate various skin and gastrointestinal symptoms.

- Avoid mast cell stimulants, such as alcohol, anticholinergics, aspirin, other NSAIDs, and morphine derivatives.
- Chemotherapy has been disappointing in cases of aggressive systemic disease.

For a more detailed discussion, see Stephen J. Galli, Ann M. Dvorak: Production, biochemistry, and function of basophils and mast cells, Chap. 79, p. 805; and Marshall A. Lichtman: Basophilopenia, basophilia, and mastocytosis, Chap. 85, p. 852, in *Williams Hematology,* 5/e, 1995.

---

47 MONOCYTOSIS AND MONOCYTOPENIA

- Monocytes in the blood are in transit. They function in the tissues, where they participate in:
  - inflammation, including granulomatous reactions and tissue repair
  - immunologic reactions, including delayed hypersensitivity
  - reactions to neoplasia and allografts
- The need for macrophages in tissues also can be met by local proliferation of macrophages, not requiring increased transit of blood monocytes.

NORMAL BLOOD MONOCYTE CONCENTRATION

- The monocyte count averages $1000/\mu l$ in neonatal life, gradually decreasing to a mean of $400/\mu l$ in adult life.
- Monocytosis (in adults): $>800/\mu l$.
- Monocytopenia: $<200/\mu l$.

HEMATOLOGIC DISORDERS ASSOCIATED WITH MONOCYTOSIS (OVER 50 PERCENT OF CASES)

Neoplastic or Clonal Monocytic Proliferations

- Myelodysplastic syndrome (preleukemic syndrome)
- Acute myelogenous leukemia (myelomonocytic or monocytic types)
- Chronic myelogenous leukemia

"Reactive" or Probably Nonclonal Monocytic Proliferations

- Neutropenic states: cyclic neutropenia; chronic granulocytopenia of childhood; familial benign neutropenia; infantile genetic agranulocytosis; chronic hypoplastic neutropenia
- Drug-induced agranulocytosis (transient monocytosis, especially in the recovery phase)
- In chlorpromazine therapy, monocytosis precedes the agranulocytosis
- Malignant lymphoma
- Hodgkin disease
- Postsplenectomy state
- Multiple myeloma

INFLAMMATORY AND IMMUNE DISORDERS ASSOCIATED WITH MONOCYTOSIS

Collagen Vascular Diseases (about 10 percent of cases)

- Rheumatoid arthritis
- Systemic lupus erythematosus

- Temporal arteritis
- Myositis
- Periarteritis nodosa

Chronic Infections

- Bacterial infections, e.g., subacute bacterial endocarditis, tonsilitis, dental infections, recurrent liver abscesses (probably *not* in typhoid fever or brucellosis)
- Tuberculosis
- Syphilis: neonatal, primary, and secondary
- Viral infections: cytomegalovirus, varicella-zoster virus

Other Inflammatory Disorders

- Sprue
- Ulcerative colitis
- Regional enteritis
- Sarcoidosis: The degree of monocytosis is inversely related to reduction in number of T lymphocytes

NONHEMOPOIETIC MALIGNANCIES

- Associated with monocytosis in about 20 percent of patients; independent of metastatic disease.

MISCELLANEOUS CONDITIONS ASSOCIATED WITH MONOCYTOSIS

- Alcoholic liver disease
- Tetrachloroethane poisoning
- Langerhans cell histiocytosis
- Parturition
- Severe depression

DISORDERS ASSOCIATED WITH MONOCYTOPENIA

- Aplastic anemia
- Hairy cell leukemia:
  - may be a helpful diagnostic clue
  - contributes to the frequent infections
- Chronic lymphocytic leukemia
- Cyclic neutropenia
- Severe thermal injury
- Rheumatoid arthritis
- Systemic lupus erythematosus

- HIV infections
- Postradiation therapy
- Following the administration of:
  - glucocorticoids
  - alpha-interferon
  - tumor necrosis factor-alpha

For a more detailed discussion, see Marshall A. Lichtman: Monocytosis and monocytopenia, Chap. 90, p. 881, in *Williams Hematology, 5/e,* 1995.

---

48 INFLAMMATORY AND MALIGNANT HISTIOCYTOSIS

The terms *macrophage* and *histiocyte* are synonyms for the mature cell of the monocyte-macrophage system.

INFLAMMATORY DISORDERS OF HISTIOCYTES

Langerhans Cell Histiocytosis

Definition and History

- Langerhans cells:
  - Macrophages with irregularly shaped nuclei present in epidermis, mucosa, lymph nodes, thymus, and spleen. Originate in marrow from common hemopoietic stem cell.
  - Identified by racquet-shaped ultrastructural inclusions (Birbeck bodies), neuroprotein S-100, neuronal-specific enolase, and surface antigen CD1.
  - Process antigens and present them to T cells.
- The term *Langerhans cell histiocytosis* includes disorders previously called histiocytosis X (eosinophilic granuloma, Letterer-Siwe disease, Hand-Schuller-Christian syndrome), self-healing histiocytosis, eosinophilic xanthomatous granuloma, pure cutaneous histiocytosis, Langerhans cell granulomatosis, and nonlipid reticuloendotheliosis.

Etiology and Pathogenesis

- Etiology unknown. Postulated atypical immunologic reaction or autoimmune disease.
- Cigarette smoking implicated in adults with primary pulmonary involvement.
- Lesions usually involve bone (especially skull and facial bones), skin, lungs, lymph nodes, spleen, thymus, pituitary, and hypothalamus.

Clinical Findings

- Inheritance and epidemiology:
  - Most cases sporadic. Some may be inherited.
  - Diagnosis made before age 10 years in 75 percent of patients; before age 30 in 90 percent. Males more frequently have limited disease. 90 percent of cases with multisystem involvement occur before age 20.
- Symptoms and signs:
  - Disease may be localized to a bone or soft tissue site, multifocal in bone only, or multifocal in bone and other sites.
  - Infants may have fever, otitis media, or mastoiditis, with enlargement of liver, spleen, and lymph nodes, or self-limited skin lesions of head and neck.

221

- Children and adolescents: pain, tenderness, swelling due to lytic bone lesion(s), bleeding from gastrointestinal tract, polydipsia, and polyuria due to hypothalamic involvement.
- Adult males: primary pulmonary involvement causes chronic nonproductive cough, chest pain, dyspnea, wheezing. High frequency of associated lung cancer.
- Young women: involvement of genital tract, localized or part of multicentric involvement; pregnancy associated with exacerbation of diabetes insipidus.

Laboratory Findings

- Blood: neutrophilia, increased erythrocyte sedimentation rate, increased serum alkaline phosphatase activity may occur.
- Biopsy of involved tissue demonstrates pathologic Langerhans cells, abundant in proliferative lesions, scarce in fibrotic lesions.

Differential Diagnosis

- Depending on site of involvement, includes chronic granulomatous infections; lymphoma; collagen vascular disease; pneumoconiosis; amyloidosis.
- Langerhans cells, most likely as reactive cells, may be present in biopsies of Hodgkin disease, malignant lymphoma, chronic lymphocytic leukemia.

Treatment

- Spontaneous remissions occur frequently. Older children and adults with multisystem disease often have a relapsing and remitting course. Glucocorticoids for pulmonary disease.
- Chemotherapy is useful in generalized disease. Vinblastine, 6-MP, methotrexate may be useful as single agents. Alkylating agents (cyclophosphamide and chlorambucil) may be successful with or without glucocorticoids.
- Bone lesions: curettage, excision, or radiation therapy.
- Blood component therapy as needed for cytopenias.
- Splenectomy for gross splenomegaly and transfusion dependence.
- Allogeneic marrow transplantation has been beneficial in some patients with multisystem disease.

Course and Prognosis

- Good prognosis is associated with isolated bone lesions.
- Poor prognosis is associated with onset of disease during first 2 years of life, fever not explained by infection, blood cytopenias, and abnormal liver function or pulmonary function tests.
- Malignancies of Langerhans cells are rare and confined to elderly patients.

Familial Hemophagocytic Histiocytosis

Definition

- Also known as familial reticulosis and familial erythrophagocytic lymphohistiocytosis.
- Affects neonates and infants; 90 percent of cases are under 2 years of age.
- Two-thirds of cases are in siblings; frequent parental consanguinity.

Clinical Findings

- In infants: fever, anorexia, vomiting, irritability.
- Enlarged liver and spleen in nearly every case.
- Lymphadenopathy, jaundice, ascites, edema may occur with progression of disease.

Laboratory Findings

- Anemia, reticulocytopenia, and thrombocytopenia in most patients; neutropenia less common; with progression of disease pancytopenia is the rule.
- Marrow: increased number of macrophages with prominent phagocytosis of blood cells (hemophagocytic histiocytes).
- Serum glutamic-oxaloacetic transaminase, glutamate-pyruvate transaminase, bilirubin and triglycerides levels often elevated.
- Increased serum concentrations of interferon-γ, tumor necrosis factor, soluble CD8, and interleukin-6 suggest relationship with cytotoxic T cells and inflammatory cytokines.
- Biopsies: lymphohistiocytic infiltrate in bone marrow, liver, spleen, lymph nodes; cytologically normal macrophages engorged with phagocytosed erythrocytes (and often leukocytes and platelets). Paracortical lymphoid depletion in lymph nodes.

Therapy

- Various combinations of therapies have been utilized, but no systematic studies have been done.
- Marrow transplantation from a histocompatible sibling can give sustained remission.

Course

- Often rapidly fatal. Less than 10 percent of patients survive more than a year.
- Death is from infection, hemorrhage, or CNS abnormalities.

Infection-, Disease-, or Drug-Induced Hemophagocytic Histiocytosis

Etiology

- Usually associated with systemic viral infection; occasionally with bacterial, fungal, or protozoal infections. Appears to be an unusual, exaggerated inflammatory reaction to infection.

- Also may be associated with malignancies, with lupus erythematosus, or after phenytoin therapy.

Clinical Findings

- Fever, severe malaise, myalgias, lethargy.
- Enlargement of liver and spleen frequent in children, less so in adults.

Laboratory Findings

- Severe anemia (<9 g/dl), leukopenia (<2500/µl), thrombocytopenia (<50,000/µl), or combination of two cytopenias in nearly all cases.
- Macrophages may be present in blood film.
- Marrow may be hypocellular, with decreased erythropoiesis and granulopoiesis. Increased macrophages, which frequently contain phagocytosed erythrocytes and erythroblasts and occasionally platelets and neutrophils.

Course

- Patients are severely ill but often recover in weeks with complete disappearance of evidence of histiocytosis in months.
- Fatal outcome likely in immunosuppressed patients.

Sinus Histiocytosis with Massive Lymphadenopathy (Rosai-Dorfman Syndrome)

Definition and History

- Benign self-limited disorder of unknown etiology.
- Usually occurs in first two decades of life, but may occur at any age.

Clinical Findings

- Massive, painless, bilateral cervical lymphadenopathy; axillary and inguinal adenopathy develops in half of patients.
- Fever is common.

Laboratory Findings

- Signs of chronic inflammation, i.e., anemia, neutrophilia, elevated erythrocyte sedimentation rate, polyclonal hypergammaglobulinemia.
- Lymphoid lesions, nodal and extranodal, widespread in the body.
- Pathologic features in lymph node:
  - Marked capsular fibrosis, distention of sinuses by phagocytic macrophages: lymphophagocytosis and erythrophagocytosis by macrophages are characteristic.

- Immunophenotyping: active phagocytes positive for S-100, CD11c, CD14, CD33, CD68, acid phosphatase, and nonspecific esterase.

Course and Prognosis

- Cases often occur in children with immunologic disorders.
- Lymph node enlargement usually progresses for weeks to months, then recedes, with no residual evidence of disease after 9 to 18 months.
- Some patients have persistent adenopathy; others may have a fatal outcome.

Therapy

- Acyclovir therapy may be effective. Herpesvirus 6 identified in 7 of 9 cases studied.
- Glucocorticoids, cytotoxic agents, radiotherapy, and antibiotics are ineffective.

Immature Sinus "Histiocytosis"

- Proliferation of monocytoid cells in expanded sinuses of lymph node paracortex in patients with toxoplasmosis and in homosexuals with lymphadenopathy.
- A misnomer: the monocytoid cells are immature B lymphocytes ("monocytoid B cells") arrested in their progression to SIgM+, SIgD+ lymphocytes.

MALIGNANT HISTIOCYTOSIS

Definition

- A rapidly fatal disorder associated with jaundice, lymphadenopathy, refractory anemia, leukopenia, and hepatosplenomegaly, originally called *histiocytic medullary reticulosis.*
- Malignant histiocytosis has been confused with large cell lymphomas in recent literature. The term malignant histiocytosis should be restricted to neoplasms of histiocytes.

Clinical Features

- Occurs in neonates, children and adults; males more frequently than females.
- Frequent symptoms: fever, weakness, weight loss, malaise, sweating, chest and back pain, and rashes.
- Signs: lymphadenopathy (local or generalized), hepatomegaly, and splenomegaly are frequent. Dermatitis, pulmonary infiltrates, soft tissue masses, bone lesions, and CNS involvement may occur. Jaundice, ascites may occur late.

Laboratory Features

- Anemia present at time of diagnosis in most patients; thrombocytopenia and leukopenia are frequent. Increased levels of serum bilirubin and lactic dehydrogenase often present.
- Diagnosis is usually made by lymph node biopsy, marrow aspiration/biopsy, or biopsy of another site. The neoplastic histiocytes are positive for nonspecific esterase cytochemically, usually express monocyte/histocyte antigens (CD11c, CD14, and CD68) and are negative for B-cell and T-cell antigens.
- In some cases, diagnosis is not made before death, despite biopsies of several sites.

Differential Diagnosis

- Infection-induced hemophagocytic syndrome: no neoplastic cells identified.
- Anaplastic large cell lymphomas: usually positive for CD30 (Ki-1), may express T cell or, less often, B cell antigens.
- Monoblastic leukemia without maturation (AML-M5A), if extramedullary involvement is present and marrow is only partially involved. Generally, marrow involvement becomes extensive and leukemia becomes obvious in a short time.

Treatment

- Multidrug regimens, similar to those used for large cell lymphomas (e.g., cyclophosphamide, doxorubicin, vincristine, and prednisone).
- Autologous marrow transplantation has been successful.

Course and Prognosis

- Remissions occur in less than half to more than two-thirds of patients but are usually short-lived.
- Although some patients remain in remission for months, and a few for years, most die within a year of onset.
- Untreated disease progresses rapidly, and is nearly uniformly fatal.

For a more detailed discussion, see Marshall A. Lichtman, Diane M. Komp: Inflammatory and malignant histiocytosis, Chap. 91, p. 885, in *Williams Hematology*, 5/e, 1995.

49 LIPID STORAGE DISEASES

In Gaucher and Niemann-Pick diseases major clinical manifestations result from accumulation of lipid in macrophages.

GAUCHER DISEASE

Etiology and Pathogenesis

- Glucocerebroside accumulates because of a deficiency of glucocerebrosidase (β-glucosidase).
- Very rarely a neuronopathic form may be due to deficiency of a glucosidase cofactor, saposin.
- Inherited as an autosomal recessive disorder, with high gene frequency among Ashkenazi Jews.
- At least 28 different mutations have been reported.

Clinical Features

- Three types of Gaucher disease are recognized:
  - Type 1 occurs in both children and adults, and is due primarily to accumulation of glucocerebroside-laden macrophages in liver, spleen, and marrow. There are no neurologic manifestations.
  - Type 2 is exceedingly rare, and is characterized by rapid neurologic deterioration and early death.
  - Type 3, or juvenile Gaucher disease, is a subacute neuronopathic disorder with later onset of symptoms and better prognosis than type 2.
- Type 1 may be asymptomatic, or symptoms may range from minimal to severe:
  - Chronic fatigue is common and some patients may develop fever.
  - Growth retardation occurs in affected children.
  - Hepatic and/or splenic enlargement may cause significant problems.
  - Skeletal lesions are often painful. "Erlenmeyer flask" deformity of the femur is common. Aseptic necrosis of femoral head and vertebral collapse often occur.

Laboratory Features

- Blood count may be normal, but normocytic, normochromic anemia with modest reticulocytosis is often found. Leukopenia and thrombocytopenia may occur and may be severe.
- Leukocytes are deficient in β-glucosidase activity.
- Gaucher cells are large cells found in marrow, spleen, and liver in varying numbers. They are characterized by small, eccentrically placed nuclei and cytoplasm with characteristic crinkles or striations. The cytoplasm stains with the periodic acid-Schiff (PAS) technique.
- Serum acid phosphatase activity is usually increased.

- Biochemical abnormalities due to severe liver disease may be found.
- Acquired coagulation factor IX deficiency has been reported, but may be artifactual.

Diagnosis

- Diagnosis is established by demonstrating β-glucosidase deficiency in leukocytes or cultured fibroblasts.
- Demonstration of specific DNA abnormalities will establish the diagnosis, but negative studies do not rule it out.
- Gaucher cells are usually readily demonstrated in the marrow, but may be few in number, and cells indistinguishable from Gaucher cells are seen in other diseases, including chronic myelogenous leukemia, Hodgkin disease, multiple myeloma, and AIDS.
- Prenatal diagnosis can be made by examination of cells obtained by amniocentesis.
- Heterozygosity may be established in many cases by assay of β-glucosidase activity in leukocytes or fibroblasts, but DNA analysis may be required.

Therapy

- Splenectomy may correct leukopenia and thrombocytopenia due to hypersplenism, but may cause more rapid deposition of lipid in liver and marrow.
- Orthopedic procedures may be necessary for complications of bony lesions.
- Enzyme replacement therapy with purified or recombinant human β-glucosidase (alglucerase) has been successful but is very expensive and is currently recommended only for patients with relatively severe disease.
- Allogeneic marrow transplantation may be curative, but its use is limited by the risk.

Course and Prognosis

- There is often great variability in expression of the disease, even among siblings.
- Severity of the disease changes little after childhood, and progression is expected to be gradual.

NIEMANN-PICK DISEASE

Etiology and Pathogenesis

- The predominant lipid accumulating in tissues is sphingomyelin, but cholesterol also accumulates.

- Sphingomyelinase deficiency is responsible in some cases (type I) but not in others (type II).
- Inherited as an autosomal recessive disorder.

Clinical Features

- Clinical picture is heterogeneous, and several classifications have been proposed. Patients may be designated as having type I if there is sphingomyelinase deficiency, or type II is sphingomyelinase activity is normal or nearly so. These two types are then divided into three forms: A (acute), S (subacute), and C (chronic).
- Type IA and IIA are afflictions of infancy with severe neurologic involvement and progressive hepatosplenomegaly.
- Type IS presents in late infancy or in childhood with hepatosplenomegaly. Type IIS has neurologic manifestations.
- Type IC and IIC present in early adult life with hepatosplenomegaly and sometimes neurologic involvement.

Laboratory Features

- Mild anemia may be present.
- Blood lymphocytes typically contain up to nine small, lipid-filled vacuoles.
- Leukocytes from patients with type I disease are deficient in sphingomyelinase activity.
- Large histiocytes containing small lipid droplets (foam cells) are demonstrable in marrow.
- Sea-blue histiocytes may be seen in marrow.

Diagnosis

- Type I disease diagnosed by demonstration that accumulated lipid is sphingomyelin and that leukocytes or cultured fibroblasts are deficient in sphingomyelinase.
- Heterozygotes for type I may be detected by measurement of sphingomyelinase activity in leukocytes or cultured fibroblasts.
- Type II disease may be diagnosed from study of uptake of cholesterol by cultured fibroblasts.

Treatment

- There is no effective treatment.

Course and Prognosis

- Patients with types IA and IIA disease usually die before the third year of life.
- Some patients with the chronic forms reach adult life.

For a more detailed discussion, see Ernest Beutler: Lipid storage diseases, Chap. 92, p. 895, in *Williams Hematology*, 5/e, 1995.

50 LYMPHOCYTOSIS AND LYMPHOCYTOPENIA

LYMPHOCYTOSIS

- Adults: absolute lymphocyte count exceeds 4000/μl.
- Normal lymphocyte count is significantly higher in childhood.
- Table 50-1 lists conditions associated with lymphocytosis.
- Examine blood film to determine if there is predominance of:
  - reactive lymphocytes, associated with infectious mononucleosis
  - large granular lymphocytes, associated with large granular lymphocyte leukemia
  - small lymphocytes and smudge cells, associated with chronic lymphocytic leukemia
  - small cleaved lymphocytes, associated with low or intermediate grade lymphomas
  - blasts, associated with acute lymphocytic leukemia
- Cell surface markers aid in distinguishing monoclonal lymphocytosis (leukemia) from polyclonal lymphocytosis (reactive).
- Immunoglobulin and T-cell-receptor in gene rearrangement studies may indicate monoclonal B-cell or T-cell proliferation, respectively.

MONOCLONAL LYMPHOCYTOSIS (see Chaps. 54, 55, 56, 57, 59)

- Neoplastic proliferation of B cells, T cells, NK cells, or immature lymphoid cells.
- Monoclonal B-cell lymphocytosis without clinical manifestations—may progress into CLL in some patients.

SECONDARY (REACTIVE) LYMPHOCYTOSIS

Infectious Mononucleosis

- Characterized morphologically by atypical lymphocytes (see Chap. 53).

Acute Infectious Lymphocytosis

- Characterized by marked lymphocytosis with morphologically normal lymphocytes that are T cells or NK cells.
- Infection of unknown etiology.
- Clinical: usually asymptomatic, but fever, abdominal pain, or diarrhea may be present for a few days.
- No enlargement of liver or spleen.
- Marrow shows variable increase in number of lymphocytes.
- Serum negative for heterophil antibodies.

Bordetella pertussis *Infection*

- Lymphocytosis of morphologically normal CD4 + T-cells, ranging from 8000 to 70,000/μl.

TABLE 50-1 Causes of Absolute Lymphocytosis

Primary lymphocytosis
Lymphocytic malignancies
  Acute lymphocytic leukemia (Chap. 54)
  Chronic lymphocytic leukemia and related disorders (Chap. 55)
    Chronic lymphocytic leukemia
    Prolymphocytic leukemia
  Hairy cell leukemia (Chap. 56)
  Adult T-cell leukemia (Chap. 59)
  Lymphoma (Chap. 59)
  Large granular lymphocytic leukemia (Chap. 57)
    NK cell leukemia
    T gamma lymphocytosis
Monoclonal B-cell lymphocytosis

Secondary (Reactive) Lymphocytosis
Mononucleosis syndromes (Chap. 53)
  Epstein-Barr virus
  Cytomegalovirus
  Toxoplasma gondii
  Human immunodeficiency virus (Chap. 52)
  Herpes simplex virus type II
  Varicella-zoster virus
  Rubella virus
  Adenovirus
  Infectious hepatitis virus
Bordetella pertussis

Stress lymphocytosis (acute)
  Cardiovascular collapse
    Acute cardiac failure
    Myocardial infarction
    Septic shock
  Drug-induced
  Hypersensitivity reactions
  Major surgery
  Sickle cell crisis
  Status epilepticus
  Trauma

Persistent lymphocytosis (chronic)
  Autoimmune disorders
  Cancer
  Cigarette smoking
  Chronic inflammation
  Hyposplenism
  Polyclonal B-cell lymphocytosis
  Sarcoidosis
  Thymoma
  Wegener granulomatosis

Source: Table 101-1 of *Williams Hematology*, 5/e, p. 964.

- Caused by failure to lymphocytes to leave the blood; a pertussis toxin inhibits the normal lymphocyte migration from blood to lymphoid tissues.

Stress Lymphocytosis

- Lymphocytosis appears promptly, due to redistribution of lymphocytes induced by adrenaline.
- Lymphocytosis, often >5,000/µl, reverts to normal or low levels within hours.
- May be associated with trauma, surgery, acute cardiac failure, septic shock, myocardial infarction, sickle cell crisis, or status epilepticus.

Persistent Lymphocytosis

- Rheumatoid arthritis
  - Increased large granular lymphocytes (<1% of RA patients) associated with neutropenia; may be a subgroup of Felty syndrome (see also Chap. 57).
- Neoplastic disease
  - In patients with thymoma, a polyclonal T-cell lymphocytosis may be due to release of thymic hormones by neoplastic thymic epithelium.
- Chronic inflammatory diseases
  - In systemic diseases associated with inflammation, e.g., sarcoidosis, Wegener granulomatosis.
- Cigarette smoking
  - In smokers, a polyclonal increase in CD4+ T cells and in B cells (some binuclear) may occur, especially in HLA-DR7-positive women.
  - Lymphocytosis may resolve with cessation of smoking.
- Hypersensitivity reactions
  - Reactions to insect bites may be associated with a large granular lymphocytic lymphocytosis and lymphadenopathy.

LYMPHOCYTOPENIA

- Absolute lymphocyte count is less than 1000/µl (1.0×10^9/l).
- Usually decrease in CD4+ (helper) T cells, because >80 percent of normal adult blood lymphocytes are T cells, two-thirds of which are CD4+.
- Table 50-2 lists the conditions associated with lymphocytopenia.
- Inherited causes: congenital immunodeficiency diseases (see Chap. 51).
  - Stem cell abnormality, either quantitative or qualitative, results in ineffective lymphopoiesis.
  - Other abnormalities, such as the Wiskott-Aldrich syndrome, result in premature destruction of T cells due to cytoskeletal abnormalities.

TABLE 50-2 Causes of Lymphocytopenia

Inherited causes
Congenital immunodeficiency disease (Chap. 51)
  Severe combined immunodeficiency disease
Aplasia of lymphopoietic stem cells
  Adenosine deaminase deficiency
  Absence of histocompatibility antigens
  Absence of CD4 + helper cells
  Thymic alymphoplasia with aleukocytosis (reticular dysgenesis)
  Ataxia-telangiectasia
  Wiskott-Aldrich syndrome
  Immunodeficiency with short-limbed dwarfism (cartilage hair hypoplasia)
  Immunodeficiency with thymoma
  Cellular immunodeficiency with immunoglobulins
  Purine nucleoside phosphorylase deficiency
  Immune deficiency with veno-occlusive disease of the liver

Acquired causes
Aplastic anemia (Chap. 4)
Infectious diseases
  Viral diseases (Chap. 52)
    AIDS
    Hepatitis
    Influenza
    Other
  Bacterial diseases
    Tuberculosis
    Typhoid fever
    Pneumonia
    Sepsis
Iatrogenic
  Immunosuppressive agents
  Antilymphocyte globulin therapy
    Glucocorticoids
    High-dose PUVA treatment
    Neoplastic chemotherapy
    Platelet apheresis procedures
    Radiation
    Surgery
    Thoracic duct drainage
Systemic disease associated
  Autoimmune diseases
    Rheumatoid arthritis
    Systemic lupus erythematosus
    Myasthenia gravis
  Hodgkin disease
  Protein-losing enteropathy
  Renal failure
  Sarcoidosis
  Thermal injury
Nutritional/dietary
  Ethanol abuse
  Zinc deficiency

Idiopathic
Idiopathic CD4 + T lymphocytopenia

Acquired Lymphocytopenia

Infectious Diseases

- AIDS; destruction of CD4 + T cells infected with HIV-1 or HIV-2.
- Other viral diseases such as hepatitis and influenza.
- Active tuberculosis; lymphocytopenia usually resolves 2 weeks after initiating appropriate therapy.

Iatrogenic

- Radiotherapy, chemotherapy, administration of antilymphocyte globulin.
- Glucocorticoid therapy: mechanism unclear, possibly redistribution as well as cell destruction.
- Postsurgery: mechanism may be redistribution of lymphocytes.
- Thoracic duct drainage: lymphocytes are lost from the body.
- Platelet apheresis: lymphocytes, as well as platelets, are removed from the body.

Systemic Disease Associated With Lymphocytopenia

- Systemic lupus erythrematosus: probably mediated by autoantibodies.
- Sarcoidosis; renal failure: probably due to impaired T-cell proliferation.
- Protein-losing enteropathy: lymphocytes may be lost from the body.
- Burns: profound T-cell lymphocytopenia due to redistribution from blood to tissues.

Nutritonal/Dietary

- Zinc deficiency: zinc is necessary for normal T-cell development and function.
- Excess alcohol intake: may impair lymphocytic proliferation.

Idiopathic CD4 + T Lymphocytopenia

- Defined by the CDC in 1993 as a CD4 + T-lymphocyte count <300/µl on two separate occasions without serologic or virologic evidence of HIV-1 or HIV-2 infection.
- Congenital immunodeficiency diseases, such as common variable immunodeficiency, must be excluded (see Chap. 51).
- Over half of reported cases had opportunistic infections indicative of cellular immune deficiency (e.g., *Pneumocystis carinii* pneumonia). Such patients are classified by WHO as having idiopathic

CD4 + lymphocytopenia and severe unexplained HIV-seronegative immune suppression. In contrast to patients infected with HIV, these patients tend to have stable CD4 + counts over time, may have reductions in other lymphocyte subgroups, and may have complete or partial spontaneous reversal of the CD4 + T lymphocytopenia.

For a more detailed discussion, see Thomas J. Kipps: Lymphocytosis and lymphocytopenia, Chap. 101, p. 963, in *Williams Hematology,* 5/e, 1995.

51 PRIMARY IMMUNODEFICIENCY SYNDROMES

- The clinical characteristics of the primary immunodeficiency states are determined by the failure of either or both the humoral and cellular arms of the immune system.
- The features of depressed humoral immunity are
  - Recurrent pyogenic bacterial infections, including sinusitis, furunculosis, and pneumonias that often terminate in bronchiectasis. These infections are responsive to antibiotics but quickly relapse.
  - The response to viral infections and organ transplant rejection are often normal.
  - Antibody response to immunization is often inadequate.
- Abnormality of cellular immunity causes
  - Susceptibility to viral, protozoal, and fungal infections.
  - Transplant rejection may be impaired. Patients are often anergic.
  - There may be a secondary defect in humoral immunity due to T-cell dysfunction.
- Autoimmune diseases such as immune-mediated thrombocytopenia and rheumatoid arthritis-like conditions occur at a higher frequency in certain primary immunodeficiency states.
- The more severe primary immune deficiencies are usually present in infancy, though common variable immunodeficiency often presents later in life.
- Major features of the primary immunodeficiency states are summarized in Table 51-1.
- Treatment with intravenous gamma-globulin (IVGG)
  - IVGG is a pooled plasma-derived preparation which contains IgG.
  - The dose for congenital immunodeficiencies is individualized, and usually starts at 200 to 800 mg/kg intravenously every 3 to 4 weeks.
  - Dose and interval are adjusted to the patient's measured immunoglobulin levels with a target of keeping the IgG above 400 to 500 mg/dl at the trough.
  - IVGG infusions should be started slowly (0.5 ml/kg/h) and slowly increased if the infusion is tolerated but no faster than 4 ml/kg/h.
  - Adverse reaction include fever, headache, nausea, vomiting, urticaria, flushing, chest tightness, and wheezing.
  - Serum sickness, transmission of viral infections, and anaphylaxis in IgA-deficient patients may occur rarely.
  - Such allergic reactions are less common when IVGG is given for other indications such as immune thrombocytopenia.

TABLE 51-1 The Major Features of the Primary Immunodeficiency States

Condition	Inheritance	Pathogenesis	Clinical features	Treatment
X-linked agamma-globuli-nemia	X-linked recessive	Mutation of atk gene	1. Humoral deficit 2. Serum IgG < 100 mg/dl, IgA and IgM undetectable 3. Absence of plasma cells and follicles in lymph nodes 4. Rheumatoid arthritis 5. Dermatomyositis and CNS infiltrates from echovirus	IVGG*
Absent IgG and IgA with increased IgM	1. X-linked recessive 2. Acquired	1. Mutation of gene for CD40 ligand 2. Inability of immunoglobulin isotype switching	1. Humoral deficit 2. Autoimmune diseases 3. Lymphatic hyperplasia	IVGG
Selective IgA deficiency	1. Complex inheritance 2. Acquired due to drugs (gold, captopril) 3. Acquired due to congenital infection with CMV, toxoplasmosis, or rubella	1. Some may have gene deletion 2. Primary defect is failure of B cells to differentiate to IgA-producing plasma cells	1. Most common primary immunodeficiency (1/700) 2. Absent IgA with normal IgM and IgG 3. 20% have IgG subclass deficiency 4. Normal immunity unless IgG subclass deficiency then humoral deficit 5. Autoimmune diseases	IVGG if subclass deficient and no anti-IgA antibody

(continued)

TABLE 51-1 (Continued)

Condition	Inheritance	Pathogenesis	Clinical features	Treatment
			6. Anaphylaxis to IgA-containing blood products if there is IgE antibody against IgA	
Selective IgG subclass deficiency	Complex	Gene deletions in some patients	1. May have normal total IgG but absence of one or more subclass 2. Many but not all have humoral deficit 3. Inability to raise IgM against polysaccharide antigens in some patients	IVGG in selected patients
Common variable immuno-deficiency	1. Congenital 2. Acquired	1. Heterogeneous 2. Decreased or absent plasma cells, but may have follicular hyperplasia 3. Decreased B cells in 25% and failure of B cells to differentiate to plasma cells in the remainder	1. Humoral deficit 2. Decreased IgG, IgM, and IgA 3. Autoimmune diseases 4. Sprue-like syndrome and giardiasis 5. Noncaseating granulomas 6. Often late onset	IVGG
Severe combined immuno-deficiency	1. X-linked recessive 2. Autosomal recessive	1. X-linked IL-2 receptor gamma chain	1. Cellular and humoral deficits	Gene therapy or bone marrow transplant

(continued)

TABLE 51-1 (Continued)

Condition	Inheritance	Pathogenesis	Clinical features	Treatment
		2. Autosomal-adenosine deaminase or nucleoside phosphorylase deficiency	2. Death in infancy 3. Lymphopenia 4. Transfusion-associated GVHD	
Ataxia-telangiectasia	Autosomal recessive	1. Thymic hypoplasia 2. Increased chromosomal breakage and DNA processing or repair defect	1. Depressed cellular immunity 3. Low IgA 3. Sinopulmonary infections 4. Ataxia and choreoathetoid movements 5. Telangiectasias 6. Increased incidence of malignancy	Antibiotics and IVGG
Wiskott-Aldrich syndrome	X-linked recessive	1. Mutation in unknown gene at Xp11.22 2. Platelets small and fragmented, lymphocytes bald, and surface sialoglycoproteins such as CD43 and gpIB on platelets are rapidly degraded	1. Thrombocytopenia with small platelets 2. Eczema 3. Progressive deterioration of thymic dependent immunity 4. Increased incidence of malignancy	1. Bone marrow transplantation 2. Splenectomy and prophylactic antibiotics have been used for thrombocytopenia 3. IVGG

(continued)

TABLE 51-1 (*Continued*)

Condition	Inheritance	Pathogenesis	Clinical features	Treatment
DiGeorge's syndrome (thymic hypoplasia)	Congenital, but not inherited	Abnormality or insult during development of third and fourth pharyngeal pouches during fetal life	1. T-cell deficit at birth which usually corrects with time 2. Susceptibility to viral, fungal, and bacterial infections 3. Hypocalcemia due to hypoparathyroidism 4. Facial and cardiovascular birth defects	Fetal thymic transplants

*IVGG, intraveneous gamma-globulin.

For a more detailed discussion, see Fred S. Rosen: Immunodeficiency diseases, Chap. 102, p. 968, in *Williams Hematology,* 5/e, 1995.

52 THE ACQUIRED IMMUNODEFICIENCY SYNDROME (AIDS)

GENERAL CONSIDERATIONS

- Primary cause is infection with the HIV-1 lentivirus.
- Usual routes of infection are sexual contact with an infected partner, perinatal exposure, parenteral drug use, or transfusions of blood or blood products.
  - Risk of HIV transmission through transfusion of a unit of red blood cells tested negative for HIV by ELISA is estimated to be 1 per 36,000 to 1 in 153,000.
  - 90 percent of those who received a contaminated unit of blood become infected.
- HIV primarily infects CD4-positive lymphocytes.
  - Monocyte-macrophages, Langerhans giant cells, follicular dendritic cells, megakaryocytes, and CD34-positive marrow progenitor cells may also be infected.
  - Heterogeneity of the gp 120 viral protein may account for strain-specific tissue tropism.
- HIV infection causes progressive loss of CD4 cells resulting in aberrant immune regulation and immunodeficiency characterized by
  - decreased lymphocyte proliferation in response to cellular antigens
  - immunological response mounted by the host against infected lymphocytes
  - exaggerated expression of inhibitors of T-cell proliferation such as TGF-β
  - impaired delayed hypersensitivity
  - decreased T-cell–mediated cytotoxicity
  - decreased helper response in immunoglobulin production
  - polyclonal B-cell activation resulting in hypergammaglobulinemia, but with blunted specific antibody responses
  - decreased gamma interferon production

CLINICAL FEATURES OF HIV INFECTION

- The clinical classification system for HIV infection and list of AIDS-defining clinical conditions are summarized in Tables 52-1 and 52-2.
- Acute retroviral syndrome is seen in 50 to 90 percent of patients beginning 1 to 3 weeks after primary infection: fatigue, malaise, headache, fever, rash, and photophobia lasting several weeks.
- Generalized adenopathy: may occur toward the end of the acute retroviral syndrome and persist indefinitely.
- Average time from acute infection to the development of symptomatic AIDS is 10 to 11 years.

TABLE 52-1 AIDS-Defining Clinical Conditions for HIV-Infected
Adolescents and Adults

Candidiasis of bronchi, trachea, or lungs
Candidiasis, esophageal
Cervical cancer, invasive*
Coccidioidomycosis, disseminated or extrapulmonary
Cryptococcosis, extrapulmonary
Cryptosporidiosis, chronic intestinal (>1 month duration)
Cytomegalovirus disease (other than liver, spleen, or nodes)
Cytomegalovirus retinitis (with loss of vision)
Encephalopathy, HIV-related
Herpes simplex: chronic ulcer(s) (>1 month duration) or bronchitis,
pneumonitis, or esophagitis
Histoplasmosis, disseminated or extrapulmonary
Isosporiasis, chronic intestinal (>1 month duration)
Kaposi sarcoma
Lymphoma, Burkitt lymphoma (or equivalent term)
Lymphoma, immunoblastic (or equivalent term)
Lymphoma, primary in brain
Mycobacterium avium complex or *M. kansasii,* disseminated or extrapul-
monary
Mycobacterium tuberculosis, any site (pulmonary* or extrapulmonary)
Pneumocystis carinii pneumonia
Pneumonia, recurrent*
Progressive multifocal leukoencephalopathy
Salmonella septicemia, recurrent
Toxoplasmosis of brain
Wasting syndrome due to HIV

*Added in the 1993 expansion of the AIDS surveillance case definition.
Source: Table 103-1 of *Williams Hematology*, 5/e, p. 976.

- Serological diagnosis of HIV infection is by ELISA with western
  blot confirmation.
  - Median time from infection to positive ELISA is 2.4 months.
  - Viral p24 antigen is detectable in plasma when HIV infection is
    active or advanced, with high rates of viral replication and heavy
    viral loads.
  - Viral RNA or proviral DNA may be detected by polymerase chain
    reaction.
- Opportunistic infections are a major clinical problem and may be
  protozoal (toxoplasmosis), fungal (*Pneumocystis carinii, Candida,*
  cryptococcus), mycobacterial (tuberculosis, *Mycobacterium avium*
  complex), bacterial (pneumonia, sinusitis), or viral (CMV).
  - Tuberculosis, candidiasis, and bacterial infections can occur early
    in the course of immunodeficiency; pneumocystis occurs in moder-
    ately advanced immunodeficiency; and *Mycobacterium avium* com-
    plex and CMV more often occur with very advanced immunodefi-
    ciency.

TABLE 52-2 Classification System for HIV Infection[1]

CD4+ T cell count	(A) Asymptomatic, acute (primary) HIV or PGL[2]	(B) Symptomatic, but not (A) or (C)	(C) AIDS-indicator conditions (Table 52-1)
	Clinical categories		
(1) ≥500/μl	A1	B1	C1[3]
(2) 200–499/μl	A2	B2	C2[3]
(3) <200/μ/l	A3[3]	B3[3]	C3[3]

[1] Criteria for HIV infection for persons over 13 years of age (a) repeatedly reactive screening test for HIV antibody (e.g., enzyme immunoassay) with specific antibody identified by supplemental tests (e.g., immunoblot, immunofluorenscence assay); (b) direct identification of virus in host tissues by virus isolation; (c) HIV antigen detection; or (d) a positive result on any other highly specified licensed test for HIV.
[2] PGL = persistent generalized lymphadenopathy.
[3] Illustrates the expanded AIDS surveillance case definition. Persons with an AIDS-indicator condition (Category C, Table 52-1) as well as those with CD4+ T-lymphocyte counts < 200/μl (Categories A3 or B3) are reportable as AIDS cases in the United States and Territories, effective January 1, 1993.
Source: Table 103-2 of Williams Hematology, 5/e, p. 976.

- Increased incidence of autoimmune phenomena.
- Neurologic manifestations: infection of microglia and macrophages in the CNS can result in dementia; painful, predominantly sensory, peripheral neuropathy; and aseptic meningitis with CSF pleocytosis and increased protein levels.
- Generalized wasting syndrome: severe cachexia due to anorexia, diarrhea, and malabsorption, increased resting energy expenditure, infections, and aberrant cytokine expression.
- Cardiac manifestations include congestive heart failure in 5 percent of HIV-infected individuals.
- Pulmonary manifestations include nonspecific interstitial pneumonitis and lymphocytic interstitial pneumonitis (typically of CD8+ cells) in addition to pneumonia.
- Renal manifestations include focal glomerulosclerosis and nephrotic syndrome leading to uremia in 10 percent of affected patients.

GENERAL TREATMENT OF HIV INFECTION

- Anticipate and treat complicating opportunistic infections (OIs)
  - Prophylaxis against OI when appropriate.
  - Consider antiretroviral therapy when CD4 counts are below 500.
  - The usual initial antiretroviral therapy is zidovudine 100 mg five times a day or 200 mg three times a day.

- Dideoxyinosine (DDI) recommended for patients intolerant of zidovudine or whose disease is progressing on zidovudine. DDI is less myelosuppressive than zidovudine.
- Zalcitabine (DDC) is also less myelosuppressive but may be less active than zidovudine. It may be useful in combination with zidovudine.
- Combination antiretroviral therapy including nonnucleoside reverse transcriptase inhibitors such as nevariapine is under study.

HEMATOLOGICAL MANIFESTATIONS

- Over 90 percent of HIV-infected patients develop cytopenias, usually in the more advanced stages of the disease, associated with low CD4 counts.
- Bone marrow is often hypercellular despite the presence of cytopenias, suggesting ineffective hemopoiesis. Dysplasia, plasmacytosis, and increased reticulin are other common marrow findings.
- Cytopenias may be exacerbated by myelosuppressive effects of drug therapy for HIV or its complications.
- Anemia:
  - Seen in 80 percent of patients at some point in their course.
  - Finding similar to anemia of chronic disease with normochromic normocytic indices, blunted erythropoietin response, low reticulocyte count, low serum iron and TIBC, and high ferritin.
  - Macrocytosis and anemia very common with zidovudine therapy. Zidovudine sometimes causes neutropenia, but thrombocytopenia only rarely.
  - Erythropoietin is useful in treating anemia secondary to zidovudine if serum erythropoietin levels are below 500 mU/ml.
  - Occasional patients have anemia, macrocytosis, and a dysplastic hypocellular marrow that does not respond to vitamin B_{12} or folate therapy.
  - Coombs test is often positive, but clinically significant hemolysis is rare.
- Leukopenia:
  - Very common; usually due to lymphopenia, but neutropenia is seen in over 50 percent of those with advanced disease.
  - Dysplastic myeloid cells and atypical lymphocytes are seen.
  - G-CSF and GM-CSF have been used to ameliorate neutropenia secondary to AIDS or associated with myelosuppressive drug therapy such as ganciclovir.
- Thrombocytopenia:
  - May occur at any stage of infection.
  - Decreased platelet production due to megakaryocyte infection and decreased platelet survival.
  - Marrow examination shows increased or normal numbers of megakaryocytes.

- Platelet-associated immunoglobulin is elevated.
- Glucocorticoid therapy may increase platelet count, but immunosuppression is undesirable.
- Splenectomy and intravenous γ-globulin are both effective treatments.
- Zidovudine may increase platelet counts, especially in those with less severe thrombocytopenia.
- Limited data suggest a role for treatment with α-interferon.
- TTP has been reported in HIV and has clinical findings and treatment similar to non-HIV–infected patients.

HIV-ASSOCIATED MALIGNANCIES

Non-Hodgkin lymphoma (NHL)

- Risk 100 times greater than general population.
- 3 percent of HIV-infected persons develop NHL. The risk of developing NHL increases with prolonged survival after the onset of symptomatic AIDS.
- Etiology:
  - Immune suppression.
  - B-cell activation and hyperplasia.
  - Dysregulation of cytokines including TNFα, IL-6, and IL-10.
  - Epstein-Barr virus may play a role, especially in primary CNS lymphoma.
  - Chronic B-cell stimulation increases the chance of chromosomal translocations and gene rearrangements.
  - c-MYC dysregulation, especially in small cell noncleaved lymphoma.
  - p53 mutations.
- Clinical features:
  - "B" symptoms (fever, night sweats, and weight loss), widespread bulky disease, and extranodal involvement are common.
  - CNS, liver, marrow, or gastrointestinal involvement is frequent.
  - Systemic lymphoma may involve leptomeninges.
- Staging evaluation: CT scans of chest, abdomen, and pelvis; marrow biopsy; and lumbar puncture. Gallium-67 scans may also be helpful at times.
- Pathology: intermediate or high-grade non-Hodgkin lymphoma; immunoblastic, large cell and small cell noncleaved cell types.
- Factors predicting poor prognosis include Karnofsky performance status less than 70 percent, marrow involvement, low CD4 count, and symptomatic AIDS prior to diagnosis of lymphoma.
- Treatment:
  - Combination chemotherapy is standard.
  - Patients with AIDS tolerate dose-intensive chemotherapy poorly.

- Intrathecal chemotherapy for CNS prophylaxis is suggested.
- Hemopoietic growth factors are used to ameliorate myelosuppression associated with chemotherapy.
- Prophylactic trimethoprim-sulfamethoxazole to prevent *Pneumocystis* infections should be given to patients receiving chemotherapy.

Primary CNS lymphoma

- Commonly seen in advanced AIDS with very low CD4 counts.
- Presents with seizures, headache, and focal neurologic findings.
- Systemic spread of CNS lymphoma is rare.
- Pathology is large cell or immunoblastic B-cell lymphoma.
- CT/MRI scan reveal mass lesions which are often large, ring enhancing, solitary, or few in number.
- Radiotherapy to brain is associated with a 20 to 50 percent CR rate, but the median survival is only 2 to 3 months, with many deaths due to opportunistic infections.

Kaposi Sarcoma (KS)

- Etiology:
  - Seen in the setting of immunosuppression from various causes including HIV.
  - There is an association with certain HLA types: DR5 and DQ1.
  - Epidemiological studies suggest, in addition to HIV, a sexually transmitted infectious cofactor which is spread by oral-fecal contact in homosexual men.
  - The action of the HIV *TAT* gene and of cytokines such as IL-6 and oncostatin-M may be important in the pathogenesis of KS.
- Clinical features:
  - Multicentric at diagnosis.
  - Discrete irregular red-violet-brown cutaneous macules, nodules, or plaques.
  - Lymphadenopathy and lymphedema common.
  - Oral and gastrointestinal involvement common; usually asymptomatic, but may cause bleeding, pain, or obstruction.
  - Pulmonary involvement denotes a poor prognosis and may cause dyspnea, fever, and infiltrates.
- The diagnosis should be confirmed by biopsy of skin lesions to rule out bacillary angiomatosis.
- Approach to therapy:
  - No available therapies are curative and complete responses are rare. Partial responses can be attained, but are brief, if unmaintained.
  - Watchful waiting is often appropriate for asymptomatic, indolent disease.
  - Local therapies include:

- surgical excision
- intralesional vinblastine, vincristine, or interferon
- cryotherapy
- radiotherapy (high incidence of oral mucositis)
- Systemic therapies include:
  - α-interferon (36 million units daily for 12 weeks, then three times a week) has a 40 percent response rate.
  - A lower response rate to interferon is seen if fever, night sweats, or weight loss, low CD4 counts, or history of opportunistic infections are present.
  - Zidovudine 500 mg/day plus α-interferon 8 to 10 million units/day gives similar response rate even with lower CD4 counts.
  - Cytotoxic chemotherapy is used for patients with rapidly progressive, visceral disease or lymphedema; patients who are thought to be poor candidates for interferon therapy; and patients whose disease progresses while receiving interferon therapy.
  - Active single agents include doxorubicin, vinblastine, vincristine, bleomycin, and etoposide.
  - Combination therapy with AVB (doxorubicin 20 mg/m^2, vincristine 2 mg, bleomycin 10 mg/m^2 every 2 weeks) is often used for visceral disease.
- Invasive cervical carcinoma is also an AIDS-defining malignancy.
- Hodgkin disease may also be seen in HIV-infected patients but is not considered AIDS defining. Extranodal disease, B symptoms are common.

For a more detailed discussion, see Alexandra M. Levine, Howard A. Liebman: The acquired immunodeficiency syndrome (AIDS), Chap. 103, p. 975, in *Williams Hematology*, 5/e, 1995.

---

53 MONONUCLEOSIS SYNDROMES

DEFINITION

- Infectious mononucleosis is used to define any blood lymphocytosis induced in response to an infectious disease.
- Pharyngeal form
  - sore throat preceded by 1 to 2 weeks of lethargy
  - Epstein-Barr virus (EBV) the cause
- Glandular form without pharyngitis
  - lymph node enlargement
  - usually due to agents other than EBV, e.g., *Toxoplasma gondii*
- Typhoidal form
  - lethargy with fever or diarrhea without pharyngitis, usually due to CMV

ETIOLOGY AND PATHOGENESIS

Epstein-Barr Virus

- Cause of most cases in developed countries.
- Transmission requires close mucocutaneous contact.
- Peak incidence teens and early twenties.
- Mononucleosis initiated by entry of EBV into epithelial cells of oropharynx or B lymphocytes of Waldeyer ring.
- Surface receptor for EBV is CD21 on B cells.
- Polyclonal B-cell proliferation occurs with a cytotoxic T-cell response.
- Most circulating atypical lymphocytes are T cells.
- Disease is usually self-limited.
- Complications:
  - idiopathic thrombocytopenic purpura (ITP) or autoimmune hemolytic anemia
  - splenic rupture
  - acute airway obstruction
  - B-cell lymphoproliferative disorder/lymphoma in immunosuppressed patients

CYTOMEGALOVIRUS (CMV)

- Common cause of typhoidal form.
- No peak age incidence.
- Atypical lymphocytosis is due to T cells reacting against CMV-infected monocytes/macrophages.

HIV

- Primary infection may manifest as heterophil-negative mononucleosis.
- High titer viremia accompanies the febrile phase.

OTHER VIRAL CAUSES

- Herpes simplex II
- Varicella zoster
- Hepatitis A or B
- Rubella
- Adenovirus

TOXOPLASMA GONDII

- Infection causes lymphadenopathy, particularly posterior auricular.
- Patients are usually afebrile.
- Pharyngitis is uncommon.

CLINICAL FEATURES

- Incubation period for EBV or CMV, 30 to 50 days.
- Pharyngitis prominent in EBV with significant tonsillar exudate.
- Exudative tonsillitis plus lymphadenopathy strongly suggests EBV.
- Rash common with EBV or CMV, worsened by ampicillin or amoxicillin.
- Hepatosplenomegaly common for both EBV and CMV.
- Various neurologic complications can occur, but Guillain-Barré syndrome is the most frequent, usually due to CMV infection.

LABORATORY FEATURES

- Principal feature: blood lymphocytosis exceeding 50 percent of the white blood count, with at least 10 percent atypical lymphocytes.
- Heterophil antibody positive: EBV only
  - 90 percent positive, 7 to 21 days into illness
  - persists for up to 1 year
  - target antigen on beef, horse, or sheep RBCs
- Autoantibodies
  - anticold agglutinins occur frequently with EBV infection
- Liver function abnormalities, usually cholestatic, are frequently present.
- Antibody tests for EBV
  - IgM and IgG virus capsid antigen (VCA): antibody appears during acute illness, IgM persists for months, IgG for life.
  - Early antigen (EA): appears slightly later than IgG anti-VCA +, persists for years.
  - Epstein-Barr nuclear antigen (EBNA) does not develop until after acute illness; persists for life.
  - Presumptive diagnosis of EBV infectious mononucleosis: anti-VCA +, anti-EBNA −.

- Antibody tests for CMV
  - Primary infection diagnosed by four-fold rise in anti-CMV antibody titer.
- Antibody for HIV
  - Primary infection, patients are HIV antibody-negative.
  - Antibodies develop after 4 to 12 weeks.
- Antibody for *Toxoplasma gondii*
  - Primary infection: high titer of IgM anti-*Toxoplasma* antibodies.

DIFFERENTIAL DIAGNOSIS

- Acute pharyngitis: β-hemolytic streptococcus, adenovirus
- Fever/splenomegaly: lymphoma

CLINICAL COURSE AND THERAPY

- Self-limited
- Prednisone (40 to 60 mg PO daily for 4 days, then taper dose over 1 week) for severe or life-threatening complications:
  - imminent upper airway obstruction
  - ITP
  - hemolytic anemia
  - CNS involvement
- Therapy required for *Toxoplasma* only if patient is pregnant or immunocompromised; or if infection involves vital organs.
  - Pyrimethamine and sulfadiazine for 2 to 4 weeks.
  - Pyrimethamine: 100 to 200 mg initially in two divided doses, then 1 mg/kg daily in a single dose.
  - Sulfadiazine 75 to 100 mg/kg daily in four divided doses.

MONONUCLEOSIS IN PREGNANCY

- Congenital infection with EBV is rare.
- Primary CMV infection in first trimester results in 25 percent rate of congenital infections; 25 percent of infected infants will have congenital abnormalities.
- Primary toxoplasmosis infection in first trimester may also result in congenital abnormalities.

For a more detailed discussion, see Robert F. Betts: Mononucleosis syndromes, Chap. 104, p. 997, in *Williams Hematology*, 5/e, 1995.

54 ACUTE LYMPHOCYTIC LEUKEMIA

DEFINITION

- Acute lymphocytic leukemia (ALL) is the result of clonal proliferation of lymphoid progenitor cells originating in the marrow. Etiology is unknown.

ETIOLOGY AND PATHOGENESIS

Incidence

- Greatest in children less than 10 years of age.
- Second most common malignancy under age 15.

Classification

- Classification by morphology uses the FAB system: L1, L2, L3 (see Table 54-1)
  - L1: most common in children
  - L2: most common in adults
- Classification by immunophenotype recognizes cells of the following types (see Table 54-2).
  - early pre-B
  - pre-B
  - B
  - T
- Immunophenotypes may be further subdivided depending on the presence of B-cell, T-cell, or myeloid markers.

TABLE 54-1 Features of the French-American-British Classification for ALL

Class	L1	L2	L3
Cell features			
Size	Small; uniform	Large; non-uniform	Large; uniform
Cytoplasm	Scanty; moderate basophilia	Variable in amount and degree of basophilia	Moderately abundant; deep basophilia; prominent vacuoles
Nucleus	Regular shape; inconspicuous nucleoli	Irregular shape; prominent nucleoli	Regular shape prominent nucleoli
Age distribution, %			
Children	85	14	1
Adults	31	60	9

Source: Table 105-1 of *Williams Hematology*, 5/e, p. 1004.

TABLE 54-2 Incidence of the Four Major Phenotypes of Childhood ALL in the United States

Leukemic cell phenotype	Percent
Early pre-B (cig⁻, sig⁻, pT⁻, E⁻, cALLa⁺ ᵒʳ ⁻)	67.2
pre-B (cig⁺, sig⁻, pT⁻, E⁻, cALLa⁺ ᵒʳ ⁻)	18.0
B (cig⁻, sig⁺, pT⁻, E⁻, cALLa⁺ ᵒʳ ⁻)	0.6
T (cig⁻, sig⁻, pT⁺, E⁺ ᵒʳ ⁻, cALLa⁺ ᵒʳ ⁻)	14.2

cig, cytoplasmic immunoglobulin (primary μ chains); sig, surface immunoglobulin; pT, pan T antigen; E, sheep erythrocyte rosette; cALLa, common acute lymphocytic leukemia antigen
Source: Table 105-2 of *Williams Hematology*, 5/e, p. 1005.

- B-cell markers: CD19, CD20
- T-cell markers: CD7, CD2
- myeloid: CD33, CD13
- Cytogenetic classification
  - Determination of the karyotype is the most powerful prognostic tool available.
  - Four major groups are recognized:

    (1) normal
    (2) pseudodiploid (46, with structural abnormalities)—more frequent in adults
    (3) hyperdiploid group I (47–50)
    (4) hyperdiploid group II ($>$50)—more frequent in children with early pre-B cell ALL

- Nonrandom translocations are clinically significant.
  - t (8;14): Consistent finding in B cell ALL (L3)
  - t (9;22): The Philadelphia chromosome (Ph+), found in 5 percent of children, and 25 percent of adults with ALL
  - t (4;11): Associated with mixed myeloid/lymphoid markers
  - t (1;19): pre-B cell ALL
  - t (11;14): T cell ALL
- Philadelphia chromosome–positive ALL (Ph+ALL): BCR/ABL fusion product is an abnormal protein (p190) with tyrosine kinase activity. Cells are usually cALLa⁺.
- Infants with ALL are likely to have 11q23 abnormalities and be cALLa⁻.

CLINICAL FEATURES

- These are most often a consequence of failure of production of normal blood cells caused by replacement of marrow by leukemic cells.
- Symptoms and signs:
  - anemia (most common presentation)
  - thrombocytopenia

- neutropenia (least common presentation)
- pain (25 percent of presentation—bone pain is the most common)
- Physical findings
  - moderate lymphadenopathy 50 to 75 percent of patients
  - splenomegaly (slight to moderate) 75 percent
  - hepatomegaly 50 to 75 percent
  - fever 50 percent
- Laboratory features
  - About 30 percent present with leukocyte counts $<5000/\mu l$.
  - Blast cells may be difficult to find in leukopenic patients.
  - Nearly all patients have anemia and thrombocytopenia.
  - Variant presentations may make diagnosis difficult:
    - Aplastic marrow with pancytopenia. In such patients common ALL may occur within 1 to 10 months of initial presentation.
    - Hypereosinophilia may be associated with ALL.
  - The leukemia cells are PAS positive, myeloperoxidase and nonspecific esterase negative, TdT positive.
  - Mediastinal mass may be seen on chest x-ray with T-cell ALL.

DIFFERENTIAL DIAGNOSIS

- Major consideration is AML versus ALL.
- Other diseases which may present similarly:
  - aplastic anemia
  - marrow infiltration by small round cell nonhemopoietic tumors, e.g., neuroblastoma, rhabdomyosarcoma, Ewing's sarcoma, small cell lung cancer
  - infectious diseases, e.g., mononucleosis, pertussis

THERAPY

- Four phases of therapy

  (1) remission induction
  (2) prophylactic treatment of CNS
  (3) consolidation
  (4) maintenance

- Several complex regimens have been developed for the treatment of childhood and adult ALL (summarized in Table 105-6 in *Williams Hematology*, 5/e).
- Sanctuary sites:
  - CNS
    - Intrathecal (IT) chemotherapy as efficacious as cranial irradiation (IT methotrexate for low-risk and intermediate risk ALL; combined IT methotrexate, hydrocortisone, cytosine arabinoside for high-risk ALL).

- CNS relapse requires systemic therapy along with treatment of CNS (cranial irradiation 24 Gy plus combined triple IT therapy).
- Testes
  - Testicular relapse in first marrow remission accounts for 6 percent of treatment failures.
  - Early testicular relapse indicates poor prognosis, usually with marrow relapse.
  - Late relapse after cessation of maintenance is compatible with subsequent long disease-free survival after treatment.
  - Treatment recommended is 20 Gy in 2-Gy fractions, and systemic reinduction.
- Allogeneic marrow transplantation is under study. May be indicated if there is an appropriate donor in the following situations:
  - refractory ALL
  - childhood ALL in second remission
  - "high-risk" adult ALL in first remission
- Autologous marrow transplantation is less well defined.
- Allopurinol is administered to patients with hyperuricemia or who appear likely to develop it.
- Patients who develop fever while receiving antileukemic therapy must be carefully evaluated for infection and receive empiric antimicrobial therapy as appropriate.

COURSE AND PROGNOSIS

- The two most important prognostic variables are initial WBC and age; higher values for either are negative prognostic factors and are a continuous variable.
  - Most favorable age is from 1 to 10.
  - Less than 25 percent of infants of less than 1 year of age will achieve disease-free survival.
  - 11q23 abnormality is common in infant ALL and is associated with poor prognosis.
  - Adolescents/adults are likely to have features indicating an unfavorable prognosis.
- Late consequences of Rx
  - Possibility of neurologic impairment from CNS prophylaxis
  - Potential for growth and development impairment
  - Risk of development of a second malignancy

For a more detailed discussion, see Alvin M. Mauer: Acute lymphocytic leukemia, Chap. 105, p. 1004, in *Williams Hematology,* 5/e, 1995.

55 CLL AND RELATED DISEASES

DEFINITION

- Chronic lymphocytic leukemia (CLL) is a neoplastic disease characterized by accumulation of small, mature-appearing lymphocytes in blood, marrow, and lymphoid tissues.
- Incidence 2.7 per 100,000 in United States.
- The most common adult leukemia in western societies.
- In 98 percent of patients, the disease is of B-cell lineage; 2 percent have T-cell lineage.

ETIOLOGY AND PATHOGENESIS

- Hereditary factors
  - Familial occurrence in some patients.
- Genetic abnormalities
  - 50 percent have clonal cytogenic abnormalities.
  - Trisomy 12 is the most common abnormality, found in 17 percent of patients. One-half of these have trisomy 12 only.
  - 15 percent of patients have structural abnormalities of 13q14, specifically hemizygous deletions of the retinoblastoma gene at 13q14, of unknown pathogenetic significance.
  - Chromosome 14 abnormalities:
    - 14q+ associated with a poorer prognosis.
    - 11:14 translocation occurs in a minority of patients, and may involve a proto-oncogene, designated *bcl*-1 or *PRAD*-1. This abnormality is rare in B-CLL, but is characteristic of mantle-cell lymphoma.
    - 14:18 translocation involves *bcl*-2 oncogene. This abnormality is rare, but high levels of expression of *bcl*-2 are found in nearly all patients with CLL, independent of the genetic rearrangement.
    - 14:19 translocation. This abnormality occurs in 10 percent of patients. It involves the oncogene *bcl*-3, and may play a pathogenetic role.
  - p53
    - 14 percent have p53 mutations, usually associated with advanced, late-stage disease.
  - Multidrug resistance (MDR) genes
    - 40 percent of patients express elevated levels of the multidrug resistance gene, *MDR*1.
- Surface antigen phenotype
  - Cells of most patients are CD19+, CD20+.
  - Monoclonal surface immunoglobulin is expressed by over 90 percent of patients: 60 percent are kappa, 40 percent are lambda.
  - IgM and IgD in over 55 percent.
  - IgM only in 25 percent.

- Cells from over 90 percent of CLL patients are CD5 +; the normal counterpart is the CD5 + B cell, which spontaneously produces polyreactive IgM autoantibodies.
- Immunologic abnormalities
  - Autoimmune diseases frequently occur in CLL.
    - Autoimmune hemolytic anemia and immune thrombocytopenia are the most common.
    - Pure red cell aplasia and autoimmune neutropenia are less common.
    - Pathogenetic autoantibodies are not produced by malignant B-cell clone.
  - Hypogammaglobulinemia
    - Develops in 75 percent during course of disease; associated with risk of infection.
  - Cellular immune defects, possibly related to high levels of TGF-β.

CLINICAL FEATURES

- 90 percent of patients are over age 50.
- Male/female ratio is 2:1.
- 25 percent of patients are asymptomatic and the disease suspected because of lymphocytosis or lymph node enlargement.
- Many patients have fatigue, reduced exercise tolerance, or malaise.
- Advanced disease presents with weight loss, recurrent infections, bleeding, and/or symptomatic anemia.
- 80 percent of patients have nontender lymphadenopathy at diagnosis.
- Lymph nodes may become very large and coalescent.
- 50 percent have mild to moderate splenomegaly at presentation.
- Extranodal involvement is frequent but not commonly symptomatic.

LABORATORY FEATURES

- Blood findings
  - Diagnosis of CLL requires sustained monoclonal lymphocytosis of greater than 5000/μl.
  - Lymphocytes are morphologically normal but smudge cells are common on peripheral blood film.
  - 20 percent have a positive Coombs test at some time in the disease. Autoimmune hemolysis occurs in 8 percent.
  - Thrombocytopenia due to antiplatelet antibodies may develop at any time. In advanced disease, thrombocytopenia may be due to marrow replacement.
- Marrow findings
  - Marrow is invariably infiltrated in one of four patterns:
    - interstitial—33 percent
    - nodular—10 percent

- mixed interstitial/nodular—25 percent
- diffuse marrow replacement—25 percent—associated with a poorer prognosis
- Lymph node findings
  - Lymph nodes are affected by diffuse infiltrate of small lymphocytes, identical to low grade, small lymphocytic lymphoma.
- Immunologic studies
  - Immunophenotyping studies recommended for all patients: B/T cell antigens, surface immunoglobulin, κ/λ light chain.
  - Protein electrophoresis
    - most common finding is hypogammaglobulinemia
    - 5 percent of patients have a serum monoclonal protein

DIFFERENTIAL DIAGNOSIS

- Monoclonal lymphocytosis versus causes of polyclonal lymphocytosis (see Chap. 50)
- Prolymphocytic leukemia (see discussion later in this chapter)
- Hairy cell leukemia (see Chap. 56)
- Lymphomas with circulating neoplastic cells (see Chap. 59)
  - small lymphocytic lymphoma
  - mantle cell lymphoma
  - lymphomas of follicular center cell origin
- Lymphoplasmacytic leukemias
  - Waldenström macroglobulinemia (see Chap. 62)
  - plasma cell myeloma (see Chap. 61)
- T cell lymphoproliferative disorders
  - T cell CLL
    - 2 percent of all cases of CLL
    - usually CD3+; may be either CD4+ or CD8+
    - clonal T-cell-receptor gene rearrangements occur
    - lymphadenopathy, marked lymphocytosis, diffuse marrow involvement, and often skin and CNS involvement
    - survival is usually less than 2 years
  - LGL leukemia (see Chap. 57)
  - T-cell prolymphocytic leukemia (see discussion later in this chapter)
  - adult T-cell leukemia/lymphoma (see Chap. 59)
  - cutaneous T-cell lymphomas (see Chap. 59)

THERAPY, COURSE, AND PROGNOSIS

- Clinical staging is helpful in defining prognosis and deciding when to initiate therapy.
  - Rai or Binet staging systems—see Tables 55-1 and 55-2
- Other prognostic indicators
  - Marrow histology: diffuse replacement carries worst prognosis
  - Leukemic cell doubling time:

TABLE 55-1 Rai Clinical Staging System

Stage	Clinical features at diagnosis	Median survival, months
0	Blood and marrow lymphocytosis	>150
I	Lymphocytosis and enlarged lymph nodes	101
II	Lymphocytosis and enlarged slpeen and/or liver	>71
III	Lymphocytosis and anemia (hemoglobin <11 g/dl)	19
IV	Lymphocytosis and thrombocyto-penia (platelets <100,000/μl)	19

Modified Rai Staging System

Stage	Initial Rai category	Median survival, months
Low risk	0	>150
Intermediate risk	I, II	90
High risk	III, IV	19

Source: Table 106-2 of Williams Hematology, 5/e, p. 1026.

- If the lymphocyte count doubles in less than 1 year, median survival is 5 years.
- If the lymphocyte count doubles only after 1 year or longer, the median survival is greater than 12 years.
- Karyotype
  - Abnormal findings are associated with shorter survival.

TABLE 55-2 Binet Clinical Staging System

Stage	Clinical features at diagnosis	Median survival, years
A	Blood and marrow lymphocytosis and less than three areas* of palpable lymphoid-tissue enlargement	>7
B	Blood and marrow lymphocytosis and three or more areas of palpable lymphoid-tissue enlargement	<5
C	Same as B with anemia (hemoglobin below 11 g/dl in men or 10 g/dl in women) or thrombocytopenia [platelets less than 100,000/μl (100 × 10^9/liter)]	<2

*An area is defined as the cervical, axillary, or inguinofemoral lymph nodes, or the liver and spleen. The liver and spleen together count as one area, as do the right and left cervical lymph nodes. However, bilateral enlargement of the axillary lymph nodes or the inguinofemoral lymph nodes each count as two areas. Thus, the number of enlarged lymphoid areas can range from one to five.
Source: Table 106-3 of Williams Hematology, 5/e, p. 1027.

TABLE 55-3 Indications for Therapy in B-Cell CLL

Anemia
Thrombocytopenia
Disease-related symptoms
Markedly enlarged or painful spleen
Symptomatic lymphadenopathy
Blood lymphocyte count doubling time < 6 months
Prolymphocytic transformation
Richter transformation
Associated autoimmune complications

Source: Table 106-4 of *Williams Hematology*, 5/e, p. 1027.

- Trisomy 12 alone has poorer prognosis than other single abnormalities.
- Multiple abnormalities in addition to trisomy 12 carry a poorer prognosis than trisomy 12 alone.
- Age
  - Less than 50 years at diagnosis is associated with a longer median survival.

Indications for Treatment (see Table 55-3)

Chemotherapy of CLL

- Glucocorticoids
  - For treatment of associated autoimmune diseases; 1 mg/kg daily, then taper.
  - Also an effective single agent for treatment of disease.
- Alkylating agents
  - Chlorambucil
    - Daily oral dose, initially 2 to 4 mg, up to 6 to 8 mg/day.
    - Intermittent schedule, total dose 0.4 to 0.7 mg/kg given over 1 to 4 days every 2 to 4 weeks.
  - Cyclophosphamide
    - As active as chlorambucil.
    - Daily oral dose, 50 to 100 mg.
    - Intermittent schedule 500 to 750 mg/m^2 given orally or intravenously every 3 to 4 weeks.
    - Fluid intake of 2 to 3 liters per day important while taking cyclophosphamide.
- Fludarabine
  - Inhibitor of adenosine deaminase (ADA).
  - Complete and partial responses achieved in 50 to 60 percent of previously treated patients, and in 70 to 90 percent of untreated patients.
  - Ability to prolong survival not established.
  - Hematologic and immunologic toxicities: immune suppression

with profoundly decreased CD4 counts associated with opportunistic infections.
- 2-Chlorodeoxyadenosine (2-CdA)
  - A purine analog resistant to adenosine deaminase, causing cell death via apoptosis.
  - 55 to 67 percent of patients respond to treatment.
  - Patients refractory to fludarabine are unlikely to respond to 2CdA.
  - Minimal side effects.
  - Thrombocytopenia may be dose-limiting.
  - Impaired cellular immunity, like fludarabine.
- Deoxycoformycin
  - Adenosine deaminase inhibitor
  - Less effective than fludarabine or 2CdA
- Combination chemotherapy
  - Chlorambucil and prednisone
    - The standard regimen when initiating treatment has been
      - chlorambucil 0.4 to 0.7 mg/kg orally on day 1
      - prednisone 80 mg orally days 1 to 5
      - repeat every 2 to 4 weeks
      - 80 percent of patients achieve partial or complete remission.
  - Chlorambucil and fludarabine
    - Uncertain if better than fludarabine alone (clinical studies in progress).
  - CVP (cyclophosphamide, vincristine, prednisone)
    - gave results not different from chlorambucil/prednisone or chlorambucil alone
  - CHOP (cyclophosphamide, doxorubicin, vincristine, prednisone)
    - has been evaluated in patients with advanced disease, but position is not established
- Splenectomy may benefit patients with hypersplenism
- Radiation therapy is effective for relieving local symptoms due to lymphadenopathy
- Experimental therapies
  - marrow or blood stem cell transplantation
  - immunotherapy and biologic response modifiers

Disease Complications

- Infection, a major cause of morbidity/mortality.
  - Susceptibility to infection correlates with hypogammaglobulinemia.
  - IV IgG decreases frequency of infection but does not improve survival.
- Autoimmune hemolytic anemia and immune thrombocytopenia.
- Increased risk for second malignancies, most frequently melanoma, sarcoma, colorectal, lung, myeloma.

Leukemic Cell Transformation

Richter transformation

- Transformation to an aggressive, large, high-grade, B-cell lymphoma
- Occurs in 3 percent of patients, at a median of 2 years after diagnosis of CLL
- Can arise from the original CLL clone
- Higher incidence of p53 mutations at transformation
- Clinical and laboratory features:
  - increased serum lactic dehydrogenase activity in 82 percent of patients
  - rapid lymph node enlargement in 64 percent
  - fever and/or weight loss in 59 percent
  - monoclonal gammopathy in 44 percent
  - extranodal disease in 41 percent
- Median survival is 5 months after transformation
- CLL/PL and prolymphocytic transformation
  - 15 percent of patients with CLL have a mixture of small lymphocytes and prolymphocytes (PL), the latter accounting for 10 to 50 percent of the lymphoid cells. These patients are considered to have CLL/PL.
  - 20 percent of patients with CLL/PL undergo prolymphocytic transformation with increase in the prolymphocyte component.
  - Progressive splenomegaly is characteristic.
  - Mean survival of 9 months after transformation.
- ALL
  - rare complication
  - can arise from same cell clone as the CLL
  - associated with high levels of expression of c-*myc* and immunoglobulin genes

PROLYMPHOCYTIC LEUKEMIA

Definition

- Clinical and morphologic variant of CLL.
  - Subacute lymphoid leukemia.
  - Incidence: 10 percent of all CLL.
  - 55 percent of circulating leukemic lymphocytes must have prolymphocytic morphology: larger size than CLL cells and a single prominent nucleolus.

Etiology and Pathogenesis

- Unknown etiology
- Cytogenetics: 60 percent have 14q+
- Cytogenesis

- 80 percent of B-cell origin
  - cells have a very high levels of surface immunoglobulin, which is usually IgM
  - only 50 percent are CD5 +
- 20 percent are of T-cell origin
  - 75 percent express CD4
  - 20 percent express CD8
  - 15 percent express both CD4 and CD8

Clinical Features

- 50 percent of patients are older than 70 years.
- Massive splenomegaly occurs in 67 percent.
- Minimal lymphadenopathy, except in patients with T-cell PLL.
- Skin infiltration found in one-third of T-cell PLL.

Laboratory Features

- Frequently find normochromic, normocytic anemia with hemoglobin levels less than 11 g/dl.
- Platelet count often <100,000/μl.
- Lymphocyte count >100,000/μl in 75 percent.
- Hypogammaglobulinemia is common, and one-third have monoclonal gammopathy.

Therapy, Course, and Prognosis

- Often have advanced disease at presentation.
- Indications for treatment:
  - disease-related symptoms
  - symptomatic splenomegaly
  - progressive marrow failure
  - lymphocyte count >200,000/μl
- Treatment is with alkylating agents similar to those used for CLL, or combinations such as CHOP.
- Fludarabine or 2CdA are effective, but experience limited.
- Splenic irradiation may be helpful.
- Median survival is 3 years; T-cell PLL survival is only 6 to 7 months.

For a more detailed discussion, see Thomas J. Kipps: Chronic lymphocytic anemia and related diseases, Chap. 106, p. 1017, in *Williams Hematology,* 5/e, 1995.

56 HAIRY CELL LEUKEMIA

DEFINITION

- Clonal B-cell malignancy associated with pancytopenia and spleno-megaly.
- Irregular cytoplasmic projections on abnormal mononuclear cells.
- Uncommon, compromising only 2 percent of all leukemias.

ETIOLOGY AND PATHOGENESIS

- Unknown etiology.
- Hairy cells are B cells in a late (pre-plasma) stage of development.
  - clonal immunoglobulin gene rearrangement
  - CD19, CD20, CD22 +
  - express plasma cell marker, PCA-1
- Express additional surface antigens uncommon on B lymphocytes
  - CD11c
  - CD25
  - CD103 (normal counterpart of hairy cells may be CD103 + B cells)
- Hairy cells elaborate cytokines such as TNFα which may be impli-cated in impaired hemopoiesis.

CLINICAL FEATURES

- Median age of onset: 50 years.
- 80 percent of patients are male.
- Presenting symptoms:
  - abdominal fullness/discomfort (25 percent)
  - fatigue, weakness, weight loss (25 percent)
  - bleeding or infection (25 percent)
  - found incidentally to have abnormal blood count and/or splenomeg-aly (25 percent)
- Splenomegaly occurs in 85 percent; in 25 percent the spleen is massive.

LABORATORY FEATURES

- Moderate to severe pancytopenia found in 67 percent.
- Rarely extreme leukocytosis (>200,000/µl); most often seen in the "hairy cell leukemia variant" (see below).
- 80 percent of patients have absolute neutropenia and monocytopenia.
- Hairy cells comprise less than 20 percent of lymphocytes in patients with low white blood cell counts, but are the predominant cell in patients whose white blood cell count is greater than 10,000/µl.
- Immunophenotypic identification depends on pattern of expression:
  - Most characteristic pattern is high levels of CD11c, CD22, CD25, and CD103.
  - Pan B-cell antigens such as CD19/CD20/CD22 may be co-expressed with CD11c, CD25, or CD103.

- Marrow biopsy shows focal or diffuse infiltrate of leukemic cells with characteristic surrounding halo of pale-staining cytoplasm.
- Marrow is usually hypercellular, occasionally hypocellular, mimicking aplastic anemia.
- Immunohistochemistry with CD103, CD20 antibodies is more sensitive than morphology in detecting residual neoplastic cells.
- Cytochemistry of hairy cells:
  - Tartrate-resistant acid phosphate activity usually present; absent in 5 percent of hairy cell cases.
- Diffuse infiltration of splenic red pulp cords and sinuses by hairy cells.
- Ribosomal-lamellar complexes on electron microscopy in about 50 percent.

DIFFERENTIAL DIAGNOSIS

- Pancytopenia with splenomegaly
  - Myeloproliferative disorders (myelofibrosis)
  - Myelodysplastic syndromes
  - Hairy cell leukemia variant:
    - high white blood cell counts, median $116,000/\mu l$
    - not associated with neutropenia or monocytopenia
    - CD25 negative
    - lack ribosomal-lamellar complex
  - Mast cell disease
  - Other B-cell lymphoproliferative disorders:
    - low-grade lymphomas
    - splenic lymphoma with circulating villous lymphocytes: has different immunophenotype

THERAPY

- Indications for treatment:
  - symptomatic splenomegaly
  - anemia (Hb level less than 10 g/dl)
  - thrombocytopenia (platelet count less than $100/000/\mu l$)
  - granulocytopenia (neutrophil count less than $1000/\mu l$) with recurrent bacterial or opportunistic infections
  - leukemic phase (white cell count greater than $20,000/\mu l$)
  - associated autoimmune complications
  - tissue infiltration with hairy cells
- 2-Chloradeoxyadenosine (2-CDA)
  - a purine analog which causes cell death by apoptosis
  - given as a 7-day continuous infusion at 0.09 mg/kg/day
  - complete remission achieved in over 75 percent of patients
  - complete remission seen in refractory cases
  - minimal toxicity

- aseptic fever in setting of neutropenia
- T-cell depletion, particularly CD4+ cells of uncertain clinical significance
- 2′-Deoxycoformycin (pentostatin)
  - A purine analog which inhibits adenosine deaminase
  - Administered as an IV bolus of 4 mg/m² every other week
  - Complete response in 50 percent of patients
  - Minimal toxicity:
    - fever, rash, conjunctivitis
    - reversible renal dysfunction
    - mild hepatic toxicity
    - depletion of CD4+ cells
- Fludarabine
  - Purine nucleoside analog that inhibits adenosine deaminase
  - Low complete response rate
- Interferon-α
  - Complete response rate 8 percent; 74 percent achieve a partial response
  - Not curative, 50 percent relapse less than 2 years after treatment.
  - Dosage schedule is 2 to 3 × 10⁶ U IFN-α/m² subcutaneously 3 times weekly for 6 to 24 months.
  - Not as effective as purine analogs.
- Splenectomy
  - Previously the treatment of choice
  - Not curative
  - Current indications:
    - massive, painful, and/or ruptured spleen
    - pancytopenia and an active infection with opportunistic pathogen (e.g., mycobacterium), that precludes immediate use of systemic chemotherapy
    - failure of systemic chemotherapy
- G-CSF
  - ameliorates neutropenia
  - adjunct to therapy

CLINICAL COURSE

- Previously median survival was 4 years.
- With improved systemic treatment, now considered curable.

For a more detailed discussion, see Thomas J. Kipps, Bruce A. Robbins: Hairy cell leukemia, Chap. 107, p. 1040, in *Williams Hematology,* 5/e, 1995.

---

57 LARGE GRANULAR LYMPHOCYTE (LGL) LEUKEMIA

DEFINITION

- T-cell large granular lymphocyte (T-LGL) leukemia is a clonal expansion of LGL with a T-cell (CD3 +) phenotype.
- Natural killer (NK)-LGL leukemia is a clonal expansion of LGL with a natural killer cell (CD3 −) phenotype.

T-LGL LEUKEMIA

Etiology

- Suggestive evidence for a role for HTLV-I/II retroviral infection in some patients.

Clinical Features

- Recurrent bacterial infections frequent.
- Splenomegaly in about one-half of patients.
- Rheumatoid arthritis that may resemble Felty syndrome in about one-quarter.

Laboratory Features

- Neutropenia, often severe.
- Anemia, thrombocytopenia less common.
- Median LGL count 4200/μl (normal: 223 ± 99/μl).
- Bone marrow infiltration in about 90 percent of patients.
- Marrow infiltration may be nodular or interstitial. If interstitial involvement, may be difficult to appreciate unless immunostaining procedures are performed.
- Serologic abnormalities:
  - positive rheumatoid factor, antinuclear antibody tests
  - polyclonal hypergammaglobulinemia
  - circulating immune complexes
- Splenic red pulp cord infiltration by leukemic LGL.
- Clonal T-cell-receptor gene rearrangement.
- Immunophenotype: CD3 +, CD8 +, CD16 +, CD56 −, CD57 +

Clinical Course

- Chronic.
- Significant morbidity/mortality from infections.
- Low-dose methotrexate 10 mg/m^2 orally once weekly or cyclophosphamide 100 mg PO daily may be effective in alleviating neutropenia/anemia.

NK-LGL LEUKEMIA

Etiology

- Molecular studies suggest a direct role for EBV in pathogenesis.

Clinical Features

- Fever, night sweats, weight loss are common.
- Massive hepatosplenomegaly typical.
- Lymphadenopathy common.

Laboratory Features

- LGL counts high, may exceed $50,000/\mu l$.
- Severe neutropenia not common.
- Anemia and thrombocytopenia very common.
- Coagulopathy frequently occurs.
- Immunophenotyping: CD3−, CD8+, CD16+, CD56+, CD57−.
- Clonal cytogenetics.

Clinical Course

- Acute presentation, aggressive course.
- Effective combination chemotherapy not reported.

For a more detailed discussion, see Thomas P. Loughran, Marshall E. Kadin: Large granular lymphocyte leukemia, Chap. 108, p. 1047, in *Williams Hematology,* 5/e, 1995.

58 HODGKIN DISEASE

DEFINITION

- Neoplasm of lymphoid tissue defined histophatologically by Reed-Sternberg cells in an appropriate cellular background.
- Four subgroups:

  (1) Lymphocyte predominant
  (2) Mixed cellularity
  (3) Nodular sclerosing
  (4) Lymphocyte depleted

ETIOLOGY AND PATHOGENESIS

- Cellular origin of Reed-Sternberg cells unknown. May be activated B or T lymphocytes.
- Reed-Sternberg cells are CD30 +, CD15 +, CD25 +.
- Nodular lymphocyte predominant a distinct type:
  - Reed-Sternberg cells are of B-cell origin; are CD20 +, lack CD15 and variably express CD30.
  - They also synthesize cytoplasmic immunoglobulin.
- EBV
  - 18 to 50 percent of patients are EBV-positive by in situ hybridization.
- Cytokine secretion may determine histologic picture:
  - TGF-β stimulates fibroblast proliferation
  - IL-5 growth factor for eosinophils
  - IL-1, IL-6, IL-9, TNFα, G-CSF, M-CSF secreted by Reed-Sternberg cells
- Immunologic dysfunction
  - All patients have multiple abnormalities of cellular immunity.
  - Some defects persist after successful treatment.

EPIDEMIOLOGY

- 7900 cases per year in the United States.
- Bimodal age distribution: peaks in the third decade and increases after age 45.
  - Nodular sclerosis predominates in young adults.
  - Mixed cellularity predominates in older ages.
- Incidence appears to be influenced by socioeconomic and environmental factors.
- Infectious etiology is suggested by evidence that serologically confirmed mononucleosis confers a three-fold risk for Hodgkin disease in young adults.
- Concept of a genetic basis supported by data showing increased risk among siblings and close relatives.

CLINICAL FEATURES

- Usual presentation is with painless lymph node enlargement.
- Constitutional symptoms may be present:
  - "B" symptoms: fever above 38°, drenching night sweats, and weight loss of more than 10 percent of baseline body weight
  - Pel-Ebstein fever: high fevers for 1 to 2 weeks alternating with afebrile periods of similar length—virtually diagnostic of Hodgkin disease
- Pruritus is not prognostically significant.
- Intrathoracic disease is present at diagnosis in 67 percent of patients.
  - Mediastinal adenopathy is common.
- Clinicopathologic correlation:
  - Lymphocyte predominance in 10 percent of patients
    - Stage I disease in 70 percent
    - Axillary nodes particularly involved
  - Nodular sclerosis in 40 to 70 percent of patients
    - Distinctive histopathology featuring the lacunar cell, a RS variant
    - In young females, frequent involvement in lower cervical, supraclavicular, and mediastinal lymph nodes
    - 70 percent have limited stage disease (see below)
  - Mixed cellularity in 30 to 50 percent of patients
    - Advanced stage disease common in both pediatric and older age groups
    - Strong association with prior EBV infection
  - Lymphocyte depleted is least frequent type
    - Patients are older and have extensive disease
    - Systemic symptoms frequent
- Staging (see Tables 58-1 and 58-2)
  - Staging laparotomy limited to patients who are candidates for management with radiotherapy only.

THERAPY COURSE AND PROGNOSIS

- Radiotherapy
  - Usual doses:
    - involved field: 4000 to 4400 cGy at 150 to 200 cGy per fraction
    - uninvolved fields (prophylactic) 3000 to 3500 cGy
  - Definition of fields:
    - mantle: cervical, supraclavicular, infraclavicular, axillary, mediastinal, and hilar nodes
    - paraaortic includes spleen or splenic pedicle
    - mantle plus paraaortic = subtotal lymphoid irradiation
    - paraaortic plus pelvic = inverted Y
    - mantle plus inverted Y = total lymphoid irradiation
- Chemotherapy
  - MOPP

TABLE 58-1 Ann Arbor Staging Classification*

Stage	Definition
I	Involvement of a single lymph node region (I) or of a single extralymphatic organ or site (I_E)
II	Involvement of two or more lymph node regions on the same side of the diaphragm (II) or localized involvement of an extra-lymphatic organ or site and of one or more lymph node regions on the same side of the diaphragm (II_E)
III	Involvement of lymph node regions on both sides of the dia-phragm (III), which may also be accompanied by involvement of the spleen (III_S) or by localized involvement of an extralym-phatic organ or site (III_E) or both (III_{SE})
IV	Diffuse or disseminated involvement of one or more extralym-phatic organs or tissues, with or without associated lymph node involvement

The absence or presence of fever, night sweats and/or unexplained loss of 10 percent or more of body weight in the 6 months preceding diagnosis are to be denoted in all cases by the suffix letters A or B, respectively.

*Adopted at the Workshop on the Staging of Hodgkin Disease held at Ann Arbor, Michigan, in April 1971.
Source: Table 110-1 of *Williams Hematology*, 5/e, p. 1063.

- 54 percent of 188 original patients with advanced disease alive and disease free after 20 years.
- ABVD
  - at least as effective as MOPP for primary therapy
  - effective for MOPP failures
  - often used together with MOPP in alternating or "hybrid" regimens
- Favorable, limited stage disease
  - Stage IA/IB or stage IIA supradiaphragmatic disease with no bulky sites and none or only one extranodal site.
  - Extended field (subtotal lymphoid) irradiation treatment of choice: 80 percent disease free survival at 15 years.
  - Combination chemotherapy also curative in 75 to 80 percent.
  - Management of stage IIB is controversial.
- Locally extensive, limited stage disease
  - Extensive mediastinal disease (greater than one-third of thoracic diameter) needs combined modality therapy: 80 percent disease-free survival compared to 50 percent with radiotherapy alone.
- Advanced disease
  - Optimal therapy for stage IIIA has been debated:
    - Radiotherapy requires total nodal irradiation.
    - Systemic chemotherapy is preferable.
  - Optimal chemotherapy is also debatable: MOPP vs. ABVD vs. MOPP/ABVD hybrids.

TABLE 58-2 Recommended Staging Procedures

All patients

Adequate surgical biopsy, reviewed by a hematopathologist

History with attention to B symptoms, pruritus, alcohol-intolerance, bone pain

Physical examination with attention to inspection of the thorax, palpation for lymphadenopathy, organomegaly, and bone tenderness

Laboratory evaluation: complete blood count, erythrocyte sedimentation rate, chemistry panel

Radiographic studies: posteroanterior and lateral chest x-ray, CT of the chest, abdomen and pelvis, bipedal lymphoangiogram

Bone marrow biopsy

Selected patients

Immunohistochemistry as needed for pathologic diagnosis

Bone scan and skeletal radiographs if bone pain or tenderness

MRI for suspected epidural disease

Exploratory laparatomy and splenectomy after assessment of risk of subdiaphragmatic disease, if radiotherapy alone is preferred management

[67]Gallium scanning may be useful to assess residual disease, especially bulky mediastinal disease

Source: Table 110-2 of *Williams Hematology*, 5/e, p. 1064.

- Treatment of recurrent disease
  - Relapse after radiotherapy: chemotherapy results in an excellent rate of cure.
  - Autologous marrow or peripheral blood stem cell transplantation is the treatment of choice for patients who fail primary induction or who relapse after chemotherapy.
- Complications of treatment
  - Secondary malignancies: AML or myelodysplasia occurs in 1 to 10 percent of patients over 10 years. The risk is proportional to cumulative dose of alkylating agents.
  - Increased risk of lymphoma, usually diffuse, aggressive, B-cell.
  - Increased risk of development of solid cancer: 18 percent at 15 years.
    - Related to radiotherapy exposure.
    - Site most often lung, stomach, bone, soft-tissue.
  - Cardiac disease may occur in recipients of mediastinal irradiation.
  - Infertility frequent after MOPP chemotherapy.
  - Radiation pneumonitis may occur depending on dose received by lung.
  - Thyroid function abnormalities in about 30 percent of patients following mantle treatment.

For a more detailed discussion, see Sandra J. Horning: Hodgkin disease, Chap. 110, p. 1057, in *Williams Hematology*, 5/e, 1995.

59 LYMPHOMAS

DEFINITION

- Solid neoplasms of the immune system (B- or T-cell), usually arising in lymph nodes.
- Currently classified according to the "Working Formulation," but new variants have been recognized (Fig. 59-1) and classification remains in flux.

ETIOLOGY AND PATHOGENESIS

- 4 percent of all cancers in the United States.
- Preadolescent peak in incidence, with a logarithmic increase with age.
- EBV implicated in etiology: 95 percent of endemic form of Burkitt's have EBV; 20 percent of nonendemic form. Inherited or acquired immunodeficiency patients also have EBV.

CLINICAL AND LABORATORY FEATURES

- Systemic symptoms (fatigue, fever, night sweats, weight loss) may occur.
- Lymph node enlargement may occur. Nodes are nontender, firm, rubbery.
- Oropharyngeal lymphoid tissue (Waldeyer's ring) may be involved.
- Extranodal involvement possible in aggressive forms.
- Evaluate for cytopenias of autoimmune etiology.
- Excisional lymph node biopsy: formalin and frozen sections.
- Staging workup (Table 59-1).
- Prognosis: poorer with
  - B symptoms: night sweats, fever, weight loss (10 percent in preceding 6 months)
  - high grade histologic subtype, best with low grade, intermediate in between
  - age > 60
  - extranodal disease
  - bulk disease (>10 cm)
  - increased levels of serum lactic dehydrogenase
- Extranodal lymphoma
  - CNS involvement in 5 to 10 percent of patients. High incidence of associated marrow involvement. Usually have aggressive histology. Presentations may be spinal cord compression, leptomeningeal spread, intracerebral mass lesions.
  - Skin: most often involved with cutaneous T-cell lymphoma and adult T-cell leukemia/lymphoma (ATL) or with anaplastic large cell lymphoma.
  - Lung involvement usually due to lymphatic spread from hilar/mediastinal nodes.

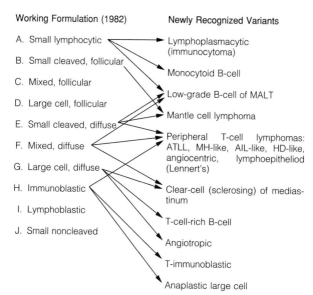

Working Formulation (1982)   Newly Recognized Variants

A. Small lymphocytic

B. Small cleaved, follicular

C. Mixed, follicular

D. Large cell, follicular

E. Small cleaved, diffuse

F. Mixed, diffuse

G. Large cell, diffuse

H. Immunoblastic

I. Lymphoblastic

J. Small noncleaved

Lymphoplasmacytic (immunocytoma)

Monocytoid B-cell

Low-grade B-cell of MALT

Mantle cell lymphoma

Peripheral T-cell lymphomas: ATLL, MH-like, AIL-like, HD-like, angiocentric, lymphoepitheliod (Lennert's)

Clear-cell (sclerosing) of mediastinum

T-cell-rich B-cell

Angiotropic

T-immunoblastic

Anaplastic large cell

FIG. 59-1 Newly recognized distinct variants of certain lymphomas (right column) are related to types in the Working Formulation (left column). The following abbreviations are used: AIL, angioimmunoblastic lymphoma; ATLL, adult T-cell leukemia/lymphoma; HD-like, Hodgkin disease-like; MALT, mucosa-associated lymphoid tissue; and MH, malignant histiocytosis. *(From Fig. 109-1 in* Williams Hematology, *5/e, 1955.)*

- Gastrointestinal tract involved in 15 percent of patients with lymphoma, usually if Waldeyer's ring also affected.
- Liver: portal tract infiltration occurs with low-grade lymphoma. Mass lesions seen with aggressive lymphoma.
- Marrow involvement common in low-grade lymphoma (follicular or small lymphoma) and in high-grade lymphoma (lymphoblastic or small noncleaved lymphoma).

LOW-GRADE LYMPHOMAS

- Small lymphocytic lymphoma
  - 5 to 10 percent of lymphomas, almost all of B-cell origin.
  - Features analogous to CLL include: surface Ig, immunoglobulin gene rearrangement, CD5+, pan-B-cell antigen positive (CD19, CD20).
  - Indolent progression, but with eventual marrow involvement.

TABLE 59-1 Staging Procedures for Lymphoma

Initial studies

History and physical examination
Pathologic diagnosis
Laboratory studies
    Blood chemistries and complete blood counts
    Bilateral posterior iliac crest marrow biopsies
Chest roentgenogram (CT if x-ray is suspicious)
CT scan of abdomen and pelvis

Subsequent studies

Ultrasonography and MRI to clarify abnormalities
Gallium scan (particularly useful to follow large masses)
Lumbar puncture if neurologic signs or symptoms or aggressive lymphoma with marrow involvement
Gastrointestinal studies if Waldeyer's ring involvement
CT or MRI of brain if neurologic signs or symptoms
Immunoglobulin and T-cell-receptor gene rearrangement studies
Polymerase chain reaction for *BCL*-1 and *BCL*-2
Flow cytometry
Immunohistochemistry
Cytogenetics

*Adapted from Table 111-1 in *Williams Hematology*, 5/e, p. 1077.

- <1 percent of T-cell origin: aggressive, inv(14)(q11;q32).
- Mucosa-associated lymphoid tissue lymphoma (MALT)
  - Hallmark is tumor cell infiltration with the formation of lymphoepithelial lesions.
  - Stomach, small intestine, lung, salivary glands, thyroid most frequently involved.
  - Indolent, local symptoms predominate.
  - Abnormal karyotypes: rearrangements of chromosome 1p; numerical abnormalities of chromosomes 3 and 7.
  - Cells are CD19 +, CD20 +, CD5 −.
  - Immunoglobulin gene rearrangement occurs.
- Monocytoid B-cell lymphoma
  - Usually disease localized to head and neck and parotid gland.
  - 15 percent of patients have Sjögren syndrome.
  - Similar to MALT immunophenotypically.
- Follicular lymphomas
  - Include follicular, small cleaved, and follicular, mixed.
  - Mature B-cell neoplasms of germinal cell origin which express monoclonal surface immunoglobulins, CD19 +, CD20 +.
  - Cells differ from CLL in that they are CD5 −, CD10 (cALLa) +.
  - Widespread at diagnosis (lymph nodes, marrow, liver, and spleen), but indolent course.

- 90 percent have t(14;18)(q32;q21) with increased expression of *BCL*-2 protein and possible inhibition of apoptosis.
- May transform to large cell lymphoma.

INTERMEDIATE-GRADE LYMPHOMAS

- Follicular, large cell
  - Mature B cells of germinal cell origin
- Diffuse, small cleaved cell
  - Counterpart of follicular, small cleaved
  - Most correspond to mantle cell lymphoma (see below)
- Mantle cell lymphoma (intermediate lymphocytic lymphoma)
  - 2 to 8 percent of all lymphomas
  - Patients are predominantly male; median age 60.
  - Generalized lymphadenopathy, hepatosplenomegaly, marrow, gastrointestinal involvement are common.
  - Comprised of small, cleaved B lymphocytes expressing C19+, CD20+, surface IgM+, and CD5+.
  - 50 percent have t(11;14)(q13;q32) causing *BCL*-1 rearrangement with overexpression of *PRAD1*/cyclin D1 gene in all cases tested.
- Diffuse, mixed small and large cell
  - Phenotypically heterogeneous: may be of B- or T-cell origin although morphologically indistinguishable.
- Diffuse, large cell
  - Heterogeneous cellular origin.
  - B-cell type of germinal cell origin
  - 20 percent of T-cell origin, morphologically indistinguishable from B-cell type
- T-cell–rich B-cell lymphoma
  - B-cell lymphoma with a predominance of reactive polyclonal T cells

HIGH-GRADE LYMPHOMAS

- Large cell, immunoblastic
  - B-cell type: plasmacytoid, CD19−, CD20−
  - T-cell type: abundant clear cytoplasm
- Lymphoblastic
  - Most common lymphoma in children.
  - Clinically and histologically related to ALL (FAB types L1 and L2).
  - Most of precursor T-cell origin, TdT+ (only lymphoma which is TdT+).
  - No detectable neoplastic cells in blood.
  - Most patients have mediastinal involvement.
- Small, noncleaved cell: Burkitt and non-Burkitt types
  - Burkitt *endemic* (African) type: occurs predominantly in male chil-

dren (5 to 10 years old); EBV implicated in 95 percent of patients. Maxilla, mandible, abdomen, and extranodal sites are affected.

- Burkitt *sporadic* type: occurs predominantly in males. EBV implicated in 20 percent of patients. Often associated with HIV infection. 9 percent have abdominal disease.
- All Burkitt types are composed of mature B cells and have immunoglobulin gene rearrangement.
- Nearly all Burkitt lymphomas have c-*MYC* translocations:
  - 75 percent have t(8;14)(q24;q32), involving c-*MYC* and the Ig heavy chain locus.
  - 25 percent have t(2;8)(q13;q24) or t(8;22)(q24;q11), involving c-*MYC* and the kappa or lambda light chain locus.
  - Malignant cells are in the blood are similar to those in ALL FAB type L3.
  - "Starry sky" appearance histologically.
- Non-Burkitt type
  - Usually occurs in adults.
  - Lymph node involvement typical, abdominal disease less frequent than in Burkitt type.
  - Cells are of mature B-cell origin.
  - t(14;18): *BCL*-2 rearrangement found in some cases.

THERAPY, COURSE, PROGNOSIS

Low-Grade Lymphoma

- Small lymphocytic lymphoma
  - Treatment is similar to CLL; not curative.
  - Initial therapy with chlorambucil; second line agents are fludarabine, 2-chlorodeoxyadenosine.
- MALT and monocytoid B-cell lymphoma
  - Local disease: treatment with surgery or radiation therapy may be curative.
  - Disseminated disease treated with alkylating agents.
- Follicular small cleaved cell lymphoma
  - Less than 20 percent are stage I/II: radiation therapy curative in 50 to 75 percent.
  - Stage III/IV treatment not curative, may "watch and wait."
  - Standard treatment is with alkylating agents (e.g., cyclophosphamide).
  - Autologous marrow transplantation being evaluated as a potentially curative modality.
- Follicular mixed lymphoma
  - 20 to 40 percent of patients with stage III/IV may be cured with CHOP regimen.
  - Autologous marrow transplantation is used for relapsed disease.

INTERMEDIATE- AND HIGH-GRADE LYMPHOMA

- All categories are treated similarly, except for lymphoblastic and Burkitt type.
- Early stage disease [stage I/II (nonbulky)]
  - 80 percent can be cured with CHOP.
  - Role of radiation therapy is uncertain.
- Advanced disease [stage II (bulky) or stage III/IV]
  - Long-term survival is one-third with CHOP.
  - More intensive regimens are equivalent to CHOP in terms of curability but are more toxic.
- Mantle cell lymphoma
  - No standard therapy.
  - Treatment is not curative.
- Lymphoblastic lymphoma
  - Regimens used for diffuse large cell lymphoma are inadequate.
  - ALL-type therapy required.
  - Because propensity for CNS involvement is similar to that in ALL CNS prophylaxis is needed.
- Small noncleaved cell lymphoma
  - Non-Burkitt type treated similarly to diffuse large cell.
  - Burkitt type needs CNS prophylaxis. Tumor-lysis syndrome precautions required.

RELAPSED OR REFRACTORY LYMPHOMA

- Chemotherapy is not curative.
- Autologous marrow transplantation employed if disease is still chemotherapy sensitive; 20 to 40 percent of patients achieve long-term, disease-free survival.

IMMUNOTHERAPY OF LYMPHOMA

- α-Interferon
  - Partial responses seen in patients with follicular small cleaved or mixed cell lymphoma.
  - Improved 5-year disease-free survival in low-grade lymphomas treated with chemotherapy plus interferon compared to chemotherapy alone.
- Anti-idiotype therapy
  - Anti-idiotype antibodies recognize a "tumor-specific" antigen.
  - Response obtained in 50 percent of patients with low-grade lymphoma.
  - Treatment is expensive, requiring generation of a unique antibody for each patient.
- Radioimmunotherapy
  - Radiolabelled monoclonal antibodies are being evaluated.

- Hematologic toxicity may require autologous marrow cell infusion.
- Immunotoxin
  - "Immunotoxins" are tumor-specific monoclonal antibodies conjugated to a toxin, such as ricin. This therapy is under evaluation.

MALIGNANT LYMPHOMAS OF T-CELL LINEAGE

Adult T-cell Leukemia/Lymphoma (ATL)

- Definition and history
  - Identified in Japan in 1977, later in the United States and the Caribbean.
- Etiology and pathogenesis
  - Linked to HTLV-I infection.
- Clinical features
  - Onset is acute.
  - Cutaneous lesions develop rapidly. May be tumors, nodules, plaques, papules, erythroderma.
  - Hypercalcemia is common and typically symptomatic.
  - Lymphadenopathy occurs in all, generalized in many, retroperitoneal in most.
  - Lung, liver, gastrointestinal tract, CNS frequently involved.
  - Opportunistic infections are common.
- Laboratory features
  - Pleomorphic lymphoid cells in the blood, with elevated WBC.
  - Malignant T cells are CD4 +, CD25 +.
- Hypercalcemia
- Therapy, course, and prognosis
  - Chemotherapy induces remission but is not curative for ATL.
  - "Smoldering ATL" more indolent with long survival without therapy.

Cutaneous T-Cell Lymphoma

- Definition and history
  - Consists of mycosis fungoides and Sézary syndrome.
  - 1500 cases per year in the United States.
  - CD4 + T cells.
- Etiology and pathogenesis
  - Role of HTLV-I (deleted variants) is under investigation.
- Clinical features
  - Epidermotrophic malignant infiltrate.
  - Epidermal clusters of convoluted cells—Pautrier microabscess.
  - Stages of skin involvement (Table 59-2) include limited plaque, generalized plaque, cutaneous tumor, and generalized erythroderma.
  - Lymphadenopathy found in 50 percent of patients.

TABLE 59-2 Survival by Skin Stage of Patients with Cutaneous T-Cell Lymphoma*

Skin stage	Mean survival, y	5-year survival, %
Limited plaque (T1)	>9	90
Generalized plaque (T2)	>7	70
Cutaneous tumor (T3)	2.5	35
Generalized erythroderma (T4)	3.5	40

*Adapted from Table 111-10 in *Williams Hematology*, 5/e, p. 1089.

- Laboratory features
  - T cells are CD4+, CD25−.
  - Mycosis fungoides cells CD7+, but not Sézary cells.
- Therapy, course, and prognosis
  - Therapeutic modalities produce remission in most patients, but cure is uncommon.
  - Topical nitrogen mustard: for early cutaneous disease, nontoxic, not curative.
  - Psoralin: 60 percent complete remission rate reported; not curative.
  - Electron-beam therapy: 80 percent complete remission rate; 20 percent disease-free at 3 years; 4 Gy/wk (total dose 36 Gy).
  - Chemotherapy: combination therapy produces 25 percent complete responses.
  - Prognosis: median survival after diagnosis is 10 years, but lymph node involvement signifies a poorer prognosis, and visceral involvement indicates poorest prognosis with median survival of less than 1 year.

Lennert Lymphoma

- Lymphoepithelial lymphoma with a multifocal epithelial histiocytic reaction.
- Neoplastic cells are mature T cells with T-cell–receptor gene rearrangement.
- Usually categorized as diffuse mixed in the Working Formulation.
- Disease usually disseminated, involving lung, spleen, lymph nodes, and marrow.

Anaplastic Large Cell Lymphoma

- Ki-1 lymphoma (CD30+).
- In the Working Formulation, usually classified as high-grade, large cell, immunoblastic.
- Incidence peaks in 3d and 7th decades.
- Lymphadenopathy: extranodal disease common, particularly in the skin.
- Usually T-cell lineage.

- t(2;5)(p23;q35) characteristic, involves a new tyrosine kinase gene.
- Histologically may be confused with carcinoma or Hodgkin disease, commonly express epithelial membrane antigen and CD45 (unlike Hodgkin).

Angiocentric Immunoproliferative Lesions

- Previously termed polymorphic reticulosis or lymphomatoid granulomatosis.
- Composed of atypical lymphoid cells with blood vessel destruction.
- Surface expression of T-cell antigens but usually not T-cell–receptor gene rearrangement.

ANGIOIMMUNOBLASTIC LYMPHADENOPATHY-LIKE LYMPHOMA

- Usually occurs in elderly patients.
- Clinical features are systemic symptoms, generalized lymphadenopathy, hepatosplenomegaly, and pruritic skin rash.
- Laboratory findings include polyclonal hypergammaglobulinemia, Coombs-positive hemolytic anemia, and eosinophilia.
- Histologically the hallmark is arborizing proliferation of small blood vessels and absence of lymphoid follicles.
- About 30 percent develop diffuse mixed or large cell immunoblastic lymphoma.

For a more detailed discussion, see Kenneth A. Foon, Richard I. Fisher: Lymphomas, Chap. 111, p. 1076, in *Williams Hematology,* 5/e, 1995.

60 PLASMA CELL NEOPLASMS: GENERAL CONSIDERATIONS AND ESSENTIAL AND SECONDARY MONOCLONAL GAMMOPATHIES

Plasma cell dyscrasias arise when a single B cell is transformed and continues to multiply and differentiate. All the progeny of the transformed B cell produce the identical whole immunoglobulin chain or chain fragment, which is evidence for monoclonality. The monoclonal protein product of this population of cells is called an *M protein*. The monoclonal B cell population may retain the ability to develop into morphologically normal-appearing plasma cells. Clinical situations characterized by the occurrence of an M protein may be malignant or nonmalignant.

LABORATORY EVALUATION OF M PROTEINS AND PLASMA CELL DYSCRASIAS

Zonal Electrophoresis

Serum Protein Electrophoresis

- A common screening test for an M protein depends on the rate of migration of proteins in an electric field.
- Molecules of each M protein have identical size and charge and thus migrate as a narrow band.
- Electrophoresis can be done on concentrated samples of urine and cerebrospinal fluid:
  - Commercial dipsticks do not detect urine free light chains, i.e., Bence Jones proteins.
  - Sulfosalicylic acid can be used to detect urine free light chains.

Immunoelectrophoresis and Immunofixation Electrophoresis

- Used to identify the exact heavy chain class and light chain type(s) in M proteins.

Analysis for Immunoglobulin Gene Rearrangements

- Specific technique to determine if a B-cell disorder is monoclonal.
- Very useful if the cells do not secrete M proteins into the serum.

Quantitative Immunoglobulin Assays

- Can be done on serum, urine, or CSF.

Serum β_2 Microglobulin (β_2M)

- β_2M is the light chain of class I HLA molecules located on the cell membranes of all nucleated cells.

- $\beta_2 M$ dissociates from cell membranes and is filtered by the glomerulus and reabsorbed in the renal tubules.
- Serum levels of $\beta_2 M$ rise in B-cell neoplasms because of increased neoplastic cell turnover.
- Serum $\beta_2 M$ levels also rise in renal dysfunction.

Serum Viscosity

- IgM and IgA M proteins most commonly form multimers and elevate the serum viscosity.
- Some IgG molecules, especially IgG_3, can increase the serum viscosity.
- The relative viscosity of normal serum in relation to distilled water is 1.8.

ESSENTIAL AND SECONDARY MONOCLONAL GAMMOPATHIES

- Monoclonal proteins that do not arise in association with B-cell or plasma-cell neoplasms may occur in the absence of associated disorders (essential monoclonal gammopathy) or in association with other disorders (secondary monoclonal gammopathy).
- A classification of monoclonal gammopathies is presented in Table 60-1.
- Monoclonal gammopathies can occur at any age. The frequency increases with age and reaches about 3 percent in people over age 70.
- The prevalence is greater among African Americans than among Caucasians.

Pathogenesis

- Caused by proliferation of a single B cell or plasma cell resulting in a population that reaches a steady state of $<1 \times 10^{11}$ cells.
- There is no bone marrow plasmacytosis as there is in multiple myeloma.
- Monoclonal gammopathy occurring in association with carcinoma is thought to be coincidental.

Clinical Features

- Usually there are no signs or symptoms related to the monoclonal cell population.
- In some patients, the monoclonal protein acts as an autoantibody and causes clinical disease, such as hemolytic anemia or acquired von Willebrand disease.
- Neuropathies with both sensory and motor involvement may occur with monoclonal gammopathies.

TABLE 60-1 Types of Benign Monoclonal Gammopathy

Essential asymptomatic monoclonal gammopathy
Types of Ig synthesized by abnormal cell clones
  Monoclonal: IgG, IgA, IgM, IgE, or IgD
  Biclonal: IgG + IgA, IgG + IgM; triclonal: IgG + IgA + IgM
  Monoclonal κ and λ light chain (Bence Jones proteinuria)

Essential symptomatic monoclonal gammopathy
Plasma protein disturbances: acquired von Willebrand disease, antierythrocyte antibodies, cryoglobulinemia, cryofibrinogenemia, acquired C1 esterase inhibitor deficiency (angioedema), acquired antithrombin, antiinsulin antibodies, antiacetylcholine receptor
Neuropathies
Renal disease

Secondary monoclonal gammopathy
Types of disease coincident with monoclonal gammopathy
  Connective tissue diseases and autoimmune diseases: e.g., rheumatoid arthritis, Crohn disease, polymyalgia rheumatica, lupus erythematosus, scleroderma, Sjögren disease, psoriatic arthritis, pernicious anemia, Hashimoto thyroiditis, myasthenia gravis
  Cutaneous diseases: e.g., pyoderma gangrenosum, psoriasis, scleromyxedema, urticaria
  Endocrine diseases: e.g., hyperparathyroidism
  Gaucher disease
  Hepatic disease: e.g., hepatitis, cirrhosis
  Infectious diseases: e.g., *Mycobacterium tuberculosis, Corynebacterium* sp., cytomegalovirus, bacterial endocarditis, purpura fulminans, AIDS
  Neoplasms of other than B cells or plasma cells
    Carcinomas: e.g., colon, lung, prostate, others
    Myeloproliferative disease: e.g., acute and chronic myelogenous leukemia, polycythemia vera, neutropenia
    T-cell lymphomas: e.g., Sézary syndrome
  After chemotherapy, radiotherapy, or marrow transplantation
  Miscellaneous diseases
    Transient and miniclonal, oligoclonal, and monoclonal immunoglobulins
    Factitious hyperferremia

Source: Adapted from Table 113-1 of *Williams Hematology*, 5/e, p. 1104.

- Secondary monoclonal gammopathies occur in a variety of diseases (Table 60-1).

Laboratory Features

- The monoclonal protein is usually IgG, but may be IgM, IgA, IgD, IgE, free urinary light chains, or bi- or triclonal gammopathy.
- In IgG monoclonal gammopathy, the concentration of M protein is usually less than 3.0 g/dl and in IgA and IgM, less than 2.5 g/dl, but there are significant exceptions to this rule.
- Features of a malignant process are absent.

- Patients with monoclonal gammopathy usually have normal poly-clonal immunoglobulin levels as opposed to patients with myeloma or macroglobulinemia.
- In essential monoclonal gammopathies
  - marrow plasma cell count is usually (<5 percent)
  - plasma cell labelling index is low (<1 percent)
  - blood T-lymphocyte subsets are normal
  - B$_2$M is not elevated

OLIGOCLONAL AND MONOCLONAL IMMUNOGLOBULINS

- Detected by high-resolution electrophoresis in patients with acute-phase reactants or polyclonal hyperglobulinemia.
  - Oligoclonal immunoglobulins are frequent in the CSF of patients with neurologic conditions, e.g., multiple sclerosis.
  - Serum oligoclonal or monoclonal immunoglobulins occur frequently in patients with AIDS.

COURSE, PROGNOSIS, AND THERAPY

- Patterns of outcome in patients with essential monoclonal gammopathy:
  - 25 percent of patients do not progress to overt multiple myeloma or macroglobulinemia, although the protein levels may rise with time.
  - 50 percent of patients die of unrelated causes.
  - 25 percent of patients progress to develop myeloma, macroglobulinemia, or lymphoma in 15 to 20 years.
  - Rarely the monoclonal protein disappears spontaneously.
- Periodic reevaluation is required to determine the clinical course.
- Therapy is generally not required for essential monoclonal gammopathy unless the monoclonal protein impairs the function of a normal plasma or tissue constituent.

For a more detailed discussion, see Stephen M. Baird: Plasma cell neoplasms: general considerations, Chap. 112, p. 1097; and Marshall A. Lichtman: Essential and secondary monoclonal gammopathies, Chap. 113, p. 1104, in *Williams Hematology,* 5/e, 1995.

61 PLASMA CELL MYELOMA

Plasma cell myeloma (multiple myeloma) is a disease of malignant plasma cells that synthesize monoclonal immunoglobulins or immuno-globulin fragments (M proteins).

ETIOLOGY AND PATHOGENESIS

- Environmental radiation and chemical exposure are associated with an increased incidence of myeloma.
- Cytogenetic and oncogene abnormalities occur in a high percentage of patients with myeloma.
  - DNA hyperdiploidy in 70 percent of patients
  - *BCL-1* and *BCL-2* gene rearrangements (15 to 20 percent of patients) and strong expression of the *BCL-2* protein
  - c-*MYC* RNA and protein overexpression (80 percent of patients)
  - *N-RAS* mutations (50 percent of patients)
  - mutations and deletions in the retinoblastoma and the p53 tumor suppressor genes in malignant plasma cells
  - multidrug resistance (MDR) gene in myeloma cells, even prior to therapy
- Cytokines are involved in the pathogenesis of myeloma:
  - IL-6 may act as an autocrine growth factor in myeloma.
  - IL-1 and TNF-β expression by myeloma cells may promote resistance of myeloma cells to treatment and cause the osteolytic bone disease in myeloma.
  - Contact with marrow stromal cells appears to be required for the complete expression of the malignant repertoire of myeloma cells.

CLINICAL FEATURES

- Pain resulting from
  - vertebral compression fractures and/or osteolytic bone lesions
  - tumor growth on nerve roots or spinal cord compression
  - amyloid (AL) deposits in various sites
- Infections
  - Bacterial, viral, or parasitic infections occur frequently because of defects in cell-mediated immunity and the humoral immune response.
- Nephropathy may develop from several causes.
  - Interstitial nephritis occurs because of deposition of light chains, usually κ, in the kidney.
  - Hypercalcemia and hypercalciuria lead to polyuria, dehydration, and prerenal azotemia.
  - Nephrotic syndrome may develop due to AL amyloidosis associated with light-chain proteinuria, usually λ light chain.
- Neuropathies
  - Nerve or spinal cord compression by tumor.

285

- Perineuronal or perivascular amyloid deposition may produce poly-neuropathies.
- Polyneuropathy may be part of the POEMS syndrome (polyneuropa-thy, organomegaly, endocrinopathy, monoclonal gammopathy, and skin changes).
- Extramedullary disease may be
  - plasma cell leukemia, often with leukemic meningitis
  - visceral organ (lymph nodes, liver, spleen, kidneys) infiltration associated with plasmablast morphology and high serum LDH activity
- Hyperviscosity occurs in <10 percent of myeloma patients and is more likely to occur with IgA myeloma than IgG. It sometimes occurs with IgG_3. (See Chap. 62.)
- Bleeding occurs in 15 percent of patients with IgG myeloma and 30 percent of patients with IgA myeloma, possibly due to anoxia and thrombosis in small capillaries, perivascular amyloid deposits, or acquired coagulopathy.
- Thrombosis due to a hypercoagulable state because of acquired protein C deficiency or a lupus anticoagulant.

LABORATORY FEATURES

- Initial evaluation requires a complete blood count, review of periph-eral blood film for rouleaux, and measurements of serum concentra-tions of electrolytes, BUN, creatinine, calcium, lactate dehydrogenase, β_2-microglobulin, serum protein electrophoresis, urinary protein ex-cretion, and marrow aspiration and biopsy. The axial skeleton should also be examined radiographically.
- Hematologic abnormalities include
  - Anemia due to marrow replacement by plasma cells and blunted response to erythropoietin.
  - Thrombocytopenia is often therapy related, and is unusual in un-treated patients, early in the disease.
  - Coagulopathy may be due to interference with fibrin formation by M proteins, acquired inhibitors of coagulation factors, e.g., factor VIII deficiency, or factor X deficiency due to AL amyloidosis.
- Detection of monoclonal immunoglobulin (see also Chap. 60).
  - M proteins in multiple myeloma are
    - 60 percent IgG
    - 20 percent IgA
    - 20 percent light chain only
    - very rarely, IgM, IgD, IgE, or more than one M protein
  - Diminished levels of uninvolved immunoglobulin classes is common.
  - Monoclonal plasma cells can be verified by immunoglobulin gene rearrangement studies of DNA from malignant plasma cells.

- Immunocytochemical and flow cytometric analysis
  - DNA aneuploidy can be demonstrated in 80 percent of patients with myeloma.
  - Myeloma cells express early and late differention markers of myeloid, monocytic, erythroid, megakaryocytic, B-cell, T-cell, and NK-cell lineage.
- A high DNA labeling index is an important negative prognostic feature.
  - The average labeling index is 1 percent. Fewer than 5 percent of patients have a labeling index of >5 percent.
- Cytogenetics are difficult to study because of low mitotic activity.
  - Abnormal karyotypes are found in 20 to 30 percent of myeloma patients, but unique myeloma-specific alterations have not been found.
  - Hypodiploidy is associated with primary drug resistance.
  - 6q- may be associated with extensive bone disease.

STAGING

- Staging criteria presented in Table 61-1 have proved useful in assessing the extent of disease in a patient.
- Other variables used to help determine prognosis

TABLE 61-1 Assessment of Tumor Mass (Durie-Salmon)

Stage I: Low tumor mass ($< 0.6 \times 10^{12}/m^2$)*
All of the following must be present:
A. Hemoglobin >10.5 g/dl or hematocrit > 32%
B. Serum calcium level normal
C. Low serum myeloma protein production rates:
  1. IgG peak < 5 g/dl
  2. IgA peak < 3 g/dl
  3. Bence Jones protein < 4 g/24 h
D. No bone lesions or osteoporosis

Stage II: Intermediate tumor mass (0.6 to 1.2 $\times 10^{12}/m^2$)*
All patients who do not qualify for high or low tumor mass categories are considered to have intermediate tumor mass

Stage III: High tumor mass (>1.2 $\times 10^{12}/m^2$)*
One of the following abnormalities must be present:
A. Hemoglobin < 8.5 g/dl, hematocrit < 25%
B. Serum calcium > 12 mg/dl
C. Very high serum or urine myeloma protein production rates:
  1. IgG peak > 7 g/dl
  2. IgA peak > 5 g/dl
  3. Bence Jones protein >12 g/24 h
D. > 3 lytic bone lession on bone survey (bone scan not acceptable)

*Estimated number of neoplastic plasma cells.
Source: Adapted from Table 114-2 of *Williams Hematology,* 5/e, p. 1118.

- Serum β_2-microglobulin concentration, which reflects neoplastic cell turnover and renal function.
- Plasma cell DNA labeling index, which reflects mitotic activity.
- C-reactive protein concentration, which reflects IL-6 activity.
- Serum lactate dehydrogenase activity, reflecting plasmablastic morphology.

DIFFERENTIAL DIAGNOSIS

- Criteria for diagnosis of plasma cell myeloma are presented in Table 61-2.
- Criteria for diagnosis of essential monoclonal gammopathy are discussed in Chap. 60.
- Evaluate for amyloidosis if patient has lymphadenopathy, hepatosplenomegaly, macroglossia, periorbital hemorrhage ("raccoon eyes"), carpal tunnel syndrome, or cardiomegaly with arrhythmias or low voltage on the ECG.

THERAPY

- Solitary plasmacytoma
  - Radiation therapy at doses of 4000 to 5000 cGy.
  - 70 percent of soft-tissue plasmacytomas are cured with radiation.
  - 30 percent of solitary plasmacytomas of bone are cured with radiation.

TABLE 61-2 Criteria for Diagnosis of Plasma Cell Myeloma*

Major criteria:
  Plasmacytomas on tissue biopsy
  Marrow plasmacytosis with > 30% plasma cells
  Monoclonal globulin spike on serum electrophoresis > 3.5 g/dl for IgG or > 2.0 g/dl for IgA; ≥1.0 g/24 h of κ or λ light-chain excretion on urine electrophoresis in the absence of amyloidosis

Minor criteria:
  Marrow plasmacytosis 10 to 30%
  Monoclonal globulin spike present, but less than the levels defined above
  Lytic bone lesions
  Concentration of normal IgM < 0.05 g/dl, IgA < 0.1 g/dl, or IgG < 0.6 g/dl

*The diagnosis of plasma cell myeloma is confirmed when at least one major and one minor criterion or at least three minor criteria are documented in symptomatic patients with progressive disease. The presence of the following features not specific for the disease supports the diagnosis, particularly if of recent onset: anemia, hypercalcemia, azotemia, bone demineralization, or hypoalbuminemia.
Source: Adapted from Table 114-3 of *Williams Hematology,* 5/e, p. 1118.

TABLE 61-3 Criteria for Diagnosis of Indolent Myeloma*

Few bone lesions (if any, <4) and no compression features

M-component levels:
 IgG < 7 g/dl
 IgA < 5 g/dl

No symptoms or associated disease features:
 Performance status > 50%
 Hemoglobin level > 10 g/dl
 Normal serum calcium levels
 Serum creatinine level < 2.0 mg/dl
 No infections

*The criteria for diagnosis of plasma cell myeloma presented in Table 61-2 must be satisfied. However, patients with indolent myeloma have all of the features listed in this table.
Source: Adapted from Table 114-5 of *Williams Hematology,* 5/e, p. 1119.

- Indolent myeloma
  - Criteria for diagnosis are presented in Table 61-3
  - Treatment is withheld until the onset of symptoms or evidence of disease progression.
- Standard treatment of symptomatic multiple myeloma
  - Melphalan and prednisone (MP) therapy controls symptoms and/ or reduces tumor burden by at least 50 percent in one-half the patients.
  - Reducing the tumor burden and stabilizing disease activity prolongs survival, compared to patients not responding to therapy.
  - There is no benefit to maintenance therapy with standard chemotherapy agents.
  - Myelodysplastic syndrome (MDS) or acute myelogenous leukemia (AML) may develop *de novo* or consequent to therapy with alkylating agents in patients with myeloma.
  - Plasma cell leukemia, meningeal disease, or transformation to plasmablastic disease with very aggressive natural history may be late manifestations of myeloma.
- Investigational therapy of symptomatic multiple myeloma
  - High-dose glucocorticoid therapy has been effective in a few patients.
  - Continuous infusion of vincristine and doxorubicin and oral decadron (VAD) may be effective in patients resistant to MP.
  - Survival rate for VAD-treated patients is the same as for patients treated with alkylating drug therapy.
  - Marrow transplantation
    - There is a dose-response curve to melphalan therapy in multiple myeloma.
    - Autologous transplantation to consolidate a remission after standard therapy yields a 50 percent complete remission rate, a median

relapse-free survival >2 years, and a median overall survival of 4 years.
  - Allogeneic transplantation may cure a small subset of myeloma patients.
- Salvage therapy for multiple myeloma
  - High-dose glucocorticoid therapy or VAD is the main salvage therapy if disease progresses after alkylator therapy.
  - Dose-intensive therapy and autologous transplantation gives a tumor response in 75 percent of patients but a complete remission rate of only 10 percent.
  - Etoposide, cisplatin, cytarabine, and dexamethasone (EDAP) is as effective as VAD for salvage therapy.
- Interferon-α (IFN-α)
  - appears to be inactive in myeloma refractory to chemotherapy but may be useful in prolonging remission after autotransplants
- Erythropoietin (EPO)
  - The anemia of myeloma responds to EPO administration in about 70 percent of patients over the course of 4 to 6 weeks.

APPROACH TO MYELOMA THERAPY TODAY

- Confirm the diagnosis.
- Consider allogeneic transplantation for all patients less than 55 years old.
  - HLA and DR type patient and siblings
- VAD as initial therapy if autologous transplant is being considered for remission consolidation.
- Patients not qualifying for transplantation because of medical reasons or advanced age (>70 years old), treat with standard alkylator chemotherapy and glucocorticoids.

Course and Prognosis

- Median survival is 30 to 36 months.
- Patients succumb to consequences of aggressive tumor growth, or to consequences of bone marrow failure (bleeding or infection), sometimes with the development of MDS or AML.

For a more detailed discussion, see Stephen M. Baird: Plasma cell neoplasms: generation considerations, Chap. 112, p. 1097; and Bart Barlogie: Plasma cell myeloma, Chap. 114, p. 1109, in *Williams Hematology,* 5/e, 1995.

---

62 MACROGLOBULINEMIA

Macroglobulinemia refers to an increase in the blood concentration of IgM, usually of a monoclonal nature. Most patients with macroglobulinemia have a lymphocytic or lymphoplasmacytic neoplasm, but about 30 percent do not have a detectable lymphoproliferative disorder and are said to have "essential macroglobulinemia" or "essential monoclonal macroglobulinemia."

DISORDERS ASSOCIATED WITH MONOCLONAL MACROGLOBULINEMIA

- Lymphoplasmacytic neoplasms (32 percent)
  - Waldenström macroglobulinemia (27 percent)
  - Extramedullary plasmacytoma (3 percent)
  - IgM myeloma (2 percent)
- B-cell neoplasms (38 percent)
  - Indolent B-cell lymphomas (31 percent)
  - B-cell chronic lymphocytic leukemia (7 percent)
- Benign monoclonal IgM proteinemias (30 percent)
  - Essential monoclonal macroglobulinemia (28 percent)
  - Cold agglutinin syndrome (2 percent)

WALDENSTRÖM MACROGLOBULINEMIA

Etiology

- Familial (genetic) factors may contribute to the development of the disease.
- Nearly all patients have chromosomal abnormalities, most frequently of chromosomes 9, 10, 11, and 12.

Pathogenesis

- The elevated concentration of IgM is responsible for
  - increased blood viscosity (hyperviscosity syndrome)
  - pancreatitis
  - leukoencephalopathy
  - demyelinating peripheral neuropathy
  - immune complex deposition
  - cryoglobulinemia and cold hypersensitivity
  - hemostatic disorders of platelets and coagulation proteins

Clinical Features

- More common in men, with a median age at diagnosis of 63.
- Presenting symptoms most commonly are fatigue, weakness, weight loss, episodic bleeding, or manifestations of the hyperviscosity syndrome.

- Physical findings include lymphadenopathy, hepatosplenomegaly, dependent purpura, mucosal bleeding, dilated tortuous retinal veins, multiple flesh-colored papules on extensor surfaces (deposits of IgM reacting to epidermal basement membrane antigens), and peripheral sensory neuropathy.

The Hyperviscosity Syndrome

- Symptoms do not develop unless the serum viscosity is > 4 times that of water.
- Frequent symptoms are headache; impaired vision; mental status changes, such as confusion or dementia; altered consciousness that may progress to coma; ataxia; and nystagmus.
- Congestive heart failure may develop.
- Ophthalmoscopic changes include link sausage appearance of retinal veins and retinal hemorrhages and papilledema.

Laboratory Findings

- Elevated serum IgM levels. The monoclonal IgM is usually IgM κ.
- Serum levels of the other immunoglobulins are normal or low.
- The serum viscosity is elevated in most patients, but only 20 percent have the hyperviscosity syndrome.
- Normocytic and normochromic anemia is present in > 80 percent of patients at diagnosis.
- MCV may be elevated spuriously by red cell aggregation.
- White blood cell counts and platelet counts are not severely depressed at diagnosis in most patients.
- The monoclonal neoplastic B cells express the usual B-cell surface antigens, i.e., CD19, CD20, CD24, but also show aberrant expression of CD5, CD10, CD11b, and CD9.
- Marrow biopsies are hypercellular, with diffuse infiltration of lymphocytes, plasmacytoid lymphocytes, and plasma cells, and with increased mast cells.
  - Lymphoid cells are neoplastic and have monoclonal surface membrane and cytoplasmic immunoglobulin.
- Thrombin time is often prolonged, and the prothrombin time and activated partial thromboplastin time may be prolonged.

Renal Abnormalities

- About one-third of patients have elevated BUN levels.
- Urine usually has small amounts of detectable light chain.
- IgM precipitation on glomerular basement membrane may occlude glomerular capillaries.

TABLE 62-1 Distinctions between Essential versus Waldenström Macroglobulinemia

	Essential macroglobulinemia	Waldenström macroglobinemia
Symptoms	Usually none, but may have peripheral neuropathy or cold sensitivity	Fatigue, weight loss, headache, epistaxis, neurologic symptoms, or cold hypersensitivity
Physical findings	Usually none	Hepatosplenomegaly, purpura, lymphadenopathy, Raynaud, neurologic signs, retinopathy
Laboratory findings		
IgM protein, g/dl	Usually <3 and stable	Often >3 and increasing
Hemoglobin, g/dl	Usually >12	<12 in 80% of patients
Serum viscosity	Normal	Increased

Source: Adapted from Table 115-1 of Williams Hematology, 5/e, p. 1130.

- Immunologic glomerulonephritis with nephrotic syndrome may develop.

Differential Diagnosis

- Essential vs. Waldenström macroglobulinemia is summarized in Table 62-1.
- Macroglobulinemia due to lymphoid neoplasms vs. Waldenström macroglobulinemia:
  - Lymphocyte morphology and immunophenotype provide differentiation.
  - Skeletal lesions or hypercalcemia indicate multiple myeloma.

Therapy, Course, and Prognosis

- Waldenström macroglobulinemia is incurable.
- Median duration of survival is 5 years.
- Asymptomatic patients may be followed without specific therapy until symptoms develop.
- Symptomatic patients should receive chemotherapy.
  - Oral alkylating agents such as chlorambucil are effective in achieving palliation of disease manifestations.
  - There is no demonstrated advantage to multiple alkylator therapy over single-drug therapy.
  - 2-Chlorodeoxyadenosine and fludarabine are effective as salvage therapy after disease progression has occurred with alkylator therapy.

- Plasmapheresis is used to help manage the hyperviscosity syndrome.
- Red cell transfusions may elevate the blood viscosity and reduce capillary blood flow, as well as exacerbate congestive heart failure in patients with Waldenström macroglobulinemia.

For a more detailed discussion, see Stephen M. Baird: Plasma cell neoplasms: general considerations, Chap. 112, p. 1097; and Thomas J. Kipps: Macroglobulinemia, Chap. 115, p. 1127, in *Williams Hematology,* 5/e, 1995.

---

63 HEAVY-CHAIN DISEASES

The heavy-chain diseases are rare B-cell lymphoproliferative disorders, characterized by the production of abnormal immunoglobulin molecules that lack light chains. α, γ, and μ heavy-chain disorders have been described. The disorders have distinct clinical features and age distributions. The salient features of these disorders are summarized in Table 63-1.

For a more detailed discussion, see Thomas J. Kipps: The heavy-chain diseases, Chap. 116, p. 1133, in *Williams Hematology,* 5/e, 1995.

TABLE 63-1 Heavy-Chain Diseases

	Disease		
	α Heavy-chain disease	γ Heavy-chain disease	μ Heavy-chain disease
Other names	Seligmann disease	Franklin disease	
Median age at diagnosis	Early-30s	Early-60s	Mid-60s
Common manifestations	Diarrhea, malabsorption, weight loss, abdominal pain, mesenteric and para-aortic adenopathy	Fever, malaise, fatigue, lymphadenopathy, palatal edema, hepatosplenomegaly	Bence Jones proteinuria, lymphadenopathy, splenomegaly, vacuolated marrow plasma cells (usually in the setting of B-cell chronic lymphocytic leukemia).
Diagnosis	Requires detection of abnormal α heavy chain without light chains, usually in urine or jejunal fluid	Requires detection of abnormal γ heavy chain without light chains, usually in urine or serum	Requires detection of abnormal μ heavy chain without light chains in serum or urine—usually requires gel filtration or ultracentrifugation.
Therapy	Intravenous hydration; antibiotics (e.g., tetracycline or metronidazole); systemic chemotherapy for refractory or advanced disease	Glucocorticoids, systemic chemotherapy directed at underlying B-cell lymphoproliferative disease	Glucocorticoids, systemic chemotherapy, irradiation of nasopharynx for palatal edema

Source: Adapted from Table 116-1 of *Williams Hematology,* 5/e, p. 1134.

64 AMYLOIDOSIS

- The term *amyloid* (AL) is used to describe a substance with a homogeneous eosinophilic appearance by light microscopy, a green birefringence on polarizing electron microscopy, and a characteristic β-pleated sheet appearance by x-ray diffraction.
- Despite the uniform appearance, there are many different types of amyloid, composed of different proteins that can be characterized biochemically and immunologically.
- Amyloid has been classified both by the associated clinical disorders and by the chemical composition of the amyloid fibrils.

CLASSIFICATION (Table 64-1)

ETIOLOGY

- Amyloid consists of long fibrils.
- Several major proteins can form amyloid fibrils:
  - AL protein (immunoglobulin light chain)
    - Usually λ light chain
    - Occurs in essential amyloidosis, plasma cell disorders, macroglobulinemia
  - AA proteins (amyloid A proteins)
    - Occurs in response to inflammation and as a familial syndrome.
  - ATTR proteins (transthyretin)
    - Occurs in several familial syndromes and in senile amyloid.
  - $A\beta_2M$ (β_2-microglobulin)
    - Occurs in chronic hemodialysis patients.
  - AP protein (P component)
    - A minor protein component of amyloid deposits.
    - Has structural homology with C-reactive protein.

PATHOGENESIS

- Each amyloid fibril protein has a precursor molecule in the serum.
- Amyloid formation involves
  - stimulus-generated change in the serum concentration or primary structure of amyloid precursor proteins
  - conversion of the precursor protein to amyloid fibrils
- Clinical manifestations arise due to amyloid deposition and interference with normal organ function.
- Organ systems often involved with amyloid are
  - kidney
    - nephrotic syndrome, renal insufficiency
  - liver and spleen
    - organ enlargement, hepatic cholestasis, traumatic rupture of enlarged spleen
  - gastrointestinal tract

TABLE 64-1 A Guide for Nomenclature and Classification of Amyloid and Amyloidosis

Amyloid protein[a]	Protein precursor	Protein type of variant	Clinical
AA[b]	apoSAA		Reactive (secondary), familial Mediterranean fever, familial amyloid nephropathy with urticaria and deafness (Muckle-Wells syndrome)
AL	κ, λ	Aκ, Aλ	Ididopathic (primary), myeloma- or macroglobulinemia-associated
AH	IgG1 (γ1)	Aγ1	
ATTR	Transthyretin	e.g., Met 30[c]	Familial amyloid polyneuropathy (Portuguese)
		e.g., Met 111	Familial amyloid cardiomyopathy (Danish)
		TTR or Ile 122	Systemic senile amyloidosis
AApoAI	apoAI	Arg26	Familial amyloid polyneuropathy (Iowa)
AGel	Gelsolin	Asn 187[c] (15)	Familial amyloidosis (Finnish)
ACys	Cystatin C	Gln 68	Hereditary cerebral hemorrhage with amyloidosis (Icelandic)
Aβ	β protein precursor	Gln 618[c] (22)	Alzheimer disease, Down syndrome
	(e.g., βPP 695[d])		Hereditary cerebral hemorrhage amyloidosis (Dutch)
Aβ₂M	β₂-microglobulin		Associated with chronic dialysis
APrP	PrP^c—cellular prion protein	PrP^sc, PrP^cjd	Creutzfeldt-Jakob disease, scrapie, kuru, Gerstmann-Straussler-Scheinker syndrome
ACal	(Pro)calcitonin	(Pro)calcitonin	Medullary carcinoma of thyroid
AANF	Atrial natriuretic factor		Isolated atrial amyloid
AIAPP	Islet amyloid polypeptide		Islets of Langerhans, diabetes type II, insulinoma

[a] Nonfibrillar protein, e.g., protein AP (amyloid P-component) excluded.
[b] Abbreviations not explained in table: AA, amyloid A protein; SAA, serum amyloid A-related protein; apo, apolipoprotein; L, immunoglobulin light chain; H, immunoglobulin heavy chain.
[c] Amino acid positions in the mature precursor protein. The position in the amyloid fibril protein is given in parentheses.
[d] Number of amino acid residues.
Source: Adapted from Table 117-1 of *Williams Hematology,* 5/e, p. 1138.

- macroglossia, obstruction, ulceration, hemorrhage, malabsorption, diarrhea
- heart
  - congestive heart failure, cardiomegaly, arrhythmias
  - low voltage on ECG, characteristic echocardiogram
- skin
  - lesions ranging from papules to large nodules, purpura
- nervous system
  - peripheral neuropathies, postural hypotension
- respiratory tract
- blood
  - coagulopathy due to depletion of fibrinogen, factor IX, and factor X

DIAGNOSIS

- Consider the diagnosis in patients with
  - unexplained kidney disease with nephrotic syndrome
  - hepatosplenomegaly in association with chronic inflammatory disorders
  - carpal tunnel syndrome
  - macroglossia
  - unexplained neuromuscular disease, congestive heart failure, or malabsorption
  - plasma cell dyscrasias
- Rectal or gingival biopsy yields the diagnosis in >80 percent of patients.
- Abdominal fat pad aspiration is also sensitive and specific.
- Tissue should be stained with alkaline Congo red and examined by polarizing microscopy.

TREATMENT, COURSE, AND PROGNOSIS

- No specific treatment is available for any type of amyloid disorder.
- Palliation is aimed at
  - decreasing the chronic antigenic stimulation that results in amyloid deposition
  - inhibiting the synthesis of amyloid fibrils
  - inhibiting the extracellular deposition of amyloid
  - Promoting the mobilization and lysis of existing amyloid fibrils
- Treating the inciting disease, e.g., osteomyelitis, may slow progression of the amyloidosis.
- Alkylating agents may reduce the number of immunoglobulin-producing B cells in AL amyloidosis.

- Colchicine prevents acute attacks of familial Mediterranean fever and thus reduces amyloid production.
- Kidney transplantation may prolong survival in patients with systemic amyloidosis and renal insufficiency.
- Average survival with generalized amyloidosis is 1 to 4 years.
- Major causes of death are from kidney failure and heart disease.

For a more detailed discussion, see Alan S. Cohen: Amyloidosis, Chap. 117, p. 1137, in *Williams Hematology,* 5/e, 1995.

---

65 THROMBOCYTOPENIA DUE TO DIMINISHED OR DEFECTIVE PLATELET PRODUCTION

HEREDITARY AND CONGENITAL THROMBOCYTOPENIAS (Table 65-1)

- Generally have a clear inheritance pattern. Since prenatal infection may be implicated, some may be congenital but not hereditary. Since Bernard-Soulier and gray platelet syndromes are primarily qualitative abnormalities, these are discussed in Chap. 70.

FANCONI ANEMIA

- Autosomal recessive severe aplastic anemia usually beginning at age 8 to 9 years.
- Homozygotes have a pathognomonic sensitivity to chromosomal breakage by DNA cross-linking agents (i.e., diepoxybutane).
- Diverse congenital abnormalities may occur, including short stature, skin pigmentation, hypoplasia of the thumb and radius, anomalies of the genitourinary, cardiac, and central nervous systems.
- Patients are at risk for acute leukemia and other malignancies.
- About half of the patients may respond to androgen therapy (few completely), but the condition is generally fatal unless corrected by allogeneic marrow transplantation.

THROMBOCYTOPENIA WITH ABSENT RADIUS (TAR) SYNDROME

- Inheritance pattern suggests autosomal recessive or double heterozygosity.
- May be acquired. Intrauterine rubella infections have been implicated in some cases.
- Noted at birth because of absence of both radii. Other skeletal anomalies are common, including absent or abnormal ulnas, bones of the shoulder girdle, feet.
- One-third of patients have congenital heart anomalies (most often tetralogy of Fallot or atrial septal defects).
- Allergy to cow's milk common.
- Platelet counts variable, typically 15,000 to 30,000/μl, lower during infancy and during periods of stress (surgery, infection).
- Megakaryocytes are diminished or absent.
- Leukemoid reactions and eosinophilia common.
- Treatment with glucocorticoids, splenectomy, and intravenous IgG are generally ineffective.
- Deaths are usually due to hemorrhage and usually occur within first year.

TABLE 65-1 Hereditary Thrombocytopenias

Syndrome	Clinical features
Autosomal recessive traits	
Fanconi syndrome	Typically fatal aplastic anemia presenting in childhood with other congenital anomalies. May present as isolated hypoplastic thrombocytopenia in adults with short stature and increased skin pigmentation.
Thrombocytopenia-absent radius (TAR)	Severe amegakaryocytic thrombocytopenia in infancy, spontaneously recovering after age 1. May cause mild, intermittent thrombocytopenia in adults with major skeletal anomalies.
Bernard-Soulier syndrome (see Chap. 70)	Giant platelets, abnormal GP Ib-IX. Heterozygotes are asymptomatic with normal platelet number and function but large platelets. Therefore, abnormal platelet size is transmitted as a dominant trait.
Gray platelet syndrome (see Chap. 70)	Large, pale platelets with diminished endogenous α-granule proteins.
Isolated thrombocytopenia	May have giant platelets. Megakaryocytes may be reduced or increased. Platelet survival may be short or normal.
Autosomal dominant traits	
May-Hegglin anomaly	Asymptomatic; giant platelets, occasional true thrombocytopenia, characteristic leukocyte inclusions.
Alport syndrome variants	Giant platelets, often severe thrombocytopenia, associated with hearing loss and interstitial nephritis. Morbidity and mortality due to progressive renal failure.
Isolated thrombocytopenia	Usually mild thrombocytopenia due to ineffective platelet production. May have giant platelets.
X-Linked	
Wiskott-Aldrich syndrome	Immune deficiency, eczema, and thrombocytopenia with very small platelets. Death due to infection, hemorrhage, or malignancy.
Isolated thrombocytopenia	Adults with moderate thrombocytopenia, possible variants of the Wiskott-Aldrich syndrome.

Source: Adapted from Table 127-1 of *Williams Hematology*, 5/e, p. 1282.

- If patient can be sustained for the first 1 to 2 years of life, the platelet count usually recovers and survival is normal.
- Platelet counts vary during adulthood but symptoms are mild.
- Patients with severe thrombocytopenia throughout childhood are candidates for allogeneic marrow transplant.

MAY-HEGGLIN ANOMALY

- Autosomal dominant inheritance of giant platelets, moderate thrombocytopenia, and inclusion bodies in neutrophils, eosinophils, and monocytes, resembling Dohle bodies seen with acute infections.
- Platelet count low but total platelet mass may be normal.
- Platelets large but ultrastructurally normal. Megakaryocytes are normal in appearance and number. Platelet survival and bleeding times are normal or slightly abnormal.
- The thrombocytopenia is rarely severe, most patients are asymptomatic, and there is no increased risk for infection.
- Usually no treatment is necessary, even for surgery or delivery.

ALPORT SYNDROME VARIANTS

- Alport syndrome is the association of hereditary nephritis and deafness. In some families, there has been associated giant platelets and thrombocytopenia (Epstein syndrome). The disorder is typically discovered in young adults, often misdiagnosed as having ITP.
  - Severe thrombocytopenia is common. The platelets are large but ultrastructurally normal. Megakaryocytes are normal. Bleeding times are normal to slightly prolonged (could be due to uremia).
  - Treatment with glucocorticoids and splenectomy is ineffective. Morbidity and mortality is due to progressive renal failure.

OTHER AUTOSOMAL DOMINANT THROMBOCYTOPENIAS

- A group of heterogeneous clinical disorders of unknown prevalence. Most have isolated thrombocytopenia with normal platelet and megakaryocyte morphology. Some have large platelets.
- Most patients discovered as adults, within minimal or no bleeding symptoms. They are often considered to have refractory ITP, but family studies demonstrate an autosomal dominant pattern.

WISKOTT-ALDRICH SYNDROME

- Triad of immunodeficiency, thrombocytopenia, and eczema.
- Rare X-linked disorder. One-third have no family history and may represent new mutations.
- A specific defect of O-glycosylation causes an abnormality of a membrane glycoprotein, CD43, present on nonerythroid hemopoietic cells that may function in T-cell activation.

- Both cellular and humoral immune responses are affected.
- Cardinal feature is very small platelet size. Megakaryocytes are normal in number and size, but ultrastructural abnormalities have been reported. Platelet survival is shortened, production is ineffective, and function is abnormal.
- Hemorrhage usually occurs in the first few months of life, commonly epistaxis and bloody diarrhea. Episodes of severe, recurrent infection and eczema begin at about 6 months of age.
- Platelets are very small and counts range between 20,000 and 100,000/μl.
- Patients have low or absent levels of anti-A and anti-B isohemagglutinins (low serum IgM), increased serum concentrations of IgA and IgE, and normal levels of IgG.
- Glucocorticoids are not effective and may exacerbate infections. Splenectomy leads to correction of both platelet number and size, but the effect may be temporary. Splenectomy may increase susceptibility to infection.
- Risk of developing malignancy is about 2 percent per year. Lymphomas are the most frequent, but AML also occurs.
- The average life-span is less than 10 years for boys with full expression of the syndrome. Death is due to infection, hemorrhage, or malignancy.
- For patients with full syndrome, allogeneic marrow transplantation is indicated and curative.

ACQUIRED THROMBOCYTOPENIAS DUE TO DECREASED PLATELET PRODUCTION

- A heterogeneous group of disorders including those caused by marrow aplasia (Chap. 4), infiltration with neoplasms (Chap. 19), treatment with chemotherapeutic agents (Chap. 3), and radiotherapy.

MEGAKARYOCYTIC APLASIA

- A rare disorder in a spectrum that includes aplastic anemia, granulocytic aplasia, and pure red cell aplasia.
- Several mechanisms may be responsible, including humoral and cellular immune disorders, and abnormal responses to cytokines.
- The natural history is unclear and treatment is empirical.

VIRAL INFECTION

- Probably the most common cause of mild thrombocytopenia.
- Reported with mumps, varicella, HIV, Epstein-Barr virus, rubella, rubeola, dengue fever, cytomegalovirus, and parvovirus.
- Decreased platelet counts are found in children receiving live attenuated measles vaccine. Megakaryocytes are reduced in number and have nuclear and cytoplasmic vacuoles.

- Severe thrombocytopenia is occasionally seen in infectious mononucleosis (<1 in 2000 patients).

DRUG AND ALCOHOL-INDUCED THROMBOCYTOPENIA

Alcohol

- In alcoholics usually the result of cirrhosis with congestive splenomegaly, or folic acid deficiency, but acute thrombocytopenia may occur in the absence of these factors.
- Alcohol ingestion for 5 to 10 days can produce sustained thrombocytopenia with decreased numbers of marrow megakaryocytes. In vitro studies suggest alcohol has an inhibitory effect on maturing megakaryocytes.
- After withdrawal of alcohol, platelet counts return to normal in 5 to 21 days and may rise above normal levels.

Drugs

- May induce thrombocytopenia as a result of direct myelotoxicity [e.g., chemotherapeutic agents (Chap. 3)], aplastic anemia (Chap. 4), or a specific effect on platelet production (e.g., diethylstilbestrol, GM-CSF).

NUTRITIONAL DEFICIENCY

- Mild thrombocytopenia occurs in about 20 percent of patients with megaloblastic anemia due to vitamin B_{12} deficiency. The frequency may be higher with folic acid deficiency because of associated alcoholism.
- Thrombocytopenia appears to be due primarily to ineffective platelet production.
- Iron deficiency typically causes thrombocytosis, but mild thrombocytopenia may occur. The platelet count returns to normal with iron replacement.

For a more detailed discussion, see James N. George: Thrombocytopenia due to diminished or defective platelet production, Chap. 127, p. 1281, in *Williams Hematology,* 5/e, 1995.

---

66 THROMBOCYTOPENIA DUE TO ENHANCED PLATELET DESTRUCTION BY NONIMMUNOLOGIC MECHANISMS

Thrombotic thrombocytopenic purpura (TTP) and hemolytic uremic syndrome (HUS) were described initially as distinct disorders but are now considered different expressions of the same disease process (Table 66-1).

IDIOPATHIC TTP-HUS

Etiology and Pathogenesis

- In adults, most episodes are sporadic and of unknown etiology, but familial occurrence has been documented, and TTP has developed in the setting of rheumatic diseases, autoimmune vasculitis, hypersensitivity reactions, paraproteinemia, and organ transplantation.
- TTP appears to be a syndrome of diverse etiologies causing diffuse endothelial damage and disseminated platelet thrombi.

Clinical Features

- There is a predominance of young women among patients with TTP.
- The classic pentad of clinical findings includes fever, thrombocyto-

TABLE 66-1 Thrombotic Thrombocytopenic Purpura–Hemolytic Uremic Syndrome (TTP-HUS): A Classification of Clinical Presentations

Idiopathic TTP-HUS
  Classic TTP of adults, also nonverotoxin-associated HUS and TTP of children

Secondary TTP-HUS
  Pregancy
    Includes syndromes of TTP, postpartum HUS, and possibly severe manifestations of preeclampsia-eclampsia
  Verotoxins of *E. coli* and *Shigella dysenteriae 1*
    Classic epidemic childhood HUS
    Epidemic TTP-HUS in adults
  Metastatic carcinoma
  Drugs
    Cancer chemotherapeutic agents: mitomycin C, cisplatin, other agents
    Immunosuppressive agents: cyclosporine, other agents
    Marrow transplantation: total body irradiation and/or intensive chemotherapy regimens
    Quinine, other drugs

Source: Adapted from Table 128-1 of *Williams Hematology*, 5/e, p. 1290.

penia, microangiopathic hemolytic anemia, neurologic abnormalities, and renal involvement.

- Recent studies have required only microangiopathic hemolytic anemia and thrombocytopenia for diagnosis; even with these minimal criteria, more than 50 percent have neurologic signs and renal disease.
- Common symptoms are hemorrhage, fatigue, abdominal pain, and neurologic changes including headache and confusion, followed by paresis, dysphasia, seizures, visual problems, and coma.
- Hemorrhagic symptoms include petechiae, epistaxis, gastrointestinal bleeding, and menorrhagia. Subarachnoid hemorrhage, intramyocardial hemorrhage, and massive hemoptysis can also occur.

Laboratory Features

- Defining features are anemia, severe thrombocytopenia, and red cell fragmentation (schistocytes). *Examination of the stained blood film is essential.*
- The white cell count is normal or elevated.
- The marrow megakaryocytes are normal in number, or increased, consistent with peripheral destruction of platelets.
- Coagulation studies are normal.
- Lactate dehydrogenase levels are often very high, consistent with severe hemolysis.
- Most patients have microscopic hematuria, casts, and proteinuria; half have an increased serum creatinine level; and some have acute, oliguric renal failure.
- The characteristic pathologic lesion is the presence of eosinophilic, granular ("hyaline") material in the lumens of arterioles and capillaries composed primarily of platelets. Renal biopsies demonstrate platelet and fibrin thrombi that may occlude glomerular capillary lumens.
- These pathologic changes are characteristic of TTP-HUS but may be identical to those seen with preeclampsia, malignant hypertension, acute scleroderma, and renal allograft rejection.

Differential Diagnosis

- Evans syndrome, both autoimmune hemolytic anemia and ITP, may be confused with TTP. The direct Coombs test is positive in Evans syndrome.
- Sepsis and disseminated intravascular coagulation (DIC) should be considered in an acutely ill patient with fever, chills, and multiple organ dysfunction. The distinction should be clear from coagulation studies, which are usually normal in TTP.
- Bacterial endocarditis can present with fever, neurologic symptoms, anemia, and thrombocytopenia.
- Other considerations include systemic lupus erythematosus with cen-

tral nervous system manifestations, paroxysmal nocturnal hemoglobinuria with thrombotic complications, and metastatic cancer.

Treatment

Plasma Exchange

- As the primary therapy, it should be started promptly. The patient's plasma is replaced with fresh frozen plasma. Plasma exchange may be effective because it removes a harmful plasma component or replaces an undefined deficiency.
- Daily plasma exchange (40 to 80 ml/kg) is performed until response is achieved, defined by resolution of neurologic symptoms, and normalization of the platelet count and serum LDH activity.
- Response is usually seen within 1 to 2 weeks, and recovery is nearly complete within 3 weeks. However, responses may take over a month.
- When the platelet count and serum LDH activity are normal for several days, exchanges are continued at gradually increasing intervals for another 1 to 2 weeks.
- Signs of TTP may return when plasma exchange is discontinued. Most relapses occur within a week of stopping the exchange, or within a month of diagnosis, and therefore treatment for a month is recommended.
- Minor allergic reactions to plasma (urticaria), nausea, and mild hypotension are common. Rarely, patients may have severe hypotension.

Glucocorticoids

- Prednisone at a dose of 1 to 2 mg/kg/day orally is frequently added to plasma exchange, but there is no proof it is of benefit.
- Prednisone alone at a dose of 200 mg/day orally may be effective in patients with minimal symptoms and no neurologic changes.

Antiplatelet Agents

- Most series include antiplatelet agents, but their role is unclear and maintenance therapy does not prevent relapses.
- The use of aspirin is appropriate if there is no response to plasma exchange and active bleeding is not present.

Splenectomy

- Successful treatment with splenectomy in combination with high-dose glucocorticoids and dextran has been reported.
- Splenectomy is usually performed late, when response to plasmapheresis is incomplete or multiple relapses have occurred.

Other Treatments

- The experience with intravenous immunoglobulin is limited, but it may be a reasonable addition to plasmapheresis therapy.
- Several reports suggest a beneficial effect of vincristine, in a regimen of 2 mg intravenously every 4 to 7 days for up to four doses.
- Other therapies include immunosuppressive agents (azathioprine, cyclophosphamide) and extracorporeal immunoadsorption.
- Platelet transfusions are appropriate with life-threatening hemorrhage but should be given with caution. Thrombocytopenia alone is not an indication for platelet transfusion.

Course and Prognosis

- Plasma exchange has improved survival to 83 percent. Half the deaths occur in the first week and most within the first month.
- Young age and previous good health are favorable features.
- Late relapses occur in 16 to 25 percent of cases. Maintenance therapy has not been effective in preventing relapses.
- Permanent sequelae from TTP are uncommon.

PREGNANCY-RELATED TTP-HUS

- TTP is more common in the second and third trimesters and HUS in the postpartum period. TTP-HUS may occur in association with preeclampsia or after a normal pregnancy and delivery.
- Distinction from preeclampsia may be impossible. The plasma antithrombin III level is low in preeclampsia and normal in TTP, and may be helpful in diagnosis.
- If thrombocytopenia and anemia are severe and the fetus is viable (>31 weeks gestation or weight >1200 g), delivery should be carried out; if not, a trial of plasma exchange is indicated.
- TTP-HUS in pregnancy responds to plasma exchange or to termination of the pregnancy. Preeclampsia does not respond to plasmapheresis.
- Subsequent pregnancies appear to carry some risk for recurrence. There is no report of transmission to the infant.

VEROTOXIN-INDUCED HEMOLYTIC UREMIC SYNDROME (CLASSIC CHILDHOOD HUS, EPIDEMIC OR ENTEROPATHIC HUS)

- Follows acute enteric infection caused by verotoxin-producing *E. coli* or *Shigella dysenteriae 1*. One to 12 percent of those infected with enteropathogenic strain of *E. coli*, O157:H7 develop HUS.
- A common source of infection is commercial heat-processed hamburger patties that are insufficiently cooked.
- Although typically a disease of young children, it can occur in adults.
- Boys and girls are equally affected. The peak age of 6 months to 4

years reflects the period of maximum exposure to enteric pathogens. 80 percent of cases occur between April and September.
- About 5 percent of children develop an atypical course that is chronic, relapsing, and often fatal, similar to idiopathic adult TTP-HUS.

Clinical and Laboratory Features

- Patients usually present with bloody diarrhea, most are oliguric, and one-third are anuric. Fever, vomiting, abdominal pain, hypertension, lethargy, and irritability are common.
- Seizures occur within the first few days and can be due to hyponatremia or to central nervous system involvement.
- Laboratory features include high serum creatinine levels, hematuria, metabolic changes of acute renal injury, microangiopathic hemolytic anemia, and thrombocytopenia. A sustained neutrophil count of $>15,000/\mu l$ is associated with a poor outcome.

Treatment, Course, and Prognosis

- Half of the patients require dialysis for 1 to 2 weeks for acute renal failure. Less than 10 percent require dialysis after 2 weeks. Chronic proteinuria, reduced glomerular filtration, and high blood pressure occur in 20 to 40 percent.
- Prospective trials have demonstrated minimal or no benefit from the use of plasma exchange.
- The mortality is 3 to 5 percent. Most deaths occur within the first week, and are usually related to central nervous system involvement, sepsis, and acute cardiac events.
- There is a substantial risk of permanently impaired renal function, and a few require renal transplantation. Other residual sequelae are unusual (e.g., neurologic impairment, cardiomyopathy) and relapses rare.

CANCER-ASSOCIATED TTP-HUS

- Microangiopathic hemolytic anemia occurs in 5 percent of patients with metastatic cancer due to widespread microvascular involvement.
- The full clinical spectrum of TTP-HUS with neurologic abnormalities can also develop in patients with metastatic cancer, but renal failure is uncommon.
- TTP-HUS is seen within a variety of carcinomas, but over half are gastric cancer.
- A leukoerythroblastic reaction indicating marrow involvement by tumor is frequently present. Evidence of DIC is generally absent in cancer-associated TTP-HUS.
- Therapy, course, and prognosis depend on the response to treatment of the metastatic carcinoma. Beneficial responses to plasmapheresis have been reported.

DRUG-INDUCED TTP-HUS

Cancer Chemotherapy

- Nearly all patients have been treated with mitomycin C. Other drugs associated with HUS are cisplatin, bleomycin, and nitrosoureas.
- The mitomycin C was usually given for gastric cancer. A high total dose of mitomycin C was generally required. HUS may occur as long as 9 months after stopping the drug.
- Microangiopathic hemolytic anemia and thrombocytopenia are constant features, renal failure is prominent, and neurologic changes are infrequent. Pulmonary edema occurs commonly and may be related to mitomycin C–induced pulmonary injury. Red cell transfusions can precipitate or exacerbate acute respiratory distress.
- Renal pathology is identical to TTP-HUS. The pulmonary pathology is fibrosing alveolitis, alveolar septal edema, and capillary congestion.
- Plasma exchange is less effective in mitomycin C–induced HUS than in TTP-HUS. Apheresis with immunoadsorption on a staphylococcal protein A column and vincristine have led to improvement in some patients.
- Most patients who develop HUS following mitomycin C therapy die of renal or respiratory failure and many of those surviving require maintenance dialysis.

Cyclosporine

- Cyclosporine, an immunosuppressive agent for organ allografts, can cause dose-related renal insufficiency and hypertension and may also cause HUS.
- In addition to the typical clinical features and renal pathologic changes of TTP-HUS, laboratory evidence of DIC can develop.
- Cyclosporine appears to damage endothelial cells and promote platelet aggregation and fibrin formation.
- The condition is almost always reversible when the drug is discontinued or the dose reduced. Plasmapheresis has been reported to be effective in some severe cases.

Marrow Transplantation

- HUS may occur after autologous and allogeneic transplant in the absence of cyclosporine therapy or graft-vs.-host disease.
- The onset is typically several months after transplantation.
- The cause appears to be radiation nephritis exacerbated by intensive chemotherapy.
- Plasma exchange, which appears to be beneficial, is rarely required; the prognosis is unclear.

Other Drugs

- Quinine-dependent antiplatelet antibodies can cause the classic features of TTP-HUS. Abdominal pain with nausea and vomiting are prominent symptoms, and some patients have severe neutropenia.
- Plasmapheresis and hemodialysis have been effective.
- Also reported with metronidazole, ticlopidine, and cocaine.

THROMBOCYTOPENIA IN PREGNANCY

Normal Pregnancy

- Thrombocytopenia found at labor may be divided into three groups: (1) incidental, 66 percent; (2) associated with obstetrical problems (e.g., premature labor, multiple births) or medical complications, 13 percent; and (3) occurring with a known cause (preeclampsia 19 percent; ITP 2 percent).
- Incidental discovery of thrombocytopenia during pregnancy has been reported in 0.3 to 4 percent of patients. The frequency at the time of labor and delivery is 4 to 8 percent, possibly related to the occurrence of subclinical DIC as part of normal parturition.
- Most patients have platelet counts >100,000/µl, there are no bleeding complications, and the platelet counts normalize within several days of delivery.
- Few infants are thrombocytopenic, and there are no bleeding problems.
- No special precautions or procedures are required.

Preeclampsia

- Pregnancy-induced hypertension and preeclampsia occur in about 5 to 10 percent of all pregnancies, more often in nulliparous women, and are the major cause of maternal and fetal morbidity and mortality.
- Pregnancy-induced hypertension develops after 20 weeks gestation and resolves after delivery.
- Preeclampsia is defined as hypertension with proteinuria and/or edema, and eclampsia has the additional feature of seizures.
- Thrombocytopenia occurs in 10 to 35 percent of patients with preeclampsia, and platelet counts are below 50,000/µl in less than 5 percent. The degree of thrombocytopenia correlates with the severity of preeclampsia. Preeclampsia causes thrombocytopenia in about 8 of 1000 deliveries.
- Overt hemolytic anemia is uncommon, but schistocytes are noted on the blood film in 15 percent of cases, and reticulocytosis is common.
- The renal lesions are comparable to TTP-HUS. DIC has been reported in some studies.

- Hepatocellular dysfunction and neurologic symptoms including headache, visual problems, apprehension, and fever may be seen.
- A severe form of preeclampsia (10 percent of patients) is termed the HELLP syndrome, an acronym for microangiopathic hemolysis (H), elevated liver function tests (EL), and low platelet (LP) counts. Platelet counts are <50,000/μl in about half of the patients. Features of liver disease may predominate, including nausea, right upper quadrant abdominal pain, ascites, and elevated serum transaminase and LDH levels.

Therapy, Course, and Prognosis

- The mainstay of management of preeclampsia, eclampsia, and the HELLP syndrome is delivery of the fetus.
- The nadir of the thrombocytopenia typically occurs the first postpartum day but may be as late as the fifth day. Platelets usually normalize within a week.
- Normal blood pressure is usually restored within 2 weeks. Hypertension or preeclampsia often recur in subsequent pregnancies.
- For patients with severe thrombocytopenia and microangiopathic hemolytic anemia, plasma exchange is indicated if the fetus cannot be delivered or if improvement does not follow delivery.

THROMBOCYTOPENIA ASSOCIATED WITH INFECTION

- Thrombocytopenia can be a complication of bacterial, viral, fungal, rickettsial, or protozoan infections.
- Most patients with bacteremia become thrombocytopenic. DIC is the underlying cause in many.
- Rickettsial infections may cause purpura and thrombocytopenia from diffuse vasculitis caused by direct infection of endothelial cells.
- Thrombocytopenia is not characteristic of disseminated fungal infections, but may occur from marrow involvement and splenomegaly.
- Viral infections and immunizations with attenuated viruses may cause thrombocytopenia from marrow suppression. In HIV infection, thrombocytopenia may result from both immunologically mediated platelet destruction and marrow failure. TTP has also been reported with HIV infection.

HEMANGIOMA-THROMBOCYTOPENIA (KASABACH-MERRITT) SYNDROME

- Thrombocytopenia associated with giant cavernous hemangiomas. The mechanism is localized or disseminated intravascular coagulation.
- The hemangiomas are usually present at birth and tumors as small as 6 cm can cause severe thrombocytopenia. The syndrome may develop in older children or adults as lesions enlarge.

- Hemangiomas are usually solitary and superficial but may occur in organs (e.g., liver, spleen, heart, GI tract).
- Trauma may provoke hemorrhage into the tumor and initiate intratumor coagulation.
- Patients may develop cardiac failure due to high volume arteriovenous shunting. A bruit may be heard over the hemangioma.
- Thrombocytopenia is usually not severe. Red cell fragmentation occurs and may be severe.
- Hemangiomas may resolve spontaneously, but treatment is often necessary. Surgery can eliminate accessible lesions, and radiation therapy is effective for multiple or unresectable lesions.
- Hemostatic abnormalities have been corrected with heparin, ϵ-aminocaproic acid, aspirin with dipyridamole, or ticlopidine. Antifibrinolytic agents may cause tumor regression by local thrombosis.

OTHER CAUSES OF DESTRUCTIVE THROMBOCYTOPENIA

- Protamine sulfate and bleomycin may cause transient thrombocytopenia.
- Venomous snake bites may cause DIC or may directly aggregate platelets.
- Patients with adult respiratory distress syndrome and severe burns are commonly thrombocytopenic, due to extensive vascular damage.
- Cardiopulmonary bypass surgery can cause thrombocytopenia due to hemodilution and turbulent extracorporeal circulation. A similar mechanism may occur in severe aortic stenosis, severe vascular disease, and pulmonary hypertension.

For a more detailed discussion, see James N. George, Mayez El-Harake: Thrombocytopenia due to enhanced platelet destruction by nonimmunologic mechanisms, Chap. 128, p. 1290, in *Williams Hematology,* 5/e, 1995.

---

67 THROMBOCYTOPENIA DUE TO ENHANCED PLATELET DESTRUCTION BY IMMUNOLOGIC MECHANISMS

Idiopathic thrombocytopenic purpura (ITP)(immune thrombocytopenic purpura, autoimmune thrombocytopenic purpura) is an acquired disease of children and adults characterized by a low platelet count, a normal marrow, and absence of evidence for other disease.

- Childhood ITP characteristically is acute in onset and resolves spontaneously within 6 months (Table 67-1).
- Adult ITP typically has an insidious onset and rarely resolves spontaneously (Table 67-1).

ADULT ITP

Etiology and Pathogenesis

- Thrombocytopenia appears to be due to splenic sequestration and destruction of platelets.
- Most patients have either normal or diminished platelet production. Antiplatelet antibodies bind to megakaryocytes and may cause ineffective thrombocytopoiesis.
- The amount of platelet surface IgG is increased in patients with ITP. Most ITP patients have antibodies to specific platelet membrane glycoproteins.
- Laboratory assays for antiplatelet antibodies have not been demonstrated to be important for clinical diagnosis and management decisions.
- Bleeding times are often shorter than expected for the platelet count, suggesting normal or enhanced platelet function.
- Autoantibodies may cause functional platelet disorders or impair platelet aggregation.
- In 15 to 20 percent of patients, thrombocytopenia is associated with an underlying disease and may be considered "secondary" ITP.
- Chronic ITP may be associated with autoimmune hemolytic anemia (Evans syndrome), and autoantibodies simultaneously affecting platelets and coagulation factors or neutrophils have been described.
- Paraproteins in patients with lymphoma, multiple myeloma, and Waldenström macroglobulinemia can cause thrombocytopenia.

Clinical Features (Table 67-1)

- Most adults present with prolonged histories (>2 months) of purpura.
- Petechiae occur most often in dependent regions. Hemorrhagic bullae in mucous membranes may occur with severe thrombocytopenia.

TABLE 67-1 Clinical Features of ITP in Children and Adults

	Children	Adults
Occurrence		
Peak age (years)	2–4	15–40
Sex (F:M)	equal	2.6:1
Prevalence per million	10–40	66
Presentation		
Onset	Acute (most with symptoms <1 week)	Insidious (most with symptoms >2 months)
Symptoms	Purpura (<10% with severe bleeding)	Purpura (typically bleeding not severe)
Platelet count	Most <20,000/μl	Most <20,000/μl[a]
Course		
Spontaneous remission	83%[b]	2%[c]
Chronic disease	24%[d]	43%[d]
Response to splenectomy	71%[e]	66%[e]
Eventual complete recovery	89%[f]	64%[f]
Complete remission with glucocorticoids	—	25%
Morbidity and mortality[g]		
Cerebral hemorrhage	<1%	3%
Hemorrhagic death	<1%	3%
Mortality of chronic, refractory disease	2%	5%

[a] Although the mean platelet counts at presentation for both children and adults were <20,000/μl in most series, some series of adults had a larger number of patients with platelet counts >30,000/μl.

[b] The frequency of spontaneous remission in children is overestimated because of the selection of patients with ITP of shorter duration and less severity for no treatment.

[c] The frequency of spontaneous remission in adults may be underestimated because in most series all patients are treated initially with glucocorticoids.

[d] Chronic disease in children is defined as thrombocytopenia persisting for longer than 6 months in most series, 12 months in two series. In adults, chronic disease is defined as the lack of a permanent complete remission with no therapy, glucocorticoids, splenectomy, and other therapy. This frequency of patients with chronic, refractory disease is an overestimate, since some of the original number of patients counted as not responding were lost to follow-up.

[e] Splenectomy in children was typically performed only if the symptomatic thrombocytopenia persisted for longer than 1 year. Many adults had splenectomy within 6 months of diagnosis.

(continued)

- Purpura, menorrhagia, epistaxis, and gingival bleeding are common, and gastrointestinal bleeding and hematuria are less so. Intracerebral hemorrhage occurs infrequently, but is the most common cause of death.
- Overt bleeding is rare unless thrombocytopenia is severe (<10,000/μl), and even at this level most patients do not experience major hemorrhage.
- A palpable spleen strongly suggests that ITP is *not* the cause for thrombocytopenia.

Laboratory Features

- Thrombocytopenia is the essential abnormality. The blood film should be reviewed to rule out pseudothrombocytopenia (see Chap. 68). The platelets present are usually of normal size but may be enlarged.
- White blood cell count and hemoglobin level are usually normal unless significant hemorrhage has occurred.
- Coagulation studies are normal.
- The bleeding time may be normal, or nearly so, and does not predict the risk of hemorrhage.
- Marrow megakaryocytes may be increased in number, with a shift to younger, less polyploid forms.

Differential Diagnosis

- Diagnosis is one of exclusion; other conditions that can mimic ITP are acute infections, myelodysplasia, chronic disseminated intravascular coagulation (DIC) and drug-induced thrombocytopenia.
- The distinction from congenital thrombocytopenia is especially important.

Therapy, Course, and Prognosis

- The results of therapy are summarized in Table 67-1. Spontaneous remissions are rare in adults but occur frequently in children.

Table 67-1 (*Continued*)
[f] "Eventual" complete recovery is strongly dependent on the duration of follow-up. One study suggests that this figure may be 80% in adults when follow-up extends for 5 to 20 years.
[g] These data are difficult to estimate. Clearly the prognosis of ITP has improved during the past 50 years. The increased morbidity and mortality in adults presumably reflects the longer course of ITP as well as the greater susceptibility of older adults for serious and fatal complications.
Source: Table 129-1 of *Williams Hematology*, 5/e, p. 1316.

Treatment: Initial Management

- Patients who are incidentally discovered to have asymptomatic mild or moderate thrombocytopenia can safely be followed with no treatment but must be evaluated for an underlying cause, such as hypersplenism.
- Patients with platelet counts over 50,000/µl usually do not have spontaneous, clinically important bleeding.

Management of Acute Bleeding Due to Severe Thrombocytopenia

- Immediate platelet transfusion is indicated for patients with hemorrhagic emergencies. Despite having a presumably short platelet survival time, some patients have substantial posttransfusion increments in their platelet counts.
- Intravenous IgG may be given as a single infusion of 0.4–1.0 g/kg followed immediately by a platelet transfusion. Intravenous IgG 1 g/kg/day for 2 days, will increase the platelet count in most patients within 3 days.
- High doses of glucocorticoids, such as 1 g of methylprednisolone daily for 3 days, may cause a rapid increase of the platelet count.
- ε-Aminiocaproic acid can be effective in controlling acute bleeding.

Glucocorticoids

- Severe thrombocytopenia may cause thinning of the microvascular endothelium, and glucocorticoid therapy may reverse this abnormality. Purpura often improves before the platelet count increases.
- Glucocorticoid therapy also decreases sequestration and destruction of antibody-sensitized platelets and may enhance platelet production.
- Glucocorticoids are also immunosuppressive in the long term.
- Prednisone, given in a dose of 1 mg/kg/day orally, is indicated for patients with symptomatic thrombocytopenia, and probably for all patients with platelet counts below 30,000 to 50,000/µl who may be at increased risk for hemorrhagic complications.
- 60 percent of patients will increase their platelet count to >50,000/µl and about one-fourth will achieve a complete recovery. Most relapse when the prednisone dose is tapered or discontinued.
- The duration of prednisone therapy prior to consideration of splenectomy depends upon the severity of the bleeding, the dose of prednisone required to maintain a response, and the risks of surgery.

Splenectomy

- Splenectomy is successful in achieving complete and permanent responses in two-thirds of patients.
- The risks of operative bleeding complications with splenectomy are low even with severe thrombocytopenia.

- Intravenous IgG can induce a transient remission of thrombocytopenia and may be used to prepare for the operation.
- Platelet transfusions should be given if bleeding is excessive during surgery.
- Most responses to splenectomy occur within several days, and responses after 10 days are unusual. Platelet counts >150,000/μl by the third postoperative day are correlated with a durable response.
- Splenectomy is associated with a small but significantly increased risk for severe infectious complications. All patients should be immunized with *Streptococcus pneumonia* and probably *Hemophilus influenzae* type B vaccines, at least 2 weeks before surgery.
- One-half of patients who relapse after an initial response to splenectomy will do so within 6 months.
- A short course of radiation therapy to the spleen may be beneficial in some patients who cannot tolerate surgery.

Removal of Accessory Spleens

- Accessory spleens are found at splenectomy in 15 to 20 percent of patients and may be present in as many as 10 percent of those refractory to splenectomy or who relapse after splenectomy.
- The absence of Howell-Jolly bodies may suggest the presence of an accessory spleen.
- An accessory spleen can be identified by imaging with ^{99m}Tc-labeled heat-damaged red cells.
- Remission after removal of an accessory spleen is unpredictable.

Treatment: Chronic Refractory ITP

- Chronic refractory ITP may be defined as (1) thrombocytopenia persisting after prior treatment with glucocorticoids and splenectomy, (2) with a patient 10 years of age or older, (3) with no concurrent illness that could cause thrombocytopenia, (4) with a platelet count <50,000/μl, and (5) with duration of ITP of >3 months.
- The treatment of chronic refractory ITP is discussed in detail in Chap. 129 of *Williams Hematology,* 5/e.
- Intravenous immunoglobulin (IV IgG) may be of benefit in chronic ITP and is used primarily when the situation requires a transient increase of the platelet count. It is believed to act by saturating phagocytic Fc receptors, or perhaps by neutralizing antiplatelet antibodies.
- The initial dose of intravenous IgG is 2 g/kg over 2 to 5 days. The complete response rate is 3 percent, and the partial response rate 71 percent. The platelet count will usually increase after several days and return to the pretreatment level in several weeks.
- In patients maintained on intermittent infusions given when counts fall below 20,000/μl, a single infusion of 60 g appears to be adequate.

- Other modalities include danazol, immunosuppressive agents, vinca alkaloids, and anti-Rh(D) antiserum.

Treatment of ITP During Pregnancy and Delivery

- One can generally assume that a pregnant patient with thrombocytopenia has ITP if she has been diagnosed previously, or if the platelet count is less than 75,000/μl with no other apparent etiology (see Chap. 66).
- Of all women who are thrombocytopenic at the time of delivery, only 2 percent will have ITP. Most will have gestational thrombocytopenia, and some will have preeclampsia, with attendant signs and symptoms.
- Early in pregnancy treatment is with prednisone as in the nonpregnant patient. Intravenous IgG is an alternative therapy that may help to delay splenectomy.
- Splenectomy should be deferred, if possible, because the platelet count may spontaneously improve after delivery, and splenectomy increases the risk of fetal death and premature labor. Early in the second trimester is considered the optimal time for splenectomy.
- 4 to 5 percent of infants of mothers with ITP have clinically important thrombocytopenia. Severe thrombocytopenia may occur in an infant born to a mother with only a history of ITP. Previous birth of a severely thrombocytopenic infant is the best evidence of risk. Neonatal thrombocytopenia can worsen or even first appear after delivery.
- Prednisone should be given only as indicated for management of the mother's thrombocytopenia.
- One recommendation is to manage the delivery in a conventional manner, with immediate platelet count monitoring of the newborn. Cesarean section should be performed only on women who have previously delivered severely thrombocytopenic infants.
- Neonatal thrombocytopenia may be successfully treated with intravenous IgG, glucocorticoids, and transfusion with irradiated platelets. Brain CT should be performed to rule out intracranial hemorrhage.

CHILDHOOD ITP

- Also referred to as postinfectious thrombocytopenia, since an infectious illness usually precedes the purpura by several weeks; however, the significance of this association is unclear.

Clinical Features (Table 67-1)

- Bruises and petechiae are nearly universal, epistaxis and gingival bleeding occur in less than a third, and hematuria and gastrointestinal bleeding in less than 10 percent. Anemia occurs in 15 percent.
- A palpable spleen is present in 12 percent (but is also present in 10 percent of normal children).

Laboratory Features

- Most children present with platelet counts <20,000/μl.
- Marrow examination is usually performed to rule out acute leukemia.

Differential Diagnosis

- Diagnosis is made on the basis of isolated thrombocytopenia with no evidence of other disease.
- Other diseases to be considered are sepsis, hemolytic-uremic syndrome, HIV infection, drug-induced thrombocytopenia, and congenital thrombocytopenia.

Therapy, Course, and Prognosis

- 83 percent of patients have a complete remission within 6 months without glucocorticoid treatment or splenectomy. Good prognostic features include a short duration of disease with an abrupt onset and mild symptoms. Most patients develop no new purpuric symptoms after the first week, and the time to a normal platelet count is typically 2 to 8 weeks.
- Purpura more than 2 to 4 weeks before diagnosis is the most important predictor of chronic thrombocytopenia. Other factors are female sex, age >10 years, and higher platelet count at presentation.
- Few children with ITP have critical complications, and even fewer die. Only 1 percent have intracerebral hemorrhage, and the mortality is <1 percent.
- Many children appear to require no specific treatment, but the issue is debatable, as is the need for hospitalization; there are conflicting data as to whether glucocorticoids hasten recovery.
- If prednisone therapy is given, the recommended dose is 1 to 2 mg/kg, although lower doses (0.25 mg/kg/day) may be equally effective.
- Intravenous IgG may be given when there is a need to increase the platelet count rapidly. The usual dose is 2 g/kg given over 2 to 5 days, and the platelet counts typically reach 50,000/μl in 2 days and are normal in 3 days.
- The great majority of patients respond to anti-Rh(D) antiserum by increasing their platelet count to >50,000/μl for several weeks. Maintenance therapy (25 to 75 μg/kg) every 5 weeks can prevent severe thrombocytopenia in children with chronic ITP.
- Splenectomy is deferred for at least 6 to 12 months following diagnosis.
- Splenectomy is recommended only for severe thrombocytopenia with significant bleeding symptoms. In such patients, splenectomy is efficacious and 71 percent achieve a continuous complete remission. Among children who have persistent thrombocytopenia after splenectomy, spontaneous remissions occur subsequently in about one-third.

- Splenectomy in children is associated with an increased risk of severe infection. All routine immunizations and those for *Streptococcus pneumonia, Hemophilus influenzae* type B and *Neisseria meningitidis* (when available), must be given >2 weeks prior to splenectomy. Penicillin prophylaxis is routinely given to splenectomized children.
- Splenectomized children and their families must be educated about the seriousness of febrile illnesses.
- Efficacy of other measures for therapy of chronic ITP in childhood is uncertain. Because the mortality is low and spontaneous remissions occur even after many years, potentially harmful agents should be used only when there is substantial risk for death or morbidity from hemorrhage.

THROMBOCYTOPENIA ASSOCIATED WITH HIV INFECTION (see also Chap. 52)

- Thrombocytopenia occurs in many patients with HIV infection, and may be the presenting sign.

Etiology and Pathogenesis

- Increased platelet destruction is assumed to be a result of immune platelet injury.
- Most patients also have decreased platelet production, possibly due to direct HIV infection of megakaryocytes.

Clinical and Laboratory Features

- Thrombocytopenia is an isolated abnormality. The marrow contains normal numbers of megakaryocytes, and the spleen is not palpable.
- Thrombocytopenia is often discovered incidentally, is mild, and may require no specific treatment and resolve spontaneously.
- Decreased levels of CD4+ lymphocytes, neutropenia, and even pancytopenia may be present. Marrow examination is required to rule out granulomatous infection or lymphoma.
- Thrombocytopenia in HIV-infected hemophiliacs may contribute to intracerebral hemorrhage and exacerbate the severe bleeding characteristic of hemophilia.

Therapy, Course, and Prognosis

- Many patients with mild thrombocytopenia respond to zidovudine, which may be effective because of its antiretroviral activity and possibly because of stimulation of megakaryocyte progenitors.
- Patients with severe and symptomatic thrombocytopenia should be managed the same as patients with severe ITP. In addition to zidovudine, prednisone is given at a dose of 1 mg/kg/day orally.
- HIV-infected patients with hemophilia should be treated more aggres-

sively, probably beginning prednisone when the platelet count drops below 50,000/μl.

- Most patients respond to glucocorticoids but will relapse when they are tapered and discontinued.
- Splenectomy is the most effective therapy and does not adversely affect the HIV infection.
- Intravenous IgG is effective in elevating the platelet count transiently.
- If zidovudine, glucocorticoids, splenectomy, and intravenous IgG are ineffective, the various agents used in chronic ITP may be beneficial (see Chap. 129 in *Williams Hematology,* 5/e).

CYCLIC THROMBOCYTOPENIA

- Occurs predominantly in young women and may be related to the menstrual cycle, but also occurs in men and postmenopausal women. In all patients, the average period of the thrombocytopenic cycle is about 30 days.
- Platelet survival time is shortened and antiplatelet antibodies have been demonstrated.
- While spontaneous remissions may occur, the cyclic occurrence of thrombocytopenia is chronic in most patients.
- Prednisone therapy is often ineffective and splenectomy has not been beneficial. Danazol provides temporary remissions in some patients. Intravenous IgG may delay the fall in platelet count but does not prevent recurrence.

DRUG-INDUCED IMMUNOLOGIC THROMBOCYTOPENIA

Etiology and Pathogenesis

- Many drugs cause acute thrombocytopenia in sensitive individuals; quinine, quinidine, sulfonamide antimicrobials, and heparin (see below) have been studied most extensively.
- Antibodies induced by quinidine and quinine bind to platelet glycoproteins. In these cases, the drug binds either to one or more components of the platelet membrane and induces a reversible structural change (cryptantigen) or forms a drug-protein complex (neoantigen) that provokes antibody.
- Occasionally, antibodies induced by a drug (e.g., gold salts, α-methyldopa) will interact with platelets even if the drug is not present.
- A few drugs (e.g., penicillin) bind covalently to platelet membranes to induce true hapten-dependent antibodies.

Drugs Implicated as Causes

- A vast number of drugs have been implicated (see Table 129-8 of *Williams Hematology,* 5/e), but only occasional patients develop the disorder. Quinine, quinidine, heparin, and gold salts are the most frequent offenders. Up to 5 percent of patients receiving gold salts may develop thrombocytopenia, and those with HLA-DRw3 appear to be at greatest risk.

- Protamine, bleomycin, ristocetin, desmopressin, and hematin appear to cause platelet destruction by nonimmunologic mechanisms.
- A 15 to 50 percent decrease in the platelet count, lasting several hours, sometimes follows intracutaneous injection of antigen or ingestion of food to which allergy has previously been manifested.
- Thrombocytopenia, often severe, occurs following anaphylaxis.

Clinical and Laboratory Features

- A careful history is crucial. In addition to prescription medications, the patient should be asked about over-the-counter drugs, soft drinks, mixers, and aperitifs that may contain quinine.
- Thrombocytopenia is common in narcotics addicts, and is often due to HIV infection in such patients, but has been associated with cocaine and also quinine used as a narcotic adulterant.
- Acute renal failure accompanied by microangiopathic hemolytic anemia and thrombocytopenia in patients taking quinine and other drugs is considered a form of drug-induced adult hemolytic uremia syndrome (see Chap. 66).
- Ingestion of a drug to which a patient is sensitive is often followed within minutes by a warm sensation, flushing, and a chill. Petechiae, purpura, hemorrhagic bullae of the oral mucosa, and often gastrointestinal bleeding and hematuria usually appear in 6 to 12 h.
- Bleeding symptoms usually disappear over a period of 3 to 4 days.
- Thrombocytopenia is often very severe initially, with platelet levels $<10,000/\mu l$ and sometimes $<1000/\mu l$.
- In the marrow the number of megakaryocytes is usually normal or elevated.
- With quinidine or quinine, drug-dependent antibodies can be detected by laboratory techniques.

Treatment and Prognosis

- In any patient with acute thrombocytopenia of unknown etiology, it is desirable to stop as many drugs as possible, especially those known to cause thrombocytopenia.
- After stopping the drug, platelets return to normal within 7 days in most instances. Gold-induced thrombocytopenia can persist for months, and dimercaprol (BAL) may speed recovery.
- Hospitalization for at least several days is advisable if the thrombocytopenia is severe.
- Glucocorticoids do not shorten the duration of thrombocytopenia, but are perhaps advisable because of their effect on vascular integrity.

- Platelet transfusions should be given for serious hemorrhage, and, in critically ill patients, plasma exchange may be helpful.
- High-dose intravenous IgG has been administered with apparent benefit.
- Antidigitoxin antibodies may be helpful if the thrombocytopenia is due to digitoxin.
- The combination of plasma exchange, intravenous IgG, platelet transfusions, and prednisone can be considered for severely thrombocytopenic patients with intracranial or other serious hemorrhage.
- Sensitivity to drugs causing immunologic thrombocytopenic purpura probably persists indefinitely and patients should be warned to avoid reexposure.

HEPARIN-ASSOCIATED THROMBOCYTOPENIA
(See also Chap. 83)

Etiology and Pathogenesis

- The mechanism is complex, but appears to involve the development of antiplatelet antibodies that require heparin (or related polyanionic molecules) for optimal interaction. Heparin appears to alter the platelet surface, facilitating the binding of antibody to antigen. IgG from patients causes platelet aggregation and secretion in the presence of heparin.

Clinical and Laboratory Features

- Thrombocytopenia can occur with any heparin preparation: unfractionated heparin, low-molecular-weight heparins, and heparin-like compounds such as pentosan (polysulfated plant polypentose) and the "heparinoid" glycosaminoglycan agent Organon 10172. Higher-molecular-weight fractions of heparin may interact more readily with platelets and thereby cause thrombocytopenia more frequently.
- Heparin isolated from beef lung appears to cause thrombocytopenia more often than heparin from pork intestinal mucosa (8 percent of patients versus 4 percent).
- Thrombocytopenia occurs more often in patients receiving high doses of heparin for treatment of thromboembolism, but has been reported with all doses and routes of administration.
- Thrombocytopenia occurs in about 5 percent (range 0 to 21 percent) of patients receiving heparin to prevent or treat thromboembolism. Severe thrombocytopenia, with platelet counts of $<50,000/\mu l$, occurs in 1 percent.
- Heparin-associated thrombocytopenia may present in one of two forms, although the distinction is often unclear.
  - Minimal thrombocytopenia, with counts $>50,000/\mu l$, may begin soon after heparin is started and may resolve even while heparin is continued.

- Severe thrombocytopenia, much less common, appears later in the course. It may be accompanied by fever, skin necrosis, DIC, and thromboses, often with catastrophic results. It may recur upon re-administration of heparin. It appears to be antibody-mediated.
- At present, assays for heparin-dependent antibodies are investigative tools and are not required for management.

Therapy, Course, and Prognosis

- Platelet counts should be obtained frequently from patients on heparin.
- The incidence of heparin-induced thrombocytopenia may be decreasing because shorter courses of heparin are now being given, and low-molecular-weight heparin is being used more often.
- Platelet counts of $<100,000/\mu l$ on two consecutive days in the absence of other causes in patients receiving heparin strongly supports the diagnosis.
- The decision to stop heparin therapy depends upon the relative risks of extension or recurrence of the thrombosis and the knowledge that many patients with counts of 50,000 to $100,000/\mu l$ spontaneously recover while continuing heparin.
- If the platelet count is $<50,000/\mu l$, and no other etiology is likely, heparin should be stopped immediately. The platelet count should improve within hours to several days.
- Discontinuation of heparin therapy for 6 to 12 h may lead to improvement in the platelet count and serve as a useful diagnostic test.
- In most patients, the thrombocytopenia is mild and self-limited and is discovered at a time in the course of therapy when heparin can be safely discontinued.
- Treatment for severe thrombocytopenia may include the use of intravenous IgG or plasmapheresis.
- Platelet transfusions could theoretically result in thrombosis and should be given with caution.

NEONATAL ALLOIMMUNE THROMBOCYTOPENIA

Etiology and Pathogenesis

- Occurs about once in 2000 to 3000 births.
- Pathogenesis is similar to erythroblastosis fetalis except that fetal platelets rather than erythrocytes provide the antigenic challenge.
- Destruction of fetal platelets is caused by transplacentally acquired maternal antibodies directed against fetal-platelet–specific antigens inherited from the father.
- The antigen, Pl^{A1} (HPA-1a), found in about 98 percent of the general population, provides the immunogenic stimulus in about half of the cases involving Caucasians.
- Other alloantigens are also implicated (see Chap. 129, *Williams Hematology,* 5/e).

Clinical and Laboratory Features

- First-born children are often affected, indicating that fetal platelets cross the placenta during gestation. Recurrence with subsequent pregnancies is common.
- Gestation and delivery are generally unremarkable.
- Severely affected infants usually have petechiae on the skin and mucosal surfaces at birth or within the first few hours. The petechiae are generalized, which helps to distinguish them from those caused by ordinary birth trauma.
- Dyspnea or neurologic changes may suggest intracranial hemorrhage.
- Jaundice and kernicterus may occur because of the limited ability of the newborn to metabolize bilirubin reabsorbed from sites of bleeding.
- In symptomatic cases, platelet levels are usually $<30,000/\mu l$ and may decrease further during the first 2 days of life. Without treatment, thrombocytopenia persists for an average of 2 weeks (range 2 to 3 days to 2 months).
- Anemia, when present, is due to bleeding.
- Marrow megakaryocytes are usually normal in number but are occasionally absent.
- Since only 2 percent of the general population lacks the Pl^{A1} platelet antigen, finding that the mother's platelets are Pl^{A1}-negative provides presumptive evidence of alloimmune origin.

Differential Diagnosis

- The diagnosis is one of exclusion unless definitive serologic tests are obtained.
- A normal platelet count in the mother and a negative history helps exclude ITP. Erythroblastosis fetalis should be excluded by a negative direct antiglobulin test.
- Viral or bacterial infection, hemangioma-thrombocytopenia syndrome, congenital absence of megakaryocytes, and thrombocytopenia with maternal drug ingestion should be considered.

Therapy, Course, and Prognosis

- May be mild and require no specific therapy.
- Although the effectiveness of glucocorticoids has not been fully established, it is reasonable to treat severely affected newborns with prednisone, 2 mg/kg daily, in the immediate postnatal period.
- Platelet transfusions are indicated for serious hemorrhage; platelets that react with the mother's antibody may be of transient benefit and are probably without hazard if given slowly.
- Compatible platelets are preferred and can be obtained by plateletpheresis of the mother. They should be washed to avoid administration of additional antibody to the infant. Maternal platelets should also be irradiated to avoid graft-vs.-host disease.

- Intravenous IgG (400 mg/kg/day for 5 days) appears to shorten the duration of thrombocytopenia, but the response is often delayed. Transfusion of compatible platelets is therefore the first therapeutic choice when there is significant risk for intracranial hemorrhage.
- Exchange transfusion is used to remove antibody in the hope of shortening the duration of thrombocytopenia. It should be reserved for infants with platelet counts of <20,000/μl who cannot be managed by other means, or who have dangerously high bilirubin levels.
- Splenectomy is not recommended.
- The mortality is about 15 percent, chiefly due to intracranial hemorrhage.

POSTTRANSFUSION PURPURA

- Acute, severe thrombocytopenia occurring 1 week after a blood transfusion associated with high-titer, platelet-specific alloantibodies. The exact prevalence is unknown.

Etiology and Pathogenesis

- Anti-Pl[A1] is present in more than 90 percent of cases.
- The Pl[A1] alloantigen appears to accumulate in plasma during storage of blood. This "soluble" alloantigen binds to Pl[A1]-negative autologous platelets to stimulate the formation of anti-Pl[A1] alloantibody. The antibody then binds to Pl[A1] antigen acquired by autologous platelets and promotes platelet destruction.
- Another potential mechanism is formation of an autoantibody which reacts with Pl[A1]-negative platelets. Patients with posttransfusion purpura often produce alloantibodies against red cells, granulocytes, and HLA antigens in addition to platelet-specific antibodies.
- Since 1 in 50 transfusion recipients is "mismatched" with respect to the Pl[A1] antigen and posttransfusion purpura is rare, it appears that only certain donor units contain sufficient amounts of soluble Pl[A1] alloantigen or only a minority of Pl[A1]-negative persons are predisposed to alloimmunization.

Clinical and Laboratory Features

- More than 90 percent of cases occur in multiparous women receiving their first blood transfusion, but it may also occur in nulliparous women and in men. The provocative transfusion is often accompanied by a febrile reaction.
- Bleeding symptoms typically occur 5 to 8 days after transfusion and are usually severe at the onset with a platelet count of <10,000/μl.
- Megakaryocytes are usually present in the marrow in normal or increased numbers.
- A potent alloantibody reactive with one or more platelet-specific antigens can be detected by appropriate serologic methods.

Therapy, Course, and Prognosis

- Patients recover spontaneously within 1 to 6 weeks; fatal intracranial hemorrhage occurs in about 10 percent.
- Improvement usually occurs with plasma exchange, presumably because of removal of antibody and antigen responsible for platelet destruction.
- Treatment with intravenous IgG, 0.4 g/kg daily for 5 days, can be effective.
- Platelet transfusions from random donors are likely to be Pl[A1]-positive and may cause severe, even life-threatening transfusion reactions.
- Glucocorticoids are commonly used but responses are probably unusual.

PASSIVELY INDUCED POST-TRANSFUSION PURPURA

- Severe thrombocytopenia occurring a few hours after transfusion of plasma-containing blood products and lasting for 1 to 2 weeks has resulted from inadvertent transfusion of antibodies specific for Pl[A1] and Br[a].
- Spontaneous recovery can be expected, but treatment with prednisone, intravenous IgG, or plasma exchange should be considered for severely affected patients.

For a more detailed discussion, see James N. George, Mayez El-Harake, Richard H. Aster: Thrombocytopenia due to enhanced platelet destruction by immunologic mechanisms, Chap. 129, p. 1315, *Williams Hematology*, 5/e, 1995.

---

68 THROMBOCYTOPENIA: PSEUDOTHROMBOCYTOPENIA, HYPERSPLENISM, AND THROMBOCYTOPENIA ASSOCIATED WITH MASSIVE TRANSFUSION

PSEUDOTHROMBOCYTOPENIA

- A false diagnosis of thrombocytopenia can occur when laboratory conditions cause platelets to clump, resulting in artificially low platelet counts as determined by automated counters.
- The blood film should always be carefully examined to confirm the presence of thrombocytopenia.

Etiology and Pathogenesis

- Platelet clumping caused by EDTA anticoagulant used for routine blood counts is the most common cause of falsely low platelet counts and occurs with a prevalence of 0.1 percent. Clumping may also be seen with other anticoagulants.
- Other mechanisms may include platelet cold agglutinins and rosetting around leukocytes.
- Clumping is usually caused by a low titer IgG antibody, presumably recognizing an epitope exposed on platelets by the in vitro conditions.

Laboratory Features

- A film made from EDTA-anticoagulated blood demonstrates more platelets than expected from the platelet count, but many are in large pools or clumps. A blood film made directly from a fingerstick sample accurately reflects the true count.
- Pseudothrombocytopenia is often accompanied by a falsely elevated white count (by 10 to 100 percent) since some platelet clumps are sufficiently large to be detected as leukocytes by an automated counter.
- Correct platelet counts can be obtained by placing fingerstick blood directly into diluting fluid at 37°C and performing counts by phase-contrast microscopy.

Clinical Features

- These platelets agglutinins have no clinical importance, except for inducing pseudothrombocytopenia.
- Platelet clumping is usually persistent but may be transient in some patients.

THROMBOCYTOPENIA DUE TO SPLENIC POOLING (HYPERSPLENISM) (See also Chap. 38)

- Pooling of platelets within the spleen (sequestration) leads to thrombocytopenia. This phenomena is often referred to as hypersplenism.

Etiology and Pathogenesis

- The spleen normally pools about one-third of the platelet mass. Reversible pooling of up to 90 percent of the platelet mass occurs in patients with hypersplenism.
- Total platelet mass and platelet production are normal, and platelet survival is often normal.
- Hypothermia has been reported to cause temporary thrombocytopenia in humans and animals, presumably because platelets are transiently sequestered in the spleen and other organs.

Clinical Features

- Thrombocytopenia associated with hypersplenism is often of no clinical importance. The degree of thrombocytopenia is modest, the total body content of platelets is normal, and platelets can be mobilized from the spleen.
- In situations such as major trauma or surgery requiring platelet transfusions, hypersplenism can be an important clinical problem, especially when compounded by the coagulopathy of liver disease.
- The most common disorder causing hypersplenism is cirrhosis, with portal hypertension and congestive splenomegaly, but any disease with an enlarged, congested spleen can be associated with thrombocytopenia.
- The spleen is usually palpable and the degree of thrombocytopenia is correlated with the size of the spleen. In some disorders, decreased platelet production may be a contributing factor.
- Although thrombocytopenia is well described in patients with hypothermia, in one report only 3 of 75 patients with hypothermia were affected.

Laboratory Features

- Rarely is the platelet count less than $50,000/\mu l$. Marrow megakaryocytes are usually normal in number and morphology.
- Patients with very large spleens and severe thrombocytopenia usually have a marrow infiltrative process and decreased platelet production as well as hypersplenism.

Treatment and Prognosis

- Since thrombocytopenia due to hypersplenism is usually not a significant problem, no treatment is generally indicated.

- Splenectomy may be appropriate in cases of severe thrombocytopenia or if it is impossible for transfusions to increase the platelet count sufficiently to achieve hemostasis.
- Splenectomy usually results in return of the platelet count to normal. Platelet counts may return to normal after portal-systemic shunting for cirrhosis.
- Therapy for thrombocytopenia of hypothermia is rewarming and documenting normalization of platelet count.

THROMBOCYTOPENIA ASSOCIATED WITH MASSIVE TRANSFUSION

- Patients receiving 15 units of red cells within 24 h regularly develop mild thrombocytopenia (47,000 to 100,000/μl), while those receiving more than 20 units may have platelet counts of 25,000 to 61,000/μl.
- The severity of the thrombocytopenia is related to the number of transfusions, but counts may be higher than predicted, due to release from the splenic pool, or lower, because of microvascular consumption.
- Severe thrombocytopenia can be prevented by giving platelet transfusions to those requiring more than 20 units of red cells within 24 h. In spite of transfusions of platelets and fresh frozen plasma, diffuse microvascular bleeding is commonly observed, with petechiae, ecchymoses, and oozing of blood from mucous membranes, catheter sites, and surgical wounds.

For a more detailed discussion, see James N. George: Thrombocytopenia: Pseudothrombocytopenia, hypersplenism, and thrombocytopenia associated with massive transfusion, Chap. 130, p. 1355, in *Williams Hematology*, 5/e, 1995.

---

69 SECONDARY THROMBOCYTOSIS

- An elevation of the platelet count above the normal upper limit of 400,000/μl in patients with various underlying disease, as outlined in Table 69-1.
- Usually due to overprotection of platelets with normal function and normal or decreased survival time.
- May be due to release of platelets from storage depots.
- Usually asymptomatic, but may cause thrombosis in elderly patients or those with atherosclerosis or immobility. Abnormal bleeding rare.
- Contrast with thrombocytosis due to myeloproliferative disorders, where complications occur frequently (see Chaps. 8 to 11).
- Treatment
  - Platelet count may be rapidly reduced by plateletpheresis.
  - Antiplatelet drugs may be useful to prevent thrombosis in high-risk patients.
- Secondary thrombocytosis of 1,000,000/μl or more is often seen after splenectomy. Most physicians do not administer heparin prophylactically in this situation, but treat thrombosis if it occurs.

TABLE 69-1 Conditions in which Elevated Platelet Counts may Be Found

Myeloproliferative disorders (see Chaps 8 to 11).
Secondary thrombocytosis*
  Malignant diseases, including hematologic malignancies
  Chronic inflammatory diseases
  Acute inflammatory diseases
  Acute blood loss
  Iron deficiency
  Hemolytic anemia
  Postoperatively, especially postsplenectomy
  In response to vincristine, epinephrine, interleukin 1b
  In response to exercise
  Upon recovery from thrombocytopenia due to myelosuppressive drugs, including alcohol
  Therapy of vitamin B_{12} deficiency
  Prematurity
  Vitamin E deficiency in infants
  Miscellaneous causes*

*Further details are presented in Table 131-1 of *Williams Hematology*, 5/e, 1995, p. 1361.

For a more detailed discussion, see William J. Williams: Secondary thrombocytosis, Chap. 131, p. 1361, in *Williams Hematology*, 5/e, 1995.

70 HEREDITARY QUALITATIVE PLATELET DISORDERS

Abnormalities of platelet function are expressed primarily by mucocutaneous bleeding (see Fig. 70-1). The most frequent laboratory abnormality is prolongation of the bleeding time. Hereditary qualitative platelet disorders may be due to abnormalities of

- platelet membrane glycoproteins
- platelet granules
- platelet coagulant activity
- signal transduction and secretion

ABNORMAL GLYCOPROTEIN (GP) IIb/IIIa ($\alpha IIb\beta_3$, CD41/CD61): GLANZMANN THROMBASTHENIA

- GP IIb/IIIa functions as receptor for fibrinogen and other adhesive glycoproteins.
- It is required for platelet aggregation induced by all agonists thought to function in vivo.
- Both IIb and IIIa are required for normal function, and defects in either component may cause thrombasthenia.
- Many different molecular biological abnormalities have been described.
- Inherited as an autosomal recessive disorder.
- Clinical features
  - Petechiae, purpura, ecchymoses
  - Menorrhagia, especially at menarche
  - Epistaxis
  - Gingival bleeding
  - Bleeding from other sites (less frequent)
  - Clinical expression does not correlate with the degree of abnormality of the laboratory findings
  - Carriers appear to be asymptomatic
- Laboratory features
  - Normal platelet count and morphology
  - Prolonged bleeding time
  - Decreased or absent clot retraction
  - Abnormal platelet aggregation to physiological stimuli
  - Many other abnormalities of platelet function of research interest
- Differential diagnosis versus the following:
  - Thrombocytopenia: platelet count normal
  - Other qualitative platelet disorders: specific laboratory findings
  - von Willebrand disease, afibrinogenemia, hemophilia, and related disorders: specific laboratory findings
  - Autoantibodies to GP IIa/IIIb: demonstrate inhibitor of platelet function by mixing studies using normal plasma and platelets

- Therapy
  - Preventive measures: dental hygiene, avoid antiplatelet drugs (see Chap. 71), hepatitis B vaccination early in life, hormone therapy to avoid menorrhagia.
  - Management of bleeding: platelet transfusion for serious hemorrhage; local therapy as appropriate, such as pressure dressings, gelfoam, dental splints, etc.; antifibrinolytic therapy may be helpful.
- Prognosis
  - Bleeding problems may be severe and frequent, but prognosis for survival is good, and has improved with increased availability of platelet transfusions.

ABNORMAL GP Ib (CD42b,c), GP IX (CD42a), and GP V: BERNARD-SOULIER SYNDROME

- GP Ib/IX complex is the platelet receptor for von Willebrand factor.
- GP Ib is also a binding site for thrombin.
- GP V appears to form noncovalent complex with GP Ib/IX.
- Several different abnormalities of these glycoproteins have been identified.
- Inherited as an autosomal recessive trait; an autosomal dominant form has also been reported.
- Clinical features
  - Ecchymoses, menometrorrhagia, gingival bleeding, and gastrointestinal bleeding are common.
  - Other bleeding sites less frequent.
- Laboratory features
  - Thrombocytopenia in nearly all patients.
  - Large platelets, some larger than lymphocytes.
  - Platelets do not aggregate in response to ristocetin. In contrast to von Willebrand disease, this abnormality is not corrected by addition of normal plasma.
  - Platelet coagulant activity may be reduced, normal, or increased.
- Treatment and prognosis are similar to Glanzmann thrombasthenia, discussed above.

ABNORMAL GP Ib (CD42b,c): PLATELET-TYPE OR PSEUDO VON WILLEBRAND DISEASE

- GP Ib/IX is receptor for von Willebrand factor.
- Abnormal form has enhanced binding of von Willebrand factor, leading to reduction in high-molecular-weight multimers in plasma, and perhaps reduction in platelet survival time.
- Specific mutations have been demonstrated in some patients.
- Inherited as an autosomal dominant trait.

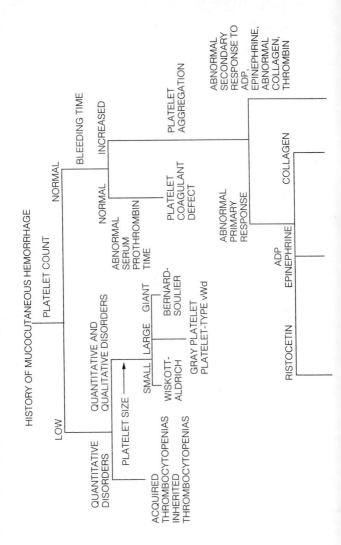

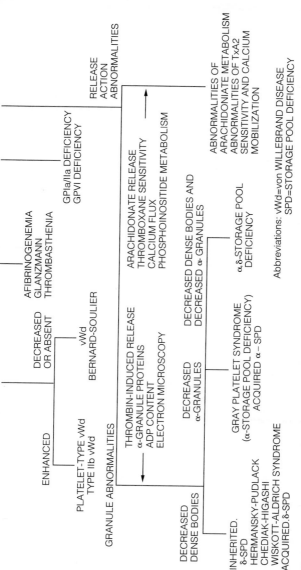

FIG. 1 Evaluation of patients with mucocutaneous hemorrhage for platelet disorders. *(From Fig. 132-1, Williams Hematology 5/e, 1995.)*

Clinical features: mild to moderate mucocutaneous bleeding.
- Laboratory features
  - Bleeding time usually prolonged.
  - Some patients have thrombocytopenia and large platelets.
  - Plasma von Willebrand factor concentration is reduced, especially the high-molecular-weight multimers.
  - Enhanced platelet aggregation in response to low concentrations of ristocetin, not corrected by normal plasma (in type II von Willebrand disease this abnormality is corrected by normal plasma).
- Therapy
  - Platelet transfusion may be beneficial.
  - Administration of von Willebrand factor may be beneficial in low doses, but can cause thrombocytopenia because of increased binding to platelets.

WISKOTT-ALDRICH SYNDROME

- Patients have thrombocytopenia, small platelets, recurrent infections, and eczema
- Inherited as an X-linked trait.
- A defect has been found in sialophorin (CD 46), a glycoprotein found on lymphocytes, neutrophils, and platelets, but it is not likely the basic abnormality because the gene coding for this protein is on chromosome 16, and the disorder is sex-linked.
- Deficiencies in GP Ib and Ia have been found in some, but not all, patients.
- Deficiency of platelet storage pool of adenine nucleotides and abnormal platelet energy metabolism are found in some patients.
- The thrombocytopenia is believed due to diminished platelet survival, but ineffective thrombopoiesis may also play a role.
- Cause of small platelets is unknown.
- Clinical features
  - Mucocutaneous bleeding
  - Recurrent infections
  - Eczema
  - Increased risk of development of lymphoma
- Laboratory features
  - Thrombocytopenia with platelets of small volume
  - Bleeding time prolonged
  - Platelet aggregation and release of dense body contents variably abnormal
  - Defects in both humoral and cellular immunity
- Treatment
  - Splenectomy improves thrombocytopenia; may lead to increased platelet size and improved function.
  - Marrow transplantation may be curative.

δ-STORAGE POOL DEFICIENCY

- A usually mild bleeding disorder with abnormalities in the second wave of platelet aggregation and deficiencies in the contents of the dense granules of platelets.
- Predisposition to hematologic malignancies in some families.
- Occurs in association with inherited multisystem disorders:
  - Hermansky-Pudlak syndrome
  - Chediak-Higashi syndrome
  - Wiskott-Aldrich syndrome (see above)
  - others less frequently
- Usually transmitted as an autosomal recessive trait, but may be autosomal dominant.
- Clinical features
  - Severe bleeding possible in patients with Hermansky-Pudlak syndrome; others mild.
  - Mucocutaneous bleeding, excessive bruising, epistaxis common.
  - Excess bleeding after surgery or trauma.
- Laboratory features
  - Bleeding time prolonged.
  - Variable abnormalities of second wave of platelet aggregation.
- Differential diagnosis (see Glanzmann thrombasthenia, above)
- Treatment
  - Avoid antiplatelet drugs.
  - Bleeding associated with surgery may be diminished by therapy with glucocorticoids.
  - Bleeding time may be diminished by therapy with desmopressin or cryoprecipitate.
  - Platelet transfusion may be helpful if bleeding is severe.

GRAY PLATELET SYNDROME (α-GRANULE DEFICIENCY)

- α-Granule membranes form abnormal vesicular structures rather than granules.
- Platelets are deficient in α-granule contents, including fibrinogen and von Willebrand factor.
- Clinical features
  - Mild hemorrhagic manifestations are usual, but severe bleeding has been reported.
- Laboratory features
  - Platelets on blood films are pale, ghost-like, oval, and larger than normal.
  - Thrombocytopenia common; may be moderately severe.
  - Platelet aggregation may be abnormal.
- Differential diagnosis (see Glanzmann thrombasthenia, above)
- Treatment

- Desmopressin or antifibrinolytic therapy may be beneficial.
- Platelet transfusion indicated for serious hemorrhage.

$\alpha\delta$-STORAGE POOL DEFICIENCY

- Moderate to severe defects in both α and δ granules
- Clinical and laboratory features similar to δ-storage pool deficiency

ABNORMALITIES OF PLATELET COAGULANT ACTIVITY

- Only a few such patients have been described; only one studied in detail.
- Leads to diminished binding of intermediates in coagulation and consequent slowing of rate of clotting.
- Clinical features
  - Bleeding occurs after trauma, post-partum, menorrhagia.
  - No mucocutaneous bledding, in contrast to other qualitative platelet disorders.
- Laboratory features
  - Bleeding time normal.
  - *Serum* prothrombin time abnormal.
  - Assays for platelet factor 3 abnormal.
- Differential diagnosis (see Glanzmann thrombasthenia, above)
- Therapy
  - Platelet transfusions for prevention and treatment.
  - Prothrombin complex concentrates may be effective, but carry risk of thrombosis and hepatitis.

ABNORMALITIES OF SIGNAL TRANSDUCTION AND SECRETION

- Usually produce only minor bleeding tendency, comparable to that induced by aspirin.
- Therapy not usually necessary.
- Defects in arachidonic acid metabolism:
  - Arachidonic acid release from phospholipids—platelets aggregate normally with arachidonic acid, but not with ADP, epinephrine, or collagen.
  - Cyclooxygenase deficiency—platelets unable to produce thromboxane; endothelium may not produce prostacyclin. Clinical manifestations may be mild bleeding disorder (platelet defect predominant) or thrombotic disease (endothelium defect predominant)
  - Thromboxane synthetase deficiency—platelets unable to convert endoperoxides to thromboxane. Usually mild bleeding disorder; prolonged bleeding time.
- Defects in platelet secretion and the second wave of platelet aggrega-

tion are found in response to epinephrine or ATP. Normal platelet aggregation is frequently observed in response to collagen or thrombin. The mechanism(s) responsible for these abnormalities remain undefined, but they are currently considered due to defects in thromboxane A_2 sensitivity, calcium mobilization and calcium responsiveness.

For a more detailed discussion, see Barry S. Coller: Hereditary qualitative platelet disorders, Chap. 132, p. 1364, in *Williams Hematology,* 5/e, 1995.

---

71 ACQUIRED QUALITATIVE PLATELET DISORDERS DUE TO DISEASES, DRUGS, AND FOODS

Acquired qualitative platelet abnormalities occur with systemic diseases, hematologic disorders, cardiopulmonary bypass, ingestion of some drugs, and consumption of certain foods. The manifestations are usually mild, but may be severe if there is an accompanying hemostatic abnormality or a predisposing local lesion. The usual laboratory abnormalities are prolongation of the bleeding time and/or abnormal platelet aggregation, but these results do not necessarily predict the risk of clinical bleeding.

ABNORMAL PLATELET FUNCTION IN UREMIA

- Platelets from uremic patients may have defects in adhesion, aggregation, or procoagulant activity due to currently unknown cause(s).
- Concurrent medications may contribute to the abnormalities, e.g., aspirin.
- Thrombocytopenia, particularly if the count is less than $100,000/\mu l$, raises the possibility of some cause other than uremia, such as multiple myeloma or drug-induced thrombocytopenia.
- Clinical features
  - Most common bleeding sites are skin, gastrointestinal, and genitourinary tracts.
  - Patients with gastrointestinal bleeding frequently have a predisposing anatomical lesion.
  - Serious bleeding may occur with surgery or trauma.
  - If bleeding occurs, initiate search for the cause without assuming uremia is responsible.
- Laboratory features
  - Bleeding time often prolonged, but does not quantitate risk of hemorrhage.
- Therapy
  - Intensive dialysis can correct bleeding time and abnormal bleeding in some patients.
  - Desmopressin (DDAVP) given intravenously or subcutaneously shortens the bleeding time in most uremic patients.
    - Dose is $0.3\ \mu g/kg$ IV over 15 to 30 min.
    - Repeat administration at intervals of 12 to 24 h; tachyphylaxis may occur.
  - Transfusion of red cells to achieve a hematocrit of 27 to 32 percent may improve the bleeding time. Combined transfusion of red cells and DDAVP may offer added benefit, but because of risks of transfusion, reserve this for emergencies.

- Conjugated estrogens will shorten the bleeding time in most patients with uremia.
  - Dose usually 0.6 mg/kg IV for 5 days.
  - Effect seen in 3 days; maximal in 5 to 7; persists for up to 14 days.
- Cryoprecipitate may shorten bleeding time and diminish bleeding, but results are uncertain and risks significant.

ANTIPLATELET ANTIBODIES

- May interfere with platelet function by binding to functional membrane components.
- Clinical features
  - Platelet dysfunction should be considered if a patient with ITP or systemic lupus erythematosus develops mucocutaneous bleeding with a platelet count above usual bleeding level.
- Laboratory features
  - Bleeding time longer than expected for platelet count.
  - Platelet aggregation absent in response to low doses of collagen, and second wave absent in response to ADP or epinephrine.
- Therapy
  - Treatment of the underlying immune thrombocytopenia.

CARDIOPULMONARY BYPASS

- Platelet dysfunction is the principal hemostatic abnormality induced by cardiopulmonary bypass.
- Platelet defect probably due to activation and membrane damage and fragmentation.
- Clinical features
  - Possible cause of excessive postoperative bleeding.
- Laboratory features
  - Prolonged bleeding time.
  - Abnormal platelet aggregation to several agonists.
  - Platelet count reduced by 50 percent during bypass and may remain low for several days.
- Therapy
  - Patients with prolonged bleeding time and excessive postoperative blood loss usually respond to platelet transfusions.
  - Such patients may also respond to DDAVP.
  - Surgical causes of bleeding must be considered, especially if response to above therapy is unsatisfactory.
  - Aprotinin (unavailable in the United States) demonstrated to be beneficial in Europe.

CHRONIC MYELOPROLIFERATIVE DISORDERS

- Multiple functional platelet abnormalities have been demonstrated.
- Clinical features

- Bleeding or thrombosis occurs in about one-third of patients.
- Laboratory features
  - Bleeding time is prolonged in some patients.
  - Thrombocytosis is common.
  - Decreased platelet aggregation and secretion in response to ADP, epinephrine, or collagen.
  - Whole blood viscosity increased in polycythemia vera.
- Therapy
  - Treatment should be reserved for symptomatic patients or those about to undergo surgery.
  - Treat underlying disorder.
  - DDAVP may benefit storage pool defects or acquired von Willebrand disease in these patients.
  - Aspirin may be helpful in patients with thrombosis but predisposes to bleeding.

LEUKEMIA AND MYELODYSPLASTIC SYNDROMES

- Thrombocytopenia is the most common cause of bleeding, but platelet dysfunction may also contribute.

Acute Myelogenous Leukemia

- Platelets may be morphologically abnormal, aggregate abnormally, and have decreased procoagulant activity.
- Bleeding usually responds to platelet transfusion and treatment of underlying disease.

Myelodysplastic Syndromes (Preleukemia)

- Abnormalities similar to those in acute myelogenous leukemia, but less severe.

Acute Lymphocytic Leukemia

- Reduced platelet aggregation may occur.

Hairy Cell Leukemia

- Thrombocytopenia is common; platelet dysfunction occurs rarely.

MULTIPLE MYELOMA AND OTHER MONOCLONAL GAMMOPATHIES

- Platelet dysfunction occurs commonly due to direct interaction of the monoclonal protein with the platelets.
- Therapy
  - Reduce plasma levels of abnormal immunoglobulins by cytoreductive therapy or plasmapheresis.
  - Acquired von Willebrand disease treated with cryoprecipitate, DDAVP, and/or plasmapheresis.

DRUGS

Table 71-1 lists drugs known to interfere with platelet function.

Aspirin

- Irreversibly inhibits cyclooxygenase and thereby interferes with normal platelet function, such as aggregation with ADP or epinephrine.
- Bleeding time prolonged in normal people to 1.5 to 2 times baseline values.
- Marked prolongation of bleeding time in patients with coagulopathies or platelet abnormalities.
- Bleeding time prolongation remains for up to 4 days after aspirin is discontinued.
- Abnormal platelet aggregation persists for up to 1 week.
- Patients taking aspirin may have increased bruising, epistaxis, and gastrointestinal blood loss.
- DDAVP infusion may correct the prolonged bleeding time.

Other NSAIDs

- Inhibit cyclooxygenase reversibly; effect short lived.
- *Piroxicam* effect may last for days due to long half-life of the drug.
- These drugs may cause transient prolongation of the bleeding time, but the clinical significance of this phenomenon is uncertain.

Antibiotics

- Most penicillins cause dose-dependent prolongation of the bleeding time, probably by binding to the platelet membrane and thereby interfering with platelet function.
- Platelet aggregation is frequently abnormal.
- Inhibition of platelet function is maximal after three days of therapy, and persists for several days after treatment is discontinued.
- Clinically significant bleeding occurs much less frequently than prolongation of bleeding time.
- Patients with coexisting hemostatic defects are particularly vulnerable.
- Some cephalosporins cause problems similar to those due to the penicillins.

Ticlopidine

- At therapeutic doses inhibits platelet function and prolongs bleeding time.
- Maximal effect in 4 to 6 days; may last 4 to 10 days after drug therapy discontinued.

Anticoagulants, Fibrinolytic Agents, and Antifibrinolytic Drugs

TABLE 71-1 Drugs That Inhibit Platelet Function*

Nonsteroidal anti-inflammatory drugs (NSAIDs)
  Aspirin, diclofenac, diflunisal, ibuprofen, indomethacin, meclofenamic
  acid, mefanamic acid, naproxen, phenylbutazone, piroxican, sulfinpyra-
  zone, sulindac, tolmetin, zompirac
Antibiotics
  Penicillins
    Ampicillin, apalcillin, azlocillin, carbenacillin, methicillin, mezlocillin, naf-
    cillin, penicillin G, piperacillin, sulbenicillin, temocillin, ticarcillin
  Cephalosporins
    Cefoperazone, cefotaxime, cephalothin, moxalactam
  Nitrofurantoin
  Miconazole
Ticlopidine
Anticoagulants, fibrinolytic agents, and antifibrinolytic agents
  Heparin
  Streptokinase, tissue plasminogen activator, urokinase, alteplase
  ϵ-Aminocaproic acid
Drugs that increase platelet cyclic AMP levels
  Dipyridamole, iloprost, prostacyclin
Cardiovascular drugs
  Diltiazem, isosorbide dinitrate, nifedipine, nimodipine, nitroglycerin, pro-
  pranolol, quinidine, sodium nitroprusside, verapamil
Volume expanders
  Dextrans, hydroxyethyl starch
Psychotropic drugs and anesthetics
  Psychotropic drugs
    Amitriptyline, chlorpromazine, flufenazine, haloperidol, imiprimine, nor-
    tryptaline, promethazine, trifluoperazine
  Anesthetics
    Local
      Butacaine, cocaine, cyclaine, dibucaine, metycaine, nepercaine,
      plaquenil, procaine, tetracaine
    General
      Halothane
Oncologic drugs
  Mithramycin, BCNU, daunorubicin
Miscellaneous agents
  Antihistamines
    Chlorpheniramine, diphenhydramine, mepyramine, pyrilamine
  Ketanserin
  Radiographic contrast agents
    Iopamidol, iothalamate, ioxalate, meglumine diatrizoate, sodium diatri-
    zoate
Foods and food activities
  ω-3 Fatty acids, ethanol, chinese black tree fungus, onion extract, ajoene,
  cumin, tumeric

*Of the drugs listed, only aspirin and ticlopidine have been demonstrated
to cause a significant increase in bleeding. The other drugs are described
as affecting platelet aggregation or the bleeding time, and for some of
the drugs, case reports have suggested an association with increased
bleeding.
Source: Table 133-2 of *Williams Hematology*, 5/e, p. 1392.

- Heparin inhibits platelet function under some circumstances, but the clinical significance of this effect is unknown.
- Similarly, platelet function may be altered during fibrinolytic therapy, but the significance of these changes is uncertain.
- Antifibrinolytic therapy with large doses of ε-aminocaproic acid can cause prolongation of the bleeding time after several days.

Cardiovascular Drugs

- Sodium nitroprusside at doses of 6 to 8 μg/kg/min increases the bleeding time about two-fold.
- Nitric oxide inhalation prolongs the bleeding time.

Volume Expanders

- Dextran interferes with platelet function by adsorption to the platelet surface but does not increase the bleeding time nor predispose to bleeding.
- Hydroxyethyl starch may prolong the bleeding time and predispose to bleeding, especially at doses exceeding 20 ml/kg of a 6% solution.

FOODS

- Diets rich in fish oils containing ω-3 fatty acids may interfere with platelet function and prolong the bleeding time.

For a more detailed discussion, see Sanford J. Shattil, Joel S. Bennett: Acquired qualitative platelet disorders due to diseases, drugs, and foods, Chap. 133, p. 1386, in *Williams Hematology,* 5/e, 1995.

---

72 THE VASCULAR PURPURAS

DEFINITIONS

- Purpura: extravasation of red cells from vasculature into skin or subcutaneous tissues.
  - Petechiae are lesions < 2 mm in diameter.
  - Purpura are lesions 2 mm to 1 cm.
  - Ecchymosis, >1 cm.
- Erythema: reddened skin due to increased capillary flow.
- Telangiectasia: dilated superficial capillaries.
  - Erythema and telangiectasia blanch with pressure, are easily demonstrable with a glass microscope slide.

PATHOPHYSIOLOGY

- Hemostatic mechanisms unable to combat basal ongoing vascular trauma.
- Vessel and surrounding tissues may be weakened structurally.
- Transmural pressure gradient may be too great.
- Palpability due to
  - extravascular coagulation and fibrin deposition
  - cellular infiltration due to inflammation or malignancy

NONPALPABLE PURPURA

Increased Transmural Pressure Gradient

- Increased intrathoracic pressure caused by coughing, vomiting, weight lifting, etc., may cause petechiae of the face, neck, and upper thorax.
- Venous valvular incompetence or tight clothing may cause petechiae on the lower extremities.

Decreased Mechanical Integrity of the Microvasculature or Supporting Tissues

- Senile purpura: red or purple irregular patches on the extensor surfaces of the forearm and hands.
- Glucocorticoid excess causes bright red purpuric lesions in thin, fragile skin on flexor and extensor surfaces of both arms and legs.
- Vitamin C deficiency (scurvy): loss of collagen and ground substance in the skin leads to follicular hyperkeratosis, petechiae, perifollicular purpura with entrapped corkscrew hairs. Large ecchymoses may develop and hemorrhagic gingivitis, stomatitis, and conjunctivitis may occur.
- Ehlers-Danlos syndrome: easy bruising is characteristic of types IV and V, but may occur with other types as well.

- Pseudoxanthoma elasticum may be associated with recurrent mucosal hemorrhages.
- Amyloidosis: infiltration of blood vessel walls may lead to increased vascular fragility and petechiae or purpura.
- Female easy bruising syndrome (purpura simplex): purpura or ecchymoses occurring predominantly in women. May be related to hormonal changes, perhaps aggravated by nonsteroidal anti-inflammatory drug ingestion.

TRAUMA

- Physical trauma can cause cutaneous bleeding. The history and shape and location of the lesions should suggest the etiology.
- Factitial purpura usually presents as medium to large ecchymoses on the lower extremities of patients who appear unconcerned about the lesions.

SUNBURN

Acute sunburn may be sufficiently severe to have a petechial component.

INFECTIONS

Purpura may occur with bacterial, fungal, viral, rickettsial, or protozoal infections or with parasitic infestations, often due to a complex, multi-factorial process. Special forms include:
- Ecthyma gangrenosum
  - May accompany infections with *Pseudomonas* sp., *Klebsiella* sp., *Aeromona hydrophilia,* or *Escherichia coli* in patients with severe granulocytopenia or immune compromise.
  - Lesions begin as erythematous or purpuric macules and progress to hemorrhagic or necrotic vesicles or bullae, then to edematous, hemorrhagic plaques, and finally to indurated painless ulcers.
- Meningococcemia
  - Erythematous papules that progress to widespread petechiae, purpura, and ecchymoses.
  - Acrocyanosis and peripheral gangrene may occur.
- Streptococcal infections
  - Scarlet fever is characterized by a diffuse, erythematous rash often with confluent petechiae in skin folds (Pastia lines).
  - Streptococcal pharyngitis without scarlet fever may also be associated with petechiae.
- Septicemia
  - Bacterial sepsis due to various organisms can cause petechial or purpuric macules or papules, hemorrhagic bullae, erosions, ulcers, or widespread ecchymoses and cutaneous infarctions (purpura fulminans, see below).

- Rickettsial infections
  - Extensive cutaneous lesions occur, beginning as urticarial macules and progressing to petechiae, ecchymoses, hemorrhagic bullae, and extensive skin necrosis.
- Lyme disease
  - The characteristic cutaneous lesion is erythema migrans, an annular, expanding plaque which may contain a purpuric macule or papule, or a hemorrhagic bulla.

EMBOLIC PURPURA

- Cholesterol crystals that embolize from atheromata in the aorta and in the lower extremities may produce petechiae and purpura, livedo reticularis, nodules, ulcers, or cyanosis and gangrene.
- Fat emboli may occur after severe trauma or after liposuction and cause petechiae of the upper extremities, thorax, and/or conjunctivae.

HYPERCALCEMIA

- Chronic hypercalcemia may lead to hemorrhagic cutaneous necrosis because of subcutaneous and vascular calcifications.

NEOPLASIA

- Petechiae or purpura may occur because of infiltration of the skin with neoplastic cells from a variety of malignancies, including Langerhans cell histiocytosis, lymphomas, leukemias, and plasma cell disorders.

PIGMENTED PURPURIC ERUPTIONS

- Include Schamberg and Majocchi diseases.
- Petechiae and purpura on background of red-brown or orange hyperpigmentation
- Similar lesions may be produced by cutaneous T-cell lymphoma, drug or chemical hypersensitivity, allergic or irritant contact dermatitis, and hyperglobulinemic purpura.

PYODERMA GANGRENOSUM

- Presents as a nodule, pustule, or hemorrhagic bulla which rapidly becomes an ulcer with an erythematous base and violaceous or blue margin surrounded by erythema.
- Most frequently associated with inflammatory bowel disease, but also seen with hematological malignancies and other disorders.

INTRAABDOMINAL HEMORRHAGE

- Purpura or ecchymoses may develop around the umbilicus (Cullen sign) or in the flanks (Grey-Turner sign) in patients with intraabdominal hemorrhage.

COUMARIN NECROSIS

- Occurs in about 1 in 500 patients receiving coumarin drugs.
- Sudden onset after 2 to 14 days of drug therapy, with painful erythematous patches which progress to hemorrhagic and necrotic plaques, nodules, and bullae.
- More common in women; most often involves thighs, buttocks, or breasts.
- More likely to occur in patients with protein C deficiency.

PURPURA FULMINANS

- May present with widespread ecchymoses, often involving the extremities, abdomen, or buttocks.
- Often seen in association with infection, but may be idiopathic or occur in infants with homozygous protein C or protein S deficiency.

PAROXYSMAL NOCTURNAL HEMOGLOBINURIA

- May be associated with erythematous cutaneous lesions with central necrosis, hemorrhagic bullae, petechiae, purpura, or ecchymoses.

ANTIPHOSPHOLIPID ANTIBODY SYNDROME

- The thrombotic tendency of this disorder may be expressed as cutaneous necrosis due to microvascular thrombi.

DRUG REACTIONS

- Reactions to any of a large number of drugs may lead to petechiae or purpura in the absence of thrombocytopenia.

AUTOERYTHROCYTE SENSITIZATION

- Painful ecchymoses appearing without explanatory trauma.
- Cause not established, but in some patients hypersensitivity to some component of the erythrocyte membrane may be responsible.
- Many patients have underlying psychiatric disorders; lesions have been factitial in some.

PALPABLE PURPURA: HENOCH-SCHOENLEIN

- A leukocytoclastic vasculitis of unknown cause involving precapillary, capillary, and postcapillary vessels.

- Lesions may be palpable purpura, urticarial papules, plaques, or hemorrhagic bullae which can progress to larger, stellate, reticulate, and necrotic lesions.
- Lesions usually symmetrical on legs and buttocks.
- Predominantly a disease of childhood.
- Arthralgias and abdominal pain in 50 percent, melena and signs of peritoneal irritation are common.
- Proteinuria and hematuria in 40 percent. Renal disease may be progressive in older children.
- Immunoglobulins and complement components may be deposited in involved vessels.
- Therapy is usually initiated with glucocorticoids, but the success rate is low. Ultimate prognosis almost uniformly good.

Acute Hemorrhagic Edema of Infancy

- Triad of fever, iris-like or medallion-like large purpuric, painful cutaneous lesions, and edema.
- Affects children age 4 months to 2 years.
- Onset is sudden, with spontaneous recovery in 5 to 11 days.
- Lesions are limited to cheeks, eyelids, ears, and extremities.
- Pathology is leukocytoclastic vasculitis with vascular deposits of immunoglobulins and complement components.

Vasculitis Associated with other Diseases

- Palpable purpura may occur in several disorders characterized by vasculitis:
  - Collagen vascular diseases
  - Systemic vasculitides
    - polyarteritis nodosa
    - Wegener granulomatosis
    - Churg-Strauss angiitis
  - Hypersensitivity vasculitis, associated with drug reactions or infections, or idiopathic.
  - Paraneoplastic, in association with any of a variety of neoplasms, including the hematological malignancies.

Cryoglobulinemia

- May be single component, IgA, IgG, or IgM, occurring in essential monoclonal gammopathy, macroglobulinemia, myeloma, or lymphoma.
- May be cold-insoluble complexes of IgG with IgM that has anti-IgG activity, or similar complexes containing other immunoglobulin components, occurring in association with a variety of diseases.
- Skin lesions occur with both types of cryoglobulin, including macular

or palpable purpura, acral hemorrhagic necrosis, livedo reticularis, or hemorrhagic bullae.

Hyperglobulinemic Purpura of Waldenström

- Usually occurs in women between ages 18 to 40, often in association with another disease.
- Crops of petechiae appear on the lower legs and ankles, recurring at intervals of days to months.
- Patients have polyclonal hypergammaglobulinemia due to elevated levels of IgA, IgG, and IgM.

Cryofibrinogenemia

- Cold-insoluble fibrinogen may be found as a primary disorder or secondary to neoplastic, thromboembolic, or infectious disorders, usually with laboratory evidence of disseminated intravascular coagulation.
- Cutaneous manifestations are similar to those described for cryoglobulinemia, above.

Primary Cutaneous Diseases

- Primary cutaneous diseases, including allergic contact dermatitis, drug eruptions, acne vulgaris, insect bites, and dermatitis herpetiformis, may present with purpuric papules and vesicles which look like septic or vasculitis lesions.

DISORDERS SIMULATING PURPURA

Telangiectasias

- Cherry angiomata
  - Papular, erythematous lesions on the trunk and extremities.
  - Occur in middle-aged men and women.
- Hereditary hemorrhagic telangiectasia
  - Autosomal dominant inheritance
  - Widespread dermal, mucosal, and visceral
  - Recurrent epistaxis most common problem, but bleeding may occur from any site.
  - Arteriovenous fistulae may occur.
- Spider telangectasias
  - Occur in chronic liver disease, CREST syndrome, and AIDS.
  - May be confused with lesions of hereditary hemorrhagic telangiectasia.
  - "Spiders" have a prominent central feeding vessel which is easily occluded, leading to blanching of the lesion.

KAPOSI SARCOMA

• Lesions may mimic petechiae, purpura, or ecchymoses on either skin or mucosae.

EXTRAMEDULLARY HEMOPOIESIS

• Cutaneous sites of extramedullary hemopoiesis appear as dark red, blue, or blue-gray macules in infants with congenital toxoplasmosis, rubella, or cytomegalovirus, and in adults with myelofibrosis.

For a more detailed discussion, see Paul Schneiderman: The vascular purpuras, Chap. 134, p. 1401, in *Williams Hematology,* 5/e, 1995.

---

73 CONGENITAL DEFICIENCIES OF COAGULATION FACTORS INCLUDING HEMOPHILIA

HEMOPHILIA A AND HEMOPHILIA B

General Aspects

- Hemophilia A and hemophilia B are caused by inherited deficiencies of factor VIII (FVIII) and factor IX (FIX), respectively.
- Both result from either decreased production of the deficient factor or production of normal amounts of a factor with decreased functional activity.
- The activated form of FIX, FIXa, is a serine protease which functions to activate factor X.
- Activated FVIII, FVIIIa, serves as a cofactor to FIX, forming a complex with FIXa on the platelet surface and dramatically accelerating the rate of factor X activation.
- Since deficiency of either FIX or FVIII causes an inability to activate factor X, the clinical characteristics and approach to treatment of hemophilia A and hemophilia B are identical and will be discussed together.
- Both are X-linked recessive disorders, affecting only males, with rare exceptions.

Laboratory Findings

- Both hemophilia A and B cause prolongation of the activated PTT (aPTT) which is corrected by the addition of normal plasma. The prothrombin time is normal.
- Hemophilia A and B can be distinguished by assays of the levels of factor VIII and IX, respectively.
- Factor VIII and IX assays are based on the aPTT and measure the activity of the factor in promoting clot formation. The normal range is between 50 and 150 percent with a mean of 100 percent.
- One unit of factor is defined as the amount of factor activity present in 1 ml of pooled normal plasma.

Clinical Findings

- Severe hemophiliacs have factor levels of 1 percent or less, moderate hemophiliacs have levels of approximately 2 to 5 percent and mild hemophiliacs have levels of 5 to 30 percent.
- Normal hemostasis is generally seen with levels in excess of 30 percent.
- The average level of carrier females is 50 percent, but occasional carriers will have levels less than 30 percent and may have bleeding with trauma or surgery.

- The factor level remains constant throughout the patient's life, and is similar in other affected members of the kindred, but varies between kindreds. One exception is hemophilia B Leyden, in which a mutation in the promoter region of the factor IX gene causes severe hemophilia at birth, which ameliorates after puberty.
- Hemophilia causes delayed, deep soft tissue bleeding.
  - Severe hemophiliacs have frequent spontaneous hemarthroses (joint bleeds) and intramuscular hematomas.
  - Moderate hemophiliacs have less frequent spontaneous bleeding but have bleeding induced by mild to moderate trauma.
  - Mild hemophiliacs do not usually have hemarthrosis or spontaneous bleeding but may have bleeding due to severe trauma or surgical procedures.
- Hemarthrosis
  - Occasionally seen in other severe congenital bleeding disorders but is characteristic of hemophilia A and B.
  - Most frequent sites are the knees, followed by the elbows, ankles, hips, and wrists.
  - Acute form is characterized by initial mild pain without physical findings, followed by more intense pain, swelling of the joint, decreased range of motion, and redness and tenseness of the overlying skin.
  - Following acute hemarthrosis, the joint develops an inflammatory reaction, resulting in a chronic synovitis, which predisposes to repeated bleeding episodes in that joint (target joint).
  - Eventually, the synovitis causes chronic end-stage arthropathy characterized by destruction of the articular cartilage, chronic pain, and an unstable dysfunctional joint.
  - Hemophilic arthropathy usually develops by the time a severe hemophiliac reaches adolescence.
- Intramuscular hematomas
  - Intramuscular hematomas occur in the large flexor muscles, especially the calf muscles, iliopsoas muscles (often presenting as back or hip pain) and forearms.
  - These hematomas may cause significant blood loss, compartment syndromes, nerve compressions, and muscle contractures.
  - The development of pseudotumors, which are large, organized encapsulated hematomas which slowly expand and compress surrounding structures, may complicate intramuscular hematomas.
- CNS hemorrhage, the most common cause of bleeding mortality, occurs spontaneously or after trauma, but onset of symptoms may be delayed by several days.
- Retroperitoneal bleeding and retropharyngeal bleeding that compromises the airway (often presenting as a complication of pharyngitis) may be life-threatening.

- Gross hematuria is common, may cause renal colic, but is seldom life-threatening.
- Postsurgical bleeding, often delayed by hours to several days, is associated with poor wound healing.

Differential Diagnosis

- Both hemophilia A and B must be distinguished from other congenital disorders of coagulation that prolong the aPTT, such as factor XI and XII deficiencies.
- Hemophilia A must be distinguished from von Willebrand disease (especially Normandy variant), an acquired inhibitor of FVIII, and combined congenital deficiency of FVIII and FV.
- Hemophilia B must be distinguished from liver disease, warfarin ingestion, vitamin K deficiency, and rarely acquired inhibitors of FIX.

Treatment

- General
  - Avoid aspirin, other antiplatelet agents, and intramuscular injections.
  - Treat bleeding episodes promptly.
  - Teach patients home infusion of factor concentrates.
  - Plan surgical procedures carefully.
- Desmopressin (DDAVP)
  - Causes release of stored endogenous FVIII and von Willebrand factor and can increase FVIII levels of many patients threefold. Often useful in the treatment of mild-moderate hemophilia A and symptomatic carrier females.
  - Dose is 0.3 µg/kg intravenously.
  - Peak effect is in 30 min and duration of action is 8 h.
  - Adverse reactions include flushing, rarely hyponatremia, and angina in patients with coronary disease.
  - Tachyphylaxis occurs with repeated doses.
  - Intranasal preparation is now available for self-administration. Usual adult dose is one spray in each nostril (300 µg).
- Replacement with factor concentrates
  - Severe hemophiliacs as well as mild-moderate hemophiliacs with serious bleeding episodes requiring maintained high-level correction should be treated with virally attenuated factor VIII concentrates.
  - Currently available concentrates include plasma-derived intermediate purity, plasma-derived monoclonally purified, and recombinant DNA-derived concentrates.
  - Viral attenuation methods include pasteurization, dry heat, and solvent-detergent treatment. No cases of HIV transmission have

been reported with currently available concentrates and they are considered generally safe from hepatitis C.

- Transmission of hepatitis A has been reported with solvent-detergent treated intermediate purity products. Parvovirus transmission has been reported with several products.
- It is uncertain which is the "best" concentrate.
- Treatment of HIV-infected hemophiliacs with monoclonally purified concentrates may be associated with a slower rate of decline in CD4 lymphocyte counts than seen with treatment with intermediate purity concentrates.

- Replacement with cryoprecipitate
  - May be given when concentrates are not available. Most bags of cryoprecipitate contain 80 to 100 U of FVIII. Cryoprecipitate is not virally attenuated.
- FVIII dosage
  - Concentrate dose may be estimated by multiplying the patient's weight in kilograms by half the needed percent correction of the factor level. For example, for a 70-kg patient with a less than 1 percent FVIII level needing a 100 percent correction, the dose would be 70(kg) $\times$ 100 percent/2 = 3500 U. The full contents of mixed factor vials should be infused.
  - The half-life of FVIII is 8 to 12 h. Factor levels may be maintained between 50 and 100 percent by giving half the loading dose every 8 to 12 h. The apparent half-life lengthens after repeated doses.
- Factor IX replacement
  - FIX is available in two classes of virally attenuated concentrates, the prothrombin complex concentrates (PCC), which contain factors II, VII, IX, and X, and the purified factor IX concentrates (Mononine and Alphanine), which contain almost exclusively FIX.
  - The volume of distribution of FIX is approximately twice that of FVIII, and the usual dose of FIX is the patient's weight in kilograms multiplied by the percent correction needed. The half-life of FIX is approximately 24 h.
  - Prothrombin complex concentrates may cause paradoxical thrombosis and disseminated intravascular coagulation due to small amounts of activated factors present in the concentrate. This risk is greatest with repeated daily doses of concentrate.
  - Purified FIX concentrates have much decreased thrombogenic potential and should be used rather than PCCs when giving repeated doses.
  - Desmopressin and cryoprecipitate are not useful for FIX replacement.
- Treatment of bleeding episodes
  - Hemarthrosis may be treated with a single dose of the appropriate

factor to raise the level to 30 to 50 percent, and repeated if necessary in 12 to 24 h. Failure to respond to two infusions should prompt evaluation to exclude inhibitor development or other diagnosis such as septic joint or fracture. Ice, analgesia, and splinting in a position of comfort are adjuncts to factor replacement.

- Superficial intramuscular hematomas are treated with 50 percent corrections.
- CNS, retroperitoneal, and retropharyngeal bleeds are treated with 100 percent corrections and maintenance of the levels between 50 and 100 percent for 7 to 10 days.
- Hematuria often subsides with rest and increased fluid intake. Persistent hematuria, minor oral bleeding, and epistaxis may be treated with single 30 percent corrections. Antifibrinolytics are contraindicated in the presence of hematuria.
- Major surgical procedures require 100 percent correction immediately prior to the procedure and maintenance of the levels between 50 and 100 percent for 7 to 10 days. If the surgery is extensive, a second intraoperative or immediate postoperative loading dose is often required.
- Joint surgery may require more prolonged replacement.
- Dental surgery and extractions may be covered with a single 100 percent correction along with ϵ-aminocaproic acid (4 g orally q 4 h) or tranexamic acid (0.25 mg/kg orally tid or qid).
- Factor levels should be monitored in life-threatening bleeding episodes and postsurgically. The aPTT is not sufficiently sensitive for this purpose.

Complications of Therapy

- development of inhibitors (see Chap. 78)
- allergic reactions (uncommon with highly purified concentrates)
- primary pulmonary hypertension
- HIV infection and chronic hepatitis in patients exposed in the past to concentrates which had not been virally attenuated

HEREDITARY FACTOR XI DEFICIENCY

- Inheritance is autosomal recessive.
- Incidence in the United States is 1 in 100,000, and is most common in Jews of Ashkenazi descent, in whom the incidence is 1/10,000.
- Homozygotes have FXI levels of 15 percent to <1 percent.
- Factor XI deficiency causes a mild and more variable bleeding disorder than the other congenital coagulopathies. There is poor correlation of symptoms to FXI levels and some patients have no bleeding despite very low levels.
- Common manifestations are epistaxis, menorrhagia, bruising, hematuria, and postpartum bleeding. Hemarthrosis is very rare.

- Only half of affected patients experience postsurgical bleeding, but the bleeding may be severe. It is more likely to occur after surgery involving areas of high fibrinolytic activity, such as the oral cavity and urinary tract. Patients who had not bled after previous surgery may be at less risk for future postsurgical hemorrhage.
- Aspirin intake increases the risk of bleeding in FXI deficient patients.
- The aPTT is prolonged, and the PT is normal. Freezing and thawing plasma may activate the contact factors including FXI, so FXI assays should be performed on fresh plasma from blood collected in plastic tubes.
- The treatment is infusion of fresh frozen plasma (10 to 20 ml/kg initially, then 5 ml/kg daily). The precise hemostatic level for surgery is not known, and a target level of 50 percent is commonly regarded as adequate.
- Antifibrinolytic therapy may be considered as an adjunct.

HEREDITARY DEFICIENCIES OF OTHER COAGULATION FACTORS

- Such deficiencies are significantly less common, ranging in prevalence from 1 per 500,000 to 1 per million.
- All are autosomal recessive.
- All may be due to either a decreased synthesis of factor protein or production of normal amounts of a factor with decreased functional activity.

Prothrombin (FII) Deficiency

- Causes a prolonged PT and PTT with a normal thrombin time.
- The differential diagnosis includes warfarin ingestion, vitamin K deficiency, liver disease, and autoantibody-induced hypoprothrombinemia associated with a lupus anticoagulant.
- The clinical severity is related to the FII level.
- Most bleeding episodes are posttraumatic.
- Treatment is with transfusions of sufficient fresh frozen plasma (10 to 20 ml/kg) to attain a FII level above 10 to 20 percent. PCCs may be used for severe bleeding episodes.

Factor V Deficiency

- Significant amounts of FV are contained in platelets.
- Deficiency causes a prolonged PT, aPTT, and bleeding time with a normal thrombin time.
- Clinical manifestations are bruising, menorrhagia, epistaxis, and rarely, hemarthrosis or deep hematomas.
- Differential diagnosis includes liver disease, DIC, combined deficiency of FV and FVIII, and acquired inhibitors to FV.

- Treatment is with transfusions of fresh frozen plasma (20 ml/kg initially, then 2 to 6 ml/kg every 12 h), and sometimes platelet transfusions. The plasma half-life is 16 h.

Factor VII Deficiency

- Severity of the bleeding is variable and does not always correlate to FVII levels. Patients with levels <1 percent will usually experience severe bleeding including hemarthoses, menorrhagia, hematuria, and mucosal bleeding.
- PT is abnormal and aPTT is normal.
- The differential diagnosis includes warfarin ingestion, vitamin K deficiency, and liver disease. Homocystinuria, Gilbert syndrome, and Dubin-Johnson syndrome are associated with decreased FVII levels.
- Treatment is with fresh frozen plasma (10 to 20 ml/kg) or PCCs. Although the half-life is only 4 h, treatment every 12 to 24 h is usually sufficient. Recombinant FVII and FVIIa concentrates are under clinical investigation.

Factor X Deficiency

- Clinical severity correlates with the FX level. Those with levels <1 percent will be severely affected, and those with levels >10 percent will be mildly affected. Severely affected patients may have hemarthroses, mucosal bleeding, or menorrhagia.
- aPTT and PT are usually both prolonged, but some mutations cause prolongation of one out of proportion to the other.
- The differential diagnosis includes liver disease, vitamin K deficiency, warfarin ingestion, and acquired FX deficiency due to amyloidosis.
- Treatment is with transfusions of fresh frozen plasma (10 to 20 ml/kg initially, then 3 to 6 ml/kg every 12 h) or PCCs.
- The plasma half-life of FX is 40 h. Levels of 50 percent are adequate for surgical hemostasis.

Deficiencies of Contact Factors (FXII, Prekallikrein, and High Molecular Weight Kininogen)

- These rare autosomal recessive disorders prolong aPTT but do not cause any clinical abnormalities of hemostasis. PT is normal.
- They must be differentiated from the other abnormalities of the intrinsic pathway which do cause bleeding.
- Factor XII deficiency has been associated with excessive thrombosis, but a specific causative relationship has not been proved.

FAMILIAL MULTIPLE COAGULATION FACTOR DEFICIENCIES (FMFD)

- Syndromes have been described in which there are deficiencies in multiple factors due to a single gene defect.

- These are usually autosomal recessive and are seen in consanguineous families.
- The pathogenesis is unknown in most cases, but may involve vitamin K metabolism or gamma carboxylation in FMFD type III.
- These syndromes have been classified according to which factors are deficient:
  - FMFD Type I—FV and FVIII
  - FMFD Type II—FVIII and FIX
  - FMFD Type III—FII, FVII, FIX, and FX
  - FMFD Type IV—FVII and FVIII
  - FMFD Type V—FVIII, FVII, and FIX
  - FMFD Type VI—FIX and FXI
- Bleeding manifestations depend upon the magnitude of individual factor deficiencies and range from severe to mild.
- Treatment is factor replacement with fresh frozen plasma and/or virally attenuated specific factor concentrates.

For a more detailed discussion, see Maureane Hoffman, Harold R. Roberts: Hemophilia and related conditions—inherited deficiencies of prothrombin (factor II), factor V, and factors VII to XII, Chap. 135, p. 1413; and Jay E. Menitove, Joan Cox Gill, Robert R. Montgomery: Preparation and clinical use of plasma and plasma fractions, Chap. 154, p. 1649, in *Williams Hematology*, 5/e, 1995.

---

74 HEREDITARY DISORDERS OF FIBRINOGEN

Hereditary disorders of fibrinogen may be

- quantitative: afibrinogenemia or hypofibrinogenemia depending on severity
- qualitative: due to structural abnormalities of fibrinogen molecules, also called dysfibrinogenemia
- Normal fibrinogen is
  - synthesized in liver
  - present in plasma at levels of 150 to 350 mg/dl (4 to 10 μM)

AFIBRINOGENEMIA

- Definition: fibrinogen concentration <20 mg/dl when measured by functional, immunological, and chemical methods.
- Inherited as autosomal recessive disorder.
- Expressed as lifelong hemorrhagic disorder in which
  - bleeding may occur without obvious cause
  - bleeding may involve any organ system
  - large ecchymoses and gastrointestinal hemorrhage are particularly common
  - hemarthroses occur in approximately 20 percent
  - early abortions are recurrent and pregnancy outcome is poor
- Laboratory tests
  - All screening tests based on development of fibrin clot are abnormal but are corrected by normal plasma.
  - Plasma and platelet fibrinogen are detected in trace amounts by immunological tests, but are absent by functional or chemical tests.
  - Mild to moderate thrombocytopenia, prolonged bleeding time, or abnormal platelet aggregation may exist.
- Differential diagnosis
  - Heparin and similar compounds, or fibrinogen/fibrin degradation products, can interfere with fibrin formation in functional coagulation assays.
  - Qualitative fibrinogen disorders can be identified by performing functional and immunological assays (see Dysfibrinogenemia, below).
  - Low fibrinogen levels occur in several familial disorders; in disseminated intravascular coagulation; in therapy with sodium valproate, asparaginase, pentoxifylline, tamoxifen, antithymocyte globulin, or high doses of glucocorticoids; and in snake bite.
- Treatment
  - Given for active bleeding or to prevent surgical bleeding.
  - Fibrinogen concentrates unavailable.
  - Cryoprecipitate contains 200 to 250 mg fibrinogen per unit and is the most practical source.

- Hemostasis requires fibrinogen levels of 50 to 100 mg/dl; 70 percent of administered fibrinogen remains in the circulation; half-life is 3 to 5 days.
- A 70-kg man with afibrinogenemia can therefore achieve a plasma fibrinogen level of 100 mg/dl with 12 U of cryoprecipitate. Additional replacement will be required every 3 to 4 days.
- Thrombosis can occur after administration of fibrinogen, and antifibrinogen antibodies may develop.
- Mortality high in infancy and childhood due to intracranial bleeding.

HYPOFIBRINOGENEMIA

- Definition: fibrinogen concentration lower than normal.
- May be heterozygous state for afibrinogenemia.
- Bleeding more likely with fibrinogen level less than 50 mg/dl.
- "Spontaneous" bleeding usually mild; postoperative bleeding often severe.
- Obstetrical complications, including spontaneous abortion, are common. Fibrinogen level at least 60 mg/dl may be required to maintain pregnancy.
- Laboratory tests of coagulation may be normal or abnormal, depending on fibrinogen level.
- Differential diagnosis—see Afibrinogenemia, above.
- Therapy
  - Replacement therapy—see Afibrinogenemia, above.
  - Danazol therapy may raise the fibrinogen level in hypofibrinogenemia.

DYSFIBRINOGENEMIA

- Definition: production of a structurally abnormal fibrinogen molecule with altered functional properties.
- Some patients have quantitatively subnormal levels of fibrinogen as well as a structural abnormality.
- Inherited as an autosomal dominant trait.
  - Most patients are heterozygotes.
  - Homozygotes usually have more significant clinical problems.
- More than 240 fibrinogen variants described, causing functional defects as follows:
  - Abnormal fibrinopeptide release: most are Aα-chain substitutions, with resulting abnormal release of fibrinopeptides A and B. Fibrinopeptide B release defects may have normal screening tests because release of fibrinopeptide A alone will cause clotting.
  - Polymerization defects: present in 70 percent of dysfibrinogens, either alone or in combination with fibrinopeptide release abnormalities.

- Stabilization defects: several variants have stabilization defects in addition to fibrinopeptide release and polymerization abnormalities.
- Biochemical abnormalities do not correlate well with clinical manifestations.
- Clinical features
  - Over one-half of all patients are asymptomatic; abnormal bleeding occurs in approximately one-third; and thrombotic manifestations in about one-sixth.
  - Bleeding usually not severe—e.g., epistaxis, menorrhagia, mild to moderate postoperative hemorrhage.
  - Excessive postpartum bleeding may occur.
  - Defective wound healing seen with several variants.
  - Thrombosis may be venous, arterial, or both.
- Laboratory features
  - Usually find prolongation of coagulation tests requiring formation of fibrin clot (e.g., prothrombin time, partial thromboplastin time, thrombin time)
  - Some variants may be detected only by abnormalities of thrombin or reptilase times.
  - Most important to compare fibrinogen concentration determined by different methods: functional, immunological, and chemical.
  - Diagnostic finding is abnormally low functional level, with normal level by chemical or immunological method.
  - In dysfibrinogenemia with hypofibrinogenemia (hypodysfibrinogenemia) reduced levels are found by all three methods. Diagnosis then made from abnormal thrombin or reptilase times.
  - Immunoelectrophoresis abnormal in about one-fourth of those tested.
  - Elevated levels of fibrin(ogen) degradation products may be found, probably due to incomplete clotting of the abnormal fibrinogen.
- Differential diagnosis
  - Must consider all causes of delayed conversion of fibrinogen to fibrin.
  - Prolonged thrombin time in infancy due to fetal fibrinogen.
  - Hypofibrinogenemia and elevated fibrin(ogen) degradation products in liver disease.
  - Acquired dysfibrinogenemia in acute pancreatitis and malignancy, including hepatic, renal cell, and lymphoma.
  - Autoantibodies which interfere with fibrin polymerization and stabilization may be found in systemic lupus erythematosis, paraproteinemias, or after therapy with isoniazid or procainamide.
  - Inhibitors of coagulation, such as heparin or fibrin(ogen) degradation products, can prolong screening tests for coagulation disorders.
  - Hypofibrinogenemia occurs with L-asparaginase and valproic acid therapy.
- Therapy

- Asymptomatic patients require no therapy.
- Patients with hemorrhage or undergoing surgery may receive replacement therapy with cryoprecipitate as a source of fibrinogen.
- Need for replacement determined from clinical picture and past medical history.
- Thrombosis treated with heparin followed by oral anticoagulants.

For a more detailed discussion, see Harvey R. Gralnick, Donald G. Connaghan: Hereditary abnormalities of fibrinogen, Chap. 136, p. 1439, in *Williams Hematology*, 5/e, 1995.

---

75 HEREDITARY AND ACQUIRED DEFICIENCIES OF FACTOR XIII

Activated factor XIII (factor XIIIa) catalyzes covalent cross-linking of fibrin monomers and polymers by forming peptide linkages between glutamic acid and lysine residues in the α and γ chains of fibrin. Cross-linking increases the mechanical stability of the clot and resistance to fibrinolysis.

HEREDITARY FACTOR XIII DEFICIENCY

- Rare disorder—only about 200 cases reported.
- Inherited as an autosomal recessive trait.
- Bleeding from umbilical stump nearly always occurs; intracerebral hemorrhage common, may bleed from any site, particularly after trauma; spontaneous abortion frequent in afflicted females; delayed wound healing common.
- Usual screening tests for coagulation abnormalities are normal.
- Detected by tests for clot solubility; diagnosis confirmed by assay of enzymatic cross-linking activity, quantitation of α- and γ-chain cross-linking, or immunologic estimates of the amount of the component chains (a,b) of factor XIII.
- Treatment is by replacement of factor XIII with fresh frozen plasma, cryoprecipitate, or concentrates of factor XIII obtained from placenta or plasma.
- Levels between 5 and 10 percent required for hemostasis.
- Factor XIII plasma half-life is 8 to 14 days.
- Prophylaxis is achieved by infusion of factor XIII–containing preparations every 4 to 6 weeks.
- Prophylaxis is effective in preventing recurrent spontaneous abortions.

ACQUIRED DEFICIENCY OF FACTOR XIII

- Inhibitors of factor XIIIa may be acquired in factor XIII deficient patients receiving replacement therapy, or in patients receiving prolonged drug therapy (isoniazid, penicillin, phenytoin).
- Inhibitors may cause massive bleeding.
- Inhibitors are detected by clot solubility testing on mixtures of normal and patient's plasma.
- Spontaneous recovery may occur, but treatment is difficult and mortality high.
- Factor XIII levels may be reduced to about 50 percent in patients with various diseases, including leukemia and inflammatory bowel disease, or after surgery. Clinical significance of this finding is uncertain.

For a more detailed discussion, see Jan McDonagh: Hereditary and acquired deficiencies of activated factor XIII, Chap. 137, p. 1455; and Jay E. Menitove, Joan Cox Gill, Robert R. Montgomery: Preparation and clinical use of plasma and plasma fractions, Chap. 154, p. 1649, in *Williams Hematology,* 5/e, 1995.

76 von WILLEBRAND DISEASE

von WILLEBRAND FACTOR (vWF)

- vWF is a plasma protein which mediates platelet adhesion to subendothelium, mediates platelet aggregation, and serves as a transport protein for factor VIII.
- The vWF gene is located on chromosome 12.
- vWF is synthesized in endothelial cells and megakaryocytes.
- vWF protein monomers form dimers through cysteine links in the carboxyl terminals, and the dimers subsequently polymerize to form high-molecular-weight multimers through links in their amino terminal ends.
- vWF is secreted constitutively and is also stored as high-molecular-weight multimers in the Weibel-Palade bodies of the endothelial cell and in platelet α granules. Stored endothelial vWF is released after stimulation by insulin, epinephrine, vasopressin, or by the modified form of vasopressin, desmopressin (DDAVP).
- vWF purified from plasma has molecular weights ranging from 500,000 to 20 million depending on the degree of multimerization. Multimers of higher molecular weight are more hemostatically competent than those of lower molecular weight.
- The structures in the subendothelium to which vWF binds are not known, although type IV collagen may play a role in veins and large arteries.
- Platelet adhesion and aggregation at high shear rates are mediated by vWF binding to glycoprotein Ib (GpIb) and to the glycoprotein IIb/IIIa (GpIIb/IIIa) complex. The platelet must be activated for vWF to bind GpIIb/IIIa.
- Binding of vWF to GpIb induces a transmembrane calcium flux which activates GpIIb/IIIa.
- Agonist-induced platelet activation causes degranulation and binding to GpIIb/IIIa of the vWF contained in platelet α granules.

LABORATORY FEATURES

- vWF antigen: vWF is measured antigenically using techniques such as ELISA or Laurell immunoelectrophoresis.
- *Ristocetin cofactor assay (R Co-F):* The activity of plasma vWF in promoting the aggregation of fixed or washed platelets is measured in response to the antibiotic ristocetin, which induces aggregation of platelets through GpIb.
- *Ristocetin induced aggregation (RIPA):* Platelet aggregation in fresh platelet-rich patient plasma induced by high and low doses of ristocetin is useful in screening for variants of vWF which cause increased aggregation, such as type IIb and platelet type vWD.
- *Factor VIII:C* activity is measured through standard factor assays.
- *Bleeding time* is best measured through the Ivy template method, which is more sensitive than the Duke bleeding time.

- *Multimeric analysis* allows the determination of the amount and size distribution of the vWF multimers through gel electrophoresis and immunostaining using anti-vWF antibodies.
- vWF levels are variable over time within a patient and vary among members of the same kindred.
- vWF is an acute-phase reactant and is increased by pregnancy, estrogen therapy, recent exercise, hyperthyroidism, uremia, and liver disease. Patients with type AB blood have significantly higher levels than those with type O.

von WILLEBRAND DISEASE-SUBTYPES

- vWD is a heterogeneous disorder caused by a decreased production or abnormal structure of vWF. Over 20 distinct subtypes have been described. Major subtypes include:
- Type I (70 percent of cases): due to decreased production of a normal vWF protein.
  - Concordant reduction in vWF antigen, R Co-F activity and F VIII:C activity, with normal multimeric patterns.
  - Inverse relationship between vWF antigen with bleeding time and clinical severity.
  - Autosomal dominant inheritance.
- Type IIa (20 percent of cases): due to a structural abnormality of vWF which causes loss of the high-molecular-weight multimers.
  - Low level of R Co-F activity compared to vWF antigen.
  - Largest multimers are absent from the plasma.
  - Autosomal dominant inheritance.
  - Increased sensitivity to proteolysis of vWF in plasma in some cases.
- Type IIb (5 percent of cases): due to point mutations in a 35 amino acid area of the protein responsible for GpIb binding, resulting in increased affinity of vWF to GpIb.
  - Increased binding of vWF to GpIb results in an absence of the higher-molecular-weight multimers in the plasma.
  - Increased RIPA.
  - Thrombocytopenia occurs due to in vivo platelet aggregation usually when the patient is under stress, but may be constant in occasional patients. Platelet aggregation does not result in thrombosis in patients.
  - No discernible clinical difference between IIb patients with and without thrombocytopenia.
  - Desmopressin may worsen thrombocytopenia in type IIb.
  - Autosomal dominant inheritance.
- Type III: Complete or almost complete absence of vWF antigen, R Co-F activity, and multimers from the plasma.
  - Severe bleeding disorder with hermarthrosis and muscle bleeding in addition to mucocutaneous bleeding.

- Factor VIII:C levels are 3 to 10 percent, with a markedly shortened plasma half-life.
- Autosomal recessive inheritance; compound heterozygosity or consanguinity.
- Platelet type von Willebrand disease: caused by a mutation in platelet GpIb resulting in increased binding of normal vWF to GpIb.
  - Decreased amounts of high-molecular-weight multimers, thrombocytopenia, and increased RIPA.
  - Laboratory abnormalities are not corrected by the addition of normal vWF.
  - Cryoprecipitate can provoke thrombocytopenia in vivo.
  - Normal platelets do not aggregate when added to patient plasma, but patient platelets aggregate when added to normal plasma.
- Normandy variant von Willebrand disease: due to point mutations in the amino terminal portion of vWF which is the binding site for FVIII:C.
  - Decreased FVIII:C levels and plasma half-life, but normal vWF antigen levels, R Co-F activity, and bleeding time.
  - Autosomal recessive inheritance.
  - Often confused with hemophilia A, and accounts for many cases of apparent female hemophiliacs.
  - Response to transfusion of purified factor VIII concentrates is suboptimal, but response to concentrates containing vWF or cryoprecipitate is appropriate.

CLINICAL MANIFESTATIONS

- The major clinical manifestation of vWD is mucocutaneous bleeding.
- Major symptoms include:
  - epistaxis (60 percent)
  - easy bruising (40 percent)
  - menorrhagia (35 percent)
  - gingival bleeding (35 percent)
  - gastrointestinal bleeding (10 percent)
  - bleeding after dental extraction (50 percent)
  - posttraumatic bleeding (35 percent)
  - postpartum bleeding (25 percent)
  - postoperative bleeding (20 percent)
- Hemarthrosis and spontaneous muscle bleeding are seen only in type III.
- With type I, expression is quite variable and penetrance incomplete. Only 65 percent of type I patients who are thought to be affected on the basis of genetic history are clinically symptomatic. Type II is more uniformly penetrant.

ACQUIRED VON WILLEBRAND DISEASE

- Acquired vWD may be due to antibody formation (see Chap. 78, Acquired Anticoagulants).
- Acquired vWD may also be due to
  - hypothroidism
  - drug therapy with valproic acid
  - adhesion of the vWF to tumor cells (Wilms tumor, lymphoma)
  - congenital or valvular heart disease which may cause depletion of high-molecular-weight multimers through high shear associated with turbulent flow; may be associated with angiodysplasia and gastrointestinal bleeding.

TREATMENT

- Goals of therapy are to correct the F VIII:C deficiency and the Ivy bleeding time during hemorrhage and periods of hemostatic stress requiring prophylaxis.
- Desmopressin, a synthetic form of vasopressin, increases FVIII:C and R Co-F three to five times above the baseline in 80 percent of patients by stimulating the release of endothelial stores of vWF. It is recommended for patients with moderate to mild vWF undergoing moderate hemostatic stress.
  - Bleeding time is corrected in a substantial proportion of patients.
  - Effect lasts 4 to 8 h.
  - Especially useful in type I vWD.
  - Response is variable in type IIa, but the multimeric pattern does not normalize.
  - Not recommended in type IIb, as it may exacerbate platelet aggregation and thrombocytopenia.
  - Ineffective in type III.
  - Response to treatment should be documented by laboratory testing and is generally reproducible in a single patient and in other members of that kindred.
  - Dose is 0.3 to 0.4 μg/kg intravenously. A concentrated nasal spray (one spray in each nostril) is available for home treatment.
  - For surgical prophylaxis the dose should be repeated every 12 h.
  - Adverse reactions include flushing, tingling, headache, and rarely dilutional hyponatremia.
  - Repeated doses may cause tachyphylaxis.
  - Useful as an adjunct in patients whose bleeding times do not correct when treated with plasma concentrates or cryoprecipitate.
- Plasma replacement therapy is needed for patients who do not respond to desmopressin or in whom the hemostatic stress is extensive.
  - Virally attenuated factor VIII concentrates known to contain vWF with the high-molecular-weight multimers present, such as Humate-P, are preferred.

- Dosing is empiric but is generally given every 12 h and is based upon the factor VIII:C content of the concentrate and the patient's weight.
- Cryoprecipitate (1 bag/10 kg body weight every 12 h) is an alternative, but it is not virally attenuated.
- It is recommended that patients receive plasma replacement therapy or desmopressin for 7 to 10 days after major surgical procedures and 3 to 5 days after minor procedures.
- Management of vWD in pregnancy:
  - vWF and F VIII levels rise during the third trimester of pregnancy.
  - Many affected patients will not bleed during labor, but levels fall to their prepregnancy levels over the first few postpartum days.
  - Hemorrhage can occur up to 1 month later and certain patients may need prolonged replacement postpartum.
  - Patients with F VIII:C levels below 30 percent require prophylactic treatment prior to delivery.
- Estrogens raise vWF levels and can be used to control menorrhagia.
- Precipitating inhibitor antibodies develop in approximately 10 percent of patients with type III vWD after transfusion (see Chap. 78). These may cause reduced therapeutic efficacy of replacement therapy and anaphylactoid reactions.
  - Treatment may include high-dose intravenous gamma globulin or extracorporeal immunoabsorption with *Staph* protein A columns.

For a more detailed discussion, see Harvey R. Gralnick, David Ginsburg: von Willebrand disease, Chap. 138, p. 1458; and Jay E. Menitove, Joan Cox Gill, Robert R. Montgomery: Preparation and clinical use of plasma and plasma fractions, Chap. 154, p. 1649, in *Williams Hematology,* 5/e, 1995.

---

77 DISORDERS OF THE VITAMIN K–DEPENDENT COAGULATION FACTORS

VITAMIN K

- May be of plant origin (vitamin K_1 or phylloquinone) or synthesized by bacteria (vitamin K_2 or menaquinone).
- Major dietary sources are vegetables, such as broccoli or spinach, and liver.
- Dietary vitamin K (phylloquinone) is actively absorbed in the small intestine, not in the colon. Bacterial vitamin K (menaquinone) is passively absorbed in the colon.
- Administration of antibiotics that kill intestinal bacteria does not interfere with vitamin K absorption but may contribute to the development of vitamin K deficiency if the patient is not eating.
- Vitamin K deficiency results in decreased plasma levels of factors II, VII, IX, and X and of proteins C and S.
- Vitamin K is a necessary cofactor for the posttranslational synthesis of γ-carboxyglutamic acid groups in precursors of coagulation factors II, VII, IX, and X and proteins C and S. The precursors are often referred to as *proteins induced by vitamin K antagonists* (PIVKA). They can be detected by immunological means in the plasma of patients with vitamin K deficiency from any cause, and they may be useful diagnostically.
- Deficiency of the vitamin K–dependent coagulation factors causes the prothrombin time to be prolonged, and in severe deficiency the partial thromboplastin time will be prolonged as well.
- Clinical disorders of the vitamin K–dependent coagulation factors are reviewed here. Disorders of proteins C and S are discussed in Chap. 81.

HEMORRHAGIC DISEASE OF THE NEWBORN

- Normal newborns have approximately 50 percent levels of vitamin K-dependent procoagulants, due to diminished synthesis *not* caused by vitamin K deficiency.
- Human milk is a poor source of vitamin K, and breast feeding may contribute to vitamin K deficiency.
- Prematurity or maternal ingestion of coumarin drugs may cause severe deficiencies which may be unresponsive to vitamin K and require replacement with fresh frozen plasma.
- Maternal ingestion of anticonvulsant drugs (phenobarbital, mysoline, phenytoin) may also cause deficiency of the vitamin K–dependent factors in the baby.
- Vitamin K (phytonadione 1 mg IM or 2 mg PO) should be given to all neonates.

GENETIC DISORDERS OF FACTORS II, VII, IX, AND X

- Congenital deficiencies of one or a combination of vitamin K–dependent procoagulants have been reported, due to a variety of mutations (see Chap. 135).

DIETARY DEFICIENCY OF VITAMIN K

- This diagnosis should be considered whenever the prothrombin time is prolonged, especially in hospitalized patients.
- Often seen in patients who are not eating well and receiving antibiotics, patients with hypoalbuminemia or renal failure, individuals of advanced age, or patients receiving parenteral nutrition.
- Some cephalosporin antibiotics (moxalactam, cefamandole, cefoperazone) may directly impair carboxylation of coagulation factor precursors.
- Differential diagnosis includes disseminated intravascular coagulation and liver disease. In vitamin K deficiency, the platelet count, fibrinogen level, and factor V activity are all normal, but are reduced in the other two disorders.
- Subcutaneous administration of phytonadione, 5 to 10 mg, usually results in complete correction of the prothrombin time in 12 to 24 h.
- Replacement therapy with fresh frozen plasma should be used only for life-threatening hemorrhage.

BILIARY OBSTRUCTION AND MALABSORPTION SYNDROMES

- Vitamin K deficiency occurs because of failure to absorb the fat-soluble vitamin.
- Therapy is with subcutaneous phytonadione, 10 mg, given daily until prothrombin time is normal.

LIVER DISEASE

- Liver disease may cause a complex hemorrhagic disorder due to reduced synthesis of coagulation factors, fibrinolysis, synthesis of abnormal fibrinogen, thrombocytopenia, and vascular abnormalities, such as esophageal varices.
- Vitamin K should be administered to ensure there is no vitamin K deficiency.
- An antifibrinolytic agent such as tranexamic acid, 10 mg/kg IV q4h, or 15 mg/kg PO q8h, may control epistaxis or gum bleeding. Larger doses may be useful if more severe hemorrhage occurs.
- Fresh frozen plasma may be helpful, but large doses are necessary and plasma exchange may be required, or plasma administration at 100 ml/h with diuretic support may be needed.

- Fibrinogen levels may be increased by administration of cryoprecipitate.
- Prothrombin-complex–rich concentrates may induce intravascular coagulation and should be used only as a last resort.

COUMARIN ANTICOAGULANTS

- These drugs interfere with reduction of vitamin K to its active form.
- The effects are influenced by the vitamin K content of the diet, malabsorption, and possibly antibiotics.
- Beware of surreptitious ingestion.
- Rodenticide (superwarfarin) ingestion may require intensive treatment with doses of 100 mg or more of phytonadione.
- Treatment with coumarin anticoagulants is reviewed in Chap. 83.

OTHER DISORDERS OF VITAMIN-K–DEPENDENT COAGULATION FACTORS

- In *amyloidosis*, factor X deficiency may occur from binding of factor X by amyloid deposits.
- In the *nephrotic syndrome* deficiency of factors II, IX, XII, or a combination of IX and XII, may occur from protein loss in the urine.
- In *Gaucher disease* deficiency of factor IX activity may be found, possibly due to an artifact of testing.

For a more detailed discussion, see Maureane Hoffman, Harold R. Roberts: Hemophilia and related conditions—inherited deficiencies of prothrombin (factor II), factor V, and factors VII to XII, Chap. 135, p. 1413; and David Green: Disorders of the vitamin K-dependent coagulation factors, Chap. 139, p. 1481, in *Williams Hematology*, 5/e, 1995.

---

78 ACQUIRED ANTICOAGULANTS

GENERAL

An anticoagulant or inhibitor is a substance, usually an immunoglobulin, which interferes with normal coagulation. An anticoagulant should be considered whenever there is an unexpected abnormal value obtained in a coagulation assay.

An anticoagulant can be differentiated from a congenital or acquired deficiency of a coagulation factor by repeating the abnormal test after the addition of an equal volume of normal plasma to determine if the abnormality is corrected. Correction of the abnormality implies a deficiency, and absence of correction implies the presence of an inhibitor. The specificity of any identified antiocoagulant must then be determined.

Coagulation factor assays can be misleading if an inhibitor interferes with the assay itself. For example, an anti-FVIII antibody can inhibit FVIII in the FIX deficient substrate plasma used in a factor IX assay, thus giving the false appearance of a FIX deficiency. This can usually be eliminated by performing the coagulation factor specific assays with more dilute plasma samples.

FACTOR VIII INHIBITORS IN HEMOPHILIA A PATIENTS

Background

- These anticoagulants are IgG antibodies, usually IgG subclass 4, which develop in hemophilia A patients after exposure to transfused factor VIII. They have a slow rate of inhibition, do not fix complement, and do not cause immunoprecipitates.
- The majority react with a small segment of the amino-terminal portion of the A2 domain or with the carboxy-terminal of the C2 domain of FVIII.
- They occur in at least 15 percent of transfused patients, have a familial predisposition, and are more likely to occur in severe hemophilia A patients with deletion or nonsense mutations.
- The development of inhibitors is most common during the first 5 to 10 years of life and appears to be related to the number of days of exposure to transfused FVIII. Inhibitor development usually occurs within the first 20 exposure days, and the development of an inhibitor is very uncommon after 100 exposure days without previous inhibitor development.
- It is controversial whether the likelihood of inhibitor formation is related to the purity of transfused FVIII. A higher than expected incidence of inhibitors was found in the clinical trials of recombinant FVIII, but a significant proportion of these were transient low-level inhibitors, which would not have been detected except for the frequency of assessment for inhibitors in these studies. The

incidence of persistent inhibitors was reported in clinical trials at 20 percent and 18 percent for recombinant FVIII, 7 percent and 20 percent for monoclonally purified FVIII, and 21 to 30 percent for intermediate purity FVIII concentrates. There are no controlled comparative trials, however.

Clinical and Laboratory Features

- Frequency and sites of bleeding episodes in hemophiliacs are not changed by the presence of an inhibitor. The life expectancy is only modestly affected by the development of an inhibitor.
- Development of an inhibitor should be suspected if a patient does not respond appropriately to FVIII infusions.
- Factor VIII inhibitors can be detected by aPTT on a mixture of equal volumes of patient plasma and normal plasma incubated for 2 h to determine if there is correction of the aPTT. The presence of some factor VIII inhibitors may be missed if the mixing study is performed without 2-h incubation.
- Inhibitor level may be quantified by the Bethesda assay in which patient plasma, both undiluted and diluted with imidazole buffer, is mixed with normal plasma, incubated for 2 h, and the FVIII level is compared to the FVIII level of normal plasma diluted with buffer alone. One Bethesda unit/ml (BU) is that amount of inhibitor which decreases the residual factor VIII activity from 100 percent to 50 percent.
- Inhibitors may have linear (type I) or nonlinear (type II) kinetics. Since type II inhibitors may have different apparent inhibitor titers at different dilutions, the Bethesda titer is reported in such cases as the titer at the dilution that most nearly gives 50 percent residual FVIII.
- Inhibitors with titers less than 0.6 BU have little clinical effect on FVIII replacement therapy.
- "Low responders" are patients who have 0.6- to 5-BU inhibitors and do not have anamnestic responses after treatment with FVIII.
- "High responders" are patients who exhibit anamnestic responses. They may have very high titer (1000 BU) inhibitors.

Treatment to Attain Hemostasis

- Human FVIII
  - Low responders can be treated by escalating the dose of FVIII. Usually inhibitors of < 10 BU can be overcome with higher doses of FVIII.
- Porcine FVIII
  - Many inhibitors do not inactivate porcine factor VIII.
  - Patients with inhibitors < 50 BU against human FVIII can often be sucessfully treated with Hyate:C, a high-purity porcine factor VIII.

- In patients with high titer antihuman FVIII inhibitors, a Bethesda assay against porcine factor VIII can be performed to help predict response to porcine FVIII, and plasma FVIII levels can be measured to monitor response to therapy after treatment with porcine FVIII.
  - The initial dose is 100 units/kg and the dose is adjusted according to factor levels achieved.
  - Adverse reactions include thrombocytopenia, hypersensitivity, and the development of inhibitor antibodies against porcine FVIII.
- Desmopressin may be used in moderate/mild hemophiliacs with inhibitors.
- Prothrombin complex concentrates (PCC) and activated PCCs
  - PCCs and activated PCCs such as FEIBA and Autoplex may be used in patients who do not respond to human FVIII or porcine FVIII.
  - Small amounts of activated FII, FX, and FVII are contained in these products and may be responsible for their ability to "bypass" the inhibitor.
  - The efficacy of these products is modest to moderate and cannot be monitored by laboratory testing. Thrombosis and DIC complicate their use.
- Recombinant factor VIIa is under clinical investigation for treatment of FVIII inhibitors.

Treatment to Eradicate the Inhibitor

- Steroids, cytotoxic agents, and immune globulin are not effective against hemophilic alloantibody inhibitors.
- Plasmapheresis and affinity chromatography that removes IgG using protein A Sepharose can transiently lower the inhibitor level to allow transfusion therapy with FVIII.
- Several immune tolerance induction regimens in which patients with inhibitors are treated daily with FVIII have been reported to eradicate inhibitors, but their application is limited by high cost.

SPONTANEOUS FVIII INHIBITORS

- Autoantibodies against FVIII may appear in patients without hemophilia. This occurs idiopathically in older adults, in pregnant and postpartum women, and in patients with immunological disorders such as systemic lupus erythematosus and rheumatoid arthritis.
- Clinical manifestations include spontaneous ecchymoses and intramuscular hemorrhages which often cause compartment syndromes. Hemarthosis is rare.
- Patients with acquired inhibitors are low responders.
- Transfusion therapy to achieve hemostasis is identical to the treatment of hemophiliacs with inhibitors.

- In contrast to hemophiliacs, most patients with spontaneous inhibitors respond to treatment to eradicate the inhibitor.
- Prednisone 1 mg/kg and oral cyclophosphamide 1 to 2 mg/kg daily have been used separately or in combination with high response rates.
- Intravenous immune globulin 1 g/kg daily for 2 days has also been shown to decrease inhibitor titers in some of these patients.

INHIBITORS TO VON WILLEBRAND FACTOR (vWF)

- Alloantibodies may develop in patients with severe von Willebrand disease who have been transfused. These inhibit ristocetin cofactor activity and form immunoprecipitates which may cause immune complex–mediated hypersensitivity reactions.
- Autoantibodies against acquired von Willebrand disease occur in patients with collagen-vascular diseases, paraproteinemias, lymphomas, or myeloproliferative disorders. The inhibitor may be monoclonal in some cases.
- Patients with acquired von Willebrand disease characteristically have decreased vWF and FVIII levels and a prolonged bleeding time. Inhibition of ristocetin cofactor activity may be difficult to demonstrate in vitro, because the antoantibody does not directly inhibit the activity but causes immunoprecipitation of vWF which is rapidly cleared in vivo. The precipitating antibody may be demonstrated in the laboratory by incubating mixtures of normal plasma and patient plasma with protein A sepharose, which depletes the mixture of the vWF-antibody complexes.
- Clinical manifestations are variable, and some patients will have only mild symptoms because platelet vWF may not be affected.
- Effective treatment of the underlying disease often eradicates the inhibitor.
- Treatment with desmopressin can increase the vWF and FVIII levels transiently.
- Infusions of cryoprecipitate or Humate-P have been used to increase the vWF and FVIII levels.
- Intravenous immunoglobulin can raise the level of vWF in some patients.

FACTOR IX INHIBITORS

- Patients with hemophilia B are liable to develop alloantibodies against FIX.
- This happens much less frequently than in hemophilia A and the incidence is thought to be 5 percent or less.
- These inhibitors can be quantified by a modified Bethesda assay.
- Treatment is with PCCs or activated PCCs.

FACTOR V INHIBITORS

- FV inhibitors occur rarely after surgery, blood transfusion, or administration of aminoglycoside antibiotics.
- They may also occur in patients who have been treated with topical bovine-thrombin preparations which contain small amounts of bovine FV, which provokes an antibody response cross-reactive with human FV.
- Most FV inhibitors are low titer and transient. Bleeding symptoms are often only minor.
- Treatment of bleeding episodes is with transfusions of plasma or with platelet transfusions, since FV in the granules of platelets is often protected from the inhibitor.

OTHER INHIBITORS OF COAGULATION FACTORS

- Antibodies to the other coagulation factors rarely have been reported and occur in the setting of alloantibodies in congenitally deficient patients.
- Patients with amyloidosis may develop an acquired factor X deficiency from the in vivo binding of the factor to the amyloid deposits. No inhibitor is demostrable in vitro, though the half-life of infused FX is short.

LUPUS-TYPE ANTICOAGULANTS

General

- Lupus-type anticoagulants are immunoglobulins, usually IgG or IgM, that prolong phospholipid-dependent in vitro coagulation assays but do not inactivate any of the known protein coagulation factors.
- The target of the lupus-type anticoagulant has been variously hypothesized as being anionic phospholipids or prothrombin present in lipid-protein complexes, or phospholipid-B2 glycoprotein I complexes.
- Anticardiolipin antibodies are related, but not identical, antiphospholipid antibodies which are detected by ELISA and other solid phase immunoassays.
- Studies of these antibodies suggest that there is a family of antibodies directed at complexes of phospholipids with different plasma proteins.
- The incidence of lupus-type anticoagulants in patients with systemic lupus erythematosis (SLE) has been estimated at 29 to 34 percent.
- The incidence of anticardiolipin antibodies is somewhat higher.
- There is little concordance in the expression of the lupus-type anticoagulant and the anticardiolipin antibody, however.
- In a series of patients with lupus-like anticoagulants, 55 percent

had SLE or related disorders, 12 percent had drug reactions, most commonly to phenothiazines, and the remainder had a mixture of diagnoses including acute infections, HIV, and lymphoproliferative disorders.
- The prevalence of lupus-type anticoagulants in the general population is 1 to 2 percent.

Clinical manifestations

- Bleeding is very unusual unless there is associated hypoprothrombinemia, thrombocytopenia, or platelet dysfunction. Surgery need not be deferred unless these associated abnormalities are present.
- Both venous and arterial thrombosis are associated with lupus-like anticoagulants. This risk is well documented in patients with SLE and lupus-like anticoagulants. However, lupus-like anticoagulants may not carry an elevated risk of thrombosis when seen in association with other clinical conditions.
- Recurrent fetal loss and intrauterine growth retardation in patients with SLE have been linked to the presence of lupus-like anticoagulants. It is unclear if this relationship exists for women who do not have SLE. While retrospective data suggest that women with idiopathic fetal loss have an increased incidence of lupus-like anticoagulants, this has not been demonstrated prospectively.

Laboratory Features

- Lupus-like anticoagulants are commonly manifested in prolonged aPTT which does not correct with addition of normal plasma.
- Coagulation factor assays usually show nonparallel curves and apparent deficiencies of multiple factors (VII, IX, XI, and XII) which correct at high dilutions of patient plasma.
- The addition of washed freeze-thawed platelets or excess phospholipid will correct the abnormal aPTT.
- If a lupus anticoagulant is suspected on clinical grounds, the dilute Russell's viper venom time and the tissue thromboplastic inhibition test are more sensitive tests than the aPTT for the presence of the anticoagulant.
- The prothrombin time is generally not prolonged by the lupus-type anticoagulant, but may be abnormal if there is associated hypoprothombinemia.

Therapy

- Most patients with lupus-like anticoagulants need no specific treatment. Prophylactic anticoagulant therapy should be considered during periods of high thrombotic stress. Long-term anticoagulant therapy decreases repeated episodes of venous thrombosis in patients who have had prior thrombosis.
- There are no controlled trials of the treatment of recurrent fetal

loss, but high-dose glucocorticoids, aspirin, and adjusted dose sub-cutaneous heparin have all been reported to be useful.

Heparin-Like Anticoagulants

• Circulating proteoglycans with heparin-like anticoagulant activity rarely cause a bleeding syndrome of variable severity in patients with malignancy. The thrombin time is prolonged and does not correct with the addition of normal plasma. The treatment is to control the underlying malignancy, and, in severe cases, treatment with protamine sulfate has also been beneficial.

For a more detailed discussion, see Leon W. Hoyer: Acquired anticoagulants, Chap. 140, p. 1485, in *Williams Hematology,* 5/e, 1995.

79 DISSEMINATED INTRAVASCULAR COAGULATION

GENERAL

Disseminated intravascular coagulation (DIC) is caused by procoagulants that are introduced into or produced in the blood and overcome the natural anticoagulant mechanisms.

In the acute form massive activation of coagulation does not allow time for a compensatory increase in the production of coagulant and anticoagulant factors. In the chronic form steady low-level or intermittent activation is variably compensated by increased production.

FEATURES OF DIC

- Tissue ischemia from microvascular thrombi, with subsequent organ dysfunction, occurs in multiple tissues, including
  - pulmonary (hypoxemia, pulmonary hemorrhage, adult respiratory distress syndrome)
  - neurologic (coma, delirium, transient focal findings)
  - renal (acute tubular necrosis, renal cortical ischemia, oliguric renal failure)
  - hepatic (jaundice)
  - cardiac (marantic endocarditis)
  - cutaneous (hemorrhagic necrosis, acral gangrene)
- Large vessel thrombosis and embolic events occasionally occur.
- Bleeding due to consumption of platelets, fibrinogen, and other coagulation factors may be manifested by petechiae, ecchymoses, oozing from venipuncture sites and catheters, and gastrointestinal, pulmonary, or CNS hemorrhage.
- Inhibitors of coagulation such as antithrombin III, protein C, and tissue factor pathway inhibitor are depleted.
- Fibrinolysis is activated with increased bleeding and production of fibrin degradation products.
- Mild microangiopathic hemolytic anemia occurs from red cells passing through capillaries partially occluded by fibrin.
- Acute DIC is often accompanied by multiorgan system dysfunction such as shock, respiratory failure, and renal failure caused directly by the inciting illness.

PATHOGENESIS OF DIC

- Production of thrombin combined with failure of the coagulation inhibitory mechanisms accounts for DIC in most instances.
- Endotoxin causes activation of factor XII, expression of tissue factor by monocytes, neutrophil adhesion and damage to endothelial cells (via cytokine activation), and shock.

- Other stimuli include activation of factor Xa by mucin-secreting adenocarcinomas, snake envenomation, and activated coagulation factors contained in prothrombin complex concentrates.

COMMON CAUSES OF DIC

Infection

- Neonates, asplenic patients, and pregnant patients are more prone to development of infection-related DIC.
- Meningococcemia, serious infections with the more common gram-negative bacteria (*E. coli, Proteus vulgaris, Pseudomonas aeruginosa*), clostridial bacteremia, and sepsis with the gram-positive organisms *Staphylococcus aureus* or pneumococcus have been associated with DIC.

Malignancy

- Solid tumors such as prostate carcinoma, pancreatic carcinoma, and mucin-producing adenocarcinomas often produce a chronic DIC in which thrombosis is more prominent than bleeding. This syndrome often responds to heparin but does not respond as well to oral anticoagulants. Full-dose intravenous heparin may be given initally, followed by long-term subcutaneous heparin.

Acute Leukemia

- Acute promyelocytic leukemia (APL) is characteristically associated with DIC because procoagulant factors are released from leukemic cells. Bleeding is usually more prominent than thrombosis.
- DIC may exacerbate during induction chemotherapy, but ameliorates with the achievement of complete remission.
- Treatment with all-*trans*-retinoic acid is less likely to exacerbate DIC.
- Additionally, APL may be associated with primary fibrinolysis.
- Some investigators have advocated routine use of heparin for APL, while others have used replacement therapy with transfusions alone.
- Acute myelogenous leukemia and acute lymphocyctic leukemia have been associated with DIC, although less commonly.

Complications of Pregnancy

- Normal pregnancy is a relatively hypercoagulable state characterized by increased levels of coagulation factors, chronic low-grade thrombin generation, and decreased fibrinolytic activity due to increased plasminogen activator inhibitor level and diminished tissue plasminogen activator levels.

- Pregnant patients are, therefore, at increased risk for DIC, which can be provoked by exposure to the procoagulant-rich uterine contents. Pregnancy-related DIC usually remits promptly after evacuation of the uterus.
- Preeclampsia and eclampsia are common causes of consumptive thrombocytopenia and microangiopathic hemolytic anemia in late (third trimester) pregnancy.
  - When these signs are seen in conjunction with hypertension, proteinuria, and edema in preeclampsia, and with seizures/coma in eclampsia, the diagnosis is straightforward and the treatment of choice is delivery of the fetus.
- The diagnosis of preeclampsia or eclampsia may be difficult to distinguish from thrombotic thrombocytopenic purpura (TTP) because of overlap in the clinical findings. Patients with these findings early in pregnancy are usually treated as TTP and patients with these findings late in pregnancy are treated as preeclamptic.
- There has been some controversy in the literature as to whether the coagulopathy in preeclampsia is due to fully expressed DIC or to a more restricted consumptive response to endothelial cell injury.
- The HELLP syndrome is characterized by *h*emolysis, *e*levated *l*iver enzymes due to fatty infiltration, and *l*ow *p*latelets from consumption in the third trimester.
  - It is associated with hypertension and is accompanied by epigastric pain and laboratory findings of DIC. Delivery of the fetus and transfusion support are indicated.
- Abruptio placentae is a sudden detachment of the placenta often accompanied by DIC and bleeding. These patients
  - are multiparous and/or hypertensive women
  - may develop hypovolemia and hypotension from retroplacental bleeding (severe cases are associated with diffuse bleeding from DIC and renal cortical necrosis)
  - are treated by correction of hypovolemia, transfusion support if the patient is bleeding, and evacuation of the uterus, which rapidly reverses the DIC
- Amniotic fluid embolism is a rare catastrophe which occurs in multiparous women undergoing difficult labors with post-mature, large fetuses.
  - Amniotic fluid, introduced through tears in the chorioamniotic membranes, rupture of the uterus, or tears of the uterine veins, obstructs the pulmonary blood vessels with fetal debris, causing acute cor pulmonale and acute cardiorespiratory failure.
  - DIC occurs in approximately one-third.
  - Pulmonary and cardiovascular support are the keys to management, and transfusion support may be required if bleeding occurs.
  - Heparin therapy may be considered if the diagnosis is recognized

early, but there are insufficient data in the literature to make firm recommendations.

- Retained dead fetus syndrome occurs several weeks after intrauterine death and is caused by tissue factor from the fetus slowly entering the maternal circulation.
  - The result is chronic DIC, which may lead to bleeding from consumption.
  - Evacuation of the uterus is the mainstay of management, along with transfusion support if the patient is bleeding.
  - If bleeding occurs, evacuation of the uterus is urgent.
  - If the patient is stable, continuous infusion of heparin has been used to interrupt DIC until platelet count and fibrinogen are normal.
  - Heparin is stopped 8 to 12 h prior to evacuation of the uterus.
- Infection and septic abortions
  - Urinary tract infections with gram-negative organisms, clostridial or gram-negative amnionitis, and endometritis are common causes of infection-related DIC in pregnant patients.

Trauma

- Patients with severe trauma may have DIC due to tissue destruction, infection, ischemia, shock, or fat embolization.
- Injury to the CNS may cause release of tissue factor, which is abundant in brain tissue.

Other Causes

- Hemolytic anemias associated with the activation of complement, such as ABO-incompatible blood transfusions, and falciparum malaria. Exposure to erythrocyte cell stroma by itself does not activate coagulation.
- Abdominal aortic aneurysms and cavernous hemangioma (Kasabach-Merritt syndrome) cause local activation of coagulation.
- Liver disease
- Burns
- Snake envenomation
- Heat stroke
- Treatment with prothrombin complex concentrates (see Chap. 73)

PURPURA FULMINANS

- Purpura fulminans is a syndrome of DIC marked by extensive venous and arterial thrombosis, extensive areas of skin and soft tissue necrosis, diffuse microthrombi, and vasculitis.
- Seen in neonates with homozygous protein C deficiency, it may also occur secondary to severe infections or following certain viral illnesses.

- Patients with secondary purpura fulminans may benefit from heparin treatment.

LABORATORY DIAGNOSIS OF DIC

- Tests usually sufficient for the diagnosis of DIC:
  - platelet count
  - prothrombin time (PT)
  - partial thromboplastin time (aPTT)
  - thrombin time (TT)
  - fibrinogen level
  - serum fibrin degradation product (FDP) level
  - plasma D-dimer concentration
  - inspection of the peripheral blood film for fragmentation of erythrocytes
- The most frequent abnormality in acute DIC is thrombocytopenia, followed in decreasing order by elevated FDP levels, prolonged PT, prolonged TT, and decreased fibrinogen concentration.
- The fibrinogen level may be normal despite consumption because of its elevation as an acute-phase reactant.
- Usually the presence of thrombocytopenia, together with three other abnormalities, confirm the diagnosis.
- Laboratory values are variable for chronic DIC. Increased production may compensate for consumption and the platelet count, clotting times and fibrinogen level may be normal, but there are usually increased concentrations of FDP and D-dimer.
- Distinguishing DIC from the coagulopathy of liver disease:
  - Latter may be difficult to distinguish from DIC since, in liver disease, thrombocytopenia may occur from hypersplenism, prolonged clotting assays and low fibrinogen levels may occur from decreased production and dysfibrinogenemia, and elevated levels of FDP may occur from decreased plasma clearance.
  - Serial assays of the coagulation profile may be useful in distinguishing the two, since the abnormalities are relatively stable over short periods in liver disease but may deteriorate rapidly in DIC.
  - An assay of factor VIII:C activity, which may be decreased in DIC and increased in liver disease, can also be helpful.
  - Additionally, patients with liver disease may be more susceptible to DIC due to decreased hemostatic reserve, high incidence of serious infection, and peritoneal-venous (Denver) shunting for ascites.
- Distinguishing DIC from primary fibrin(ogen)olysis:
  - Primary fibrin(ogen)olysis occurs when excess plasmin is produced in the absence of DIC and has been noted most frequently in the setting of thrombolytic therapy, although it may also occur idiopathically or with malignancy.

- Characteristically, FDP levels are significantly elevated in the face of normal platelet counts and D-dimer levels in primary fibrin(ogen)olysis.
- Additionally, there is often rapid whole blood clot lysis and shortened euglobulin lysis times.

TREATMENT OF DIC

- Acute DIC usually is secondary to serious primary illness.
  - Rapid and appropriate treatment of the underlying disorder is of utmost importance, including antibiotics for infection, surgical debridement of necrotic tissues, chemotherapy of acute leukemia, evacuation of a dead fetus.
  - Since a majority of patients with acute DIC are critically ill, appropriate supportive care including fluids, pressors, dialysis, and respiratory and ventilator management are essential.
- There is no convincing evidence that transfusion support "fuels the fire," and patients with documented deficiencies who are bleeding or require surgical or invasive procedures should receive transfusion support with platelets for thrombocytopenia, fresh frozen plasma for coagulation factor depletion, and occasionally cryoprecipitate for hypofibrinogenemia.
- In most forms of acute DIC, heparin treatment has not been shown to be effective in decreasing the mortality rate.
  - Although heparin treatment may be associated with improvement in laboratory parameters, its use may aggravate bleeding, and it is therefore not routinely indicated.
  - Specific indications for heparin treatment include purpura fulminans, dead fetus syndrome, aortic aneurysms, migratory thrombophlebitis due to malignancy, and DIC with large vessel thrombosis.
  - Some, but not all, authorities believe that patients with APL may benefit from heparin therapy.
  - Less established indications for heparin therapy include skin necrosis and acral gangrene, amniotic fluid embolism, ABO-mismatched blood transfusion, and septic abortion.
  - For chronic DIC, a heparin dose of 500 to 750 U/h via continuous infusion without a loading bolus may be sufficient.
  - For acute DIC, a heparin bolus of 10,000 U followed by 1000 U/h may be used.
  - The decision to use heparin must be individualized, and the risks and benefits considered carefully.
- Small studies using antithrombin III concentrates have shown laboratory findings, but no change in mortality.
- Antifibrinolytic therapy is generally contraindicated in DIC because it may provoke increased thrombosis and microvascular occulsion.

- It may be considered when primary fibrin(ogen)olysis, rather than DIC, is the major process.
- In such cases, the patient should have bleeding that has not responded to transfusion therapy and also shortened whole blood clot lysis and euglobulin lysis times.

For a more detailed discussion, see: Uri Seligsohn: Disseminated intravascular coagulation, Chap. 141, p. 1497, in *Williams Hematology*, 5/e, 1995.

80 HYPERFIBRINOLYSIS AND THERAPY WITH ANTIFIBRINOLYTIC AGENTS

HYPERFIBRINOLYSIS

- Pathophysiology
  - Local activation of the fibrinolytic system accompanies the formation of the hemostatic plug and is important in repair of injury and reestablishment of blood flow.
  - Excessive local or systemic fibrinolysis can disrupt hemostasis and lead to significant bleeding.
  - Inhibition or deficient activation of fibrinolysis can lead to local or systemic thrombosis.
- Systemic hyperfibrin(ogen)olysis
  - Endothelial cell plasminogen activator may be released in pathological states in sufficient amounts to convert plasma plasminogen to plasmin.
  - A hemorrhagic state may ensure with the following laboratory features:
    - shortened euglobulin lysis time
    - decreased levels of fibrinogen and plasminogen
    - elevated levels of fibrin(ogen) degradation products
    - normal platelet count
- Localized fibrinolysis may also cause abnormal bleeding in patients with either normal or defective hemostasis.

THERAPY WITH ANTIFIBRINOLYTIC AGENTS

- Table 80-1 lists disorders that have been treated with antifibrinolytic therapy.
- The two drugs currently in use in the United States are ϵ-aminocaproic acid and tranexamic acid, synthetic lysine analogs which block plasmin activity by occupying the lysine-binding site of the enzyme.
- EACA or ϵ-aminocaproic acid
  - Peak plasma levels achieved by 2 h after oral dose.
  - 80 percent of intravenous dose cleared unchanged within 3 h.
  - Excreted for 12 to 36 h because of large volume of distribution.
  - Administered as intravenous priming dose of about 0.1 g/kg body weight over 20 to 30 min, followed by continuous intravenous infusion of 0.5 to 1 g/h, or equivalent intermittent dose either intravenously or orally every 1, 2, or 4 h.
- Tranexamic acid
  - Plasma half-life approximately 1 to 2 h
  - More than 90 percent excreted unchanged in urine within 24 h.
  - Oral dosage is 25 mg/kg 3 or 4 times daily.
  - Intravenous dose is 10 mg/kg 3 or 4 times daily.

TABLE 80-1 Antifibrinolytic Therapy with EACA or Tranexamic Acid in Bleeding States

Clinical bleeding state	Experience with antifibrinolytic agents	Comment
	Systemic hyperfibrinolysis	
Spontaneous	Usually a self-limited disease; treatment seldom required	Contraindicated if DIC also present
Therapeutic (thrombolytic agents)	Usually not necessary	May be useful if bleeding is serious, especially during or just after therapy
Extracorporeal bypass surgery	Bleeding reduced, especially in cyanotic heart disease and prolonged pump time	Intrapleural or intrapericardial clots resistant to lysis may occur
Congenital α_2-antiplasmin or plasminogen activator inhibitor-1 deficiency	Life-long bleeding state, controlled with inhibitors	Rare autosomal recessive trait
Acquired antiplasmin deficiency	Treatment controls the acute bleeding state	Predisposing states include acute promyelocytic leukemia and amyloidosis
Liver transplantation	Commonly encountered, protracted oozing can be better controlled	Preexisting hyperfibrinolytic state with hepatocellular dysfunction
Malignancy (solid tumor)	Useful if bleeding due to hyperfibrinolysis alone	Hypercoagulable state may be "unmasked" by antifibrinolytic treatment
Acute promyelocytic leukemia	May reduce bleeding manifestations	Coexistent thrombotic state may preclude use
	Localized fibrinolysis with defective hemostasis	
Hemophilia	Proven use for dental extractions, probable usefulness after other surgical procedures	Not effective as prophylaxis for hemarthrosis
Anticoagulated patients	Dental surgery blood loss decreased, with administration as mouthwash	Potential usefulness in management of other bleeding episodes

(*continued*)

TABLE 80-1 (*Continued*)

Clinical bleeding state	Experience with antifibrinolytic agents	Comment
Thrombocytopenia	Controlled trials fail to show benefit	May be useful in selected patients
Renal	Effective, but usually considered only as an alternative to surgery	Risk of clots in the renal collecting system
Menorrhagia	Effectively reduces blood loss	Evaluate for underlying pathology
Subarachnoid hemorrhage	Incidence of rebleeding reduced but vasospasm is accentuated	No reduction in mortality
Upper gastrointestinal	Useful adjunctive measure to reduce bleeding	Carefully evaluate underlying lesion
Ulcerative colitis	May reduce blood loss but no effect on underlying disease	Unresponsive cases only
Traumatic hyphema	Reduces the incidence of early rebleeding	Long-term benefit not established
Posttonsillectomy	Incidence of rebleeding can be reduced	May be useful in selected cases

Source: Table 142-1 of *Williams Hematology*, 5/e, p. 1519.

- Side effects
  - Infrequently thrombosis, myonecrosis, or hypersensitivity reaction.
  - Thrombosis risk most significant when there is an associated thrombogenic process, such as occult disseminated intravascular coagulation (DIC).
  - In patients with upper urinary tract bleeding antifibrinolytic therapy can lead to obstructing clots in the urinary collecting system.

For a more detailed discussion, see Victor J. Marder, Charles W. Francis: Hyperfibrinolysis and therapy with antifibrinolytic agents, Chap. 142, p. 1517, in *Williams Hematology,* 5/e, 1995.

81 HYPERCOAGULABLE STATES

GENERAL

- Hypercoagulable states may be a result of an inherited abnormality or may be acquired.
- Laboratory markers for the activation of coagulation include
  - fragment F_{1-2}: activation peptide released by the action of factor Xa on prothrombin
  - fibrinopeptide A: activation peptide released by the action of thrombin on fibrinogen
  - protein C activation peptide: released by action of thrombin-thrombomodulin on protein C
  - activated protein C

INHERITED HYPERCOAGULABLE STATES

- Clinical features suggesting the presence of an inherited hypercoagulable state:
  - thrombosis at an early age
  - family history of thrombosis
  - unusual sites of thrombosis, such as hepatic or mesenteric veins
  - recurrent thrombosis, with or without precipitating factors
  - recurrent thrombosis, despite adequate therapy
  - warfarin-induced skin necrosis
- Venous thrombosis occurs more commonly in hypercoagulable states than arterial thrombosis.
- Testing for the hypercoagulable state:
  - Perform when the patient is stable, not during acute thrombotic event.
  - Patients should not be receiving anticoagulant therapy as heparin decreases antithrombin III (AT III) levels, and warfarin decreases protein C and S levels.
  - Diagnostic yield higher in patients with suggestive clinical features as listed above.
  - Functional assays are preferable to antigenic assays.
  - Repeated testing and family studies are helpful in confirming the diagnosis.
  - Recommended screening studies include:
    - functional AT III levels (heparin cofactor assay)
    - immunological and functional protein C levels
    - immunological total and free protein S and functional protein S levels
    - testing for dysfibrinogenemia with immunological and functional fibrinogen levels and thrombin time

AT III DEFICIENCY

- Autosomal dominant inheritance of thrombophilia.
- Prevalence in general population: 1 in 350.

- Type I deficiency is due to reduced synthesis of the AT III protein.
- Type II deficiency is due to production of an AT III protein with abnormal function.
- Two functional AT III assays are available:
  - The antithrombin III–heparin cofactor assay measures the ability of AT-III to inactivate serine proteases in the presence of heparin.
  - The progressive AT III assay quantifies the inhibitory activity in the absence of heparin.
- The normal range is narrow, with a lower limit of 70 percent of the mean. Values below are considered to be deficient.
- Some patients may be normal in one functional assay but abnormal in the other.
  - Heterozygous patients with deficient heparin cofactor activity but normal progressive AT III activity appear to have thrombotic events infrequently.
  - Those with deficient progressive AT III activity, combined functional deficiency, or type I deficiency have higher risk for thrombosis.
- 55 percent of biochemically affected individuals develop venous thrombosis, occurring spontaneously, or more frequently, related to stress such as pregnancy, oral contraceptive use, surgery, or trauma.
- Risk of thrombosis increases with age.
- Acquired causes of low AT III levels: heparin therapy, disseminated intravascular coagulation (DIC), liver disease, nephrotic syndrome, oral contraceptive use, L-asparaginase therapy, acute thrombosis, eclampsia, and other hypertensive disorders of pregnancy.

TREATMENT OF AT III DEFICIENCY

- Acute thrombosis in the AT-III–deficient patient is treated similarly to thrombosis in a patient not AT III deficient.
- Higher than usual doses of heparin may be required, but most patients can be successfully anticoagulated.
- Role of AT III concentrates used with heparin not well defined.
- Long-term oral anticoagulation indicated for recurrent thrombotic events.
- Subcutaneous heparin or AT III concentrates should be used instead of warfarin during pregnancy.
- The number, severity, and precipitating factors of thrombotic events, the pattern of thrombosis in the family, the patient's lifestyle, sex, and child-bearing potential should be considered in the decision to initiate or withhold long-term anticoagulation after a single thrombotic event or for prophylaxis in the asymptomatic patient.
- Anticoagulation usually not needed in asymptomatic individuals, except during periods of thrombotic stress.
- Prophylactic anticoagulation or AT III concentrates should be given during perioperative periods.

PROTEIN C DEFICIENCY

- Autosomal dominant inheritance of thrombophilia.
- Affected heterozygotes have protein C levels of approximately 50 percent.
- Type I deficiency is due to decreased synthesis of a normal protein.
- Type II deficiency is due to production of an abnormally functioning protein.
- Clinical features are similar to AT III deficiency.
- About 75 percent of affected individuals have venous thrombosis, most often spontaneous.
  - A minority have nonhemorrhagic stroke.
  - Usual onset is in young adulthood.
  - Risk of thrombosis increases with age.
- Warfarin-induced skin necrosis more likely to occur in patients with protein C deficiency, though its absolute incidence remains low (see Chap. 83).
- Neonatal purpura fulminans occurs in homozygotes with protein C levels below 5 percent.
- Acquired causes of low protein C levels: neonates (especially if premature), liver disease, DIC, sepsis, L-asparaginase therapy, breast cancer chemotherapy with cyclophosphamide, methotrexate, and flurorouracil, vitamin K deficiency, or treatment with oral anticoagulants.
- Treatment of protein C deficiency
  - General management is similar to AT III deficiency.
  - Because of the risk of warfarin-induced skin necrosis, oral anticoagulaltion is given with concomitant heparin therapy, and heavy loading doses of warfarin should be avoided.
  - Neonatal purpura fulminans is treated by replacement of protein C, using either plasma infusions or protein C concentrate. Heparin therapy is ineffective, but long-term warfarin has been used after initial replacement therapy.

PROTEIN S DEFICIENCY

- Autosomal dominant inheritance of thrombophilia.
- Clinical features are similar to protein C deficiency, including warfarin-induced skin necrosis and purpura fulminans in homozygotes.
- Protein S in plasma is both bound to C4b-binding protein and in an unbound (free) form. Only the free form is active.
- Free protein S antigen and functional activities are generally more severely decreased than bound protein S.
- Protein S levels increase with age and are higher in men than women.
- Acquired causes of low protein S levels include liver disease, L-asparaginase therapy, DIC, acute thrombosis, pregnancy, and oral contraceptive use.

- C4b-binding protein is an acute-phase reactant; inflammation causes a decline in free protein S levels due to a shift to bound form.
- There is no agreement on what level of protein S is diagnostic of hereditary protein S deficiency, but levels of 30 percent or less are consistent with hereditary deficiency.
- Therapy for protein S deficiency is similar to that for protein C deficiency.

INHERITED RESISTANCE TO ACTIVATED PROTEIN C

- Recently described syndrome of familial thrombophilia associated with a poor response of patient's plasma to activated protein C in a PTT-based assay.
  - Autosomal dominant inheritance.
  - May be the most common inherited thrombophilia.
  - Appears to be due to abnormality of coagulation factor V.
- Patients with protein C deficiency who co-inherit resistance to activated protein C may be more prone to thrombosis than those with protein C deficiency alone.

ABNORMALITIES OF FIBRINOGEN AND FIBRINOLYSIS

- Inherited abnormalities of fibrinogen rarely may result in thrombosis due to resistance to fibrinolysis (see Chap. 74).
- Inherited dysplasminogenemia or hypoplasminogenemia are also associated with thrombophilia, but the correlation between deficiency and thrombosis in family members is weak.

ACQUIRED HYPERCOAGULABLE STATES

- Venous stasis: immobilization, pregnancy, congestive heart failure, previous thrombosis, obesity
- Malignancy: Trousseau syndrome (migratory thrombophlebitis), marantic endocarditis, thrombosis associated with chronic DIC, and related to chemotherapy treatment (L-asparaginase, mitomycin)
- Associated with lupus anticoagulants (see Chap. 78)
- Hyperestrogenic states: pregnancy and post partum, DES treatment of prostate cancer, oral contraceptive use
- Prothrombin complex concentrate therapy (see Chap. 73)
- Postoperative state
- Myeloproliferative diseases (see Chap. 9, 10, and 11)
- Paroxysmal nocturnal hemoglobinuria (see Chap. 5)
- Hyperlipidemia

- Diabetes mellitus
- Homocystinuria
- Hyperviscosity syndrome (see Chap. 62)
- Cigarette smoking
- Sickle cell disease (see Chap. 26)
- Nephrotic syndrome

For a more detailed discussion, see Kenneth A. Bauer: The hypercoagulable states, Chap. 144, p. 1531, in *Williams Hematology,* 5/e, 1995.

---

82 ANTIPLATELET THERAPY

THE ROLE OF PLATELETS IN THROMBOSIS

- Properties which make platelets useful in the arrest of hemorrhage also allow platelets to form thrombi in vessels, and on heart valves, artificial membranes, and prosthetic devices.
- Circulating platelets do not adhere to each other or to endothelium unless activated, which occurs after platelet exposure to injured or denuded endothelium, such as following rupture of an atherosclerotic plaque.
- Adherent platelets secrete mediators, including thromboxane A_2 and ADP, which activate and recruit other platelets to the forming thrombus. The surfaces of activated platelets and platelet microparticles also accelerate the formation of thrombin, leading to fibrin deposition.
- Additionally, platelets secrete mediators involved in vasospasm, atherogenesis, proliferative responses, and inflammation.
- In contrast to veins, the flow conditions in arteries favor the displacement of platelets away from the axial stream toward the vessel wall, accounting, in part, for the greater role of platelets in arterial thrombosis.
- Drugs which inhibit platelet function may, therefore, have clinical application in the treatment and prevention of thrombosis.

ANTIPLATELET DRUGS

Drugs which inhibit platelet function include the following.

Aspirin

- Most widely used antiplatelet agent.
- Inhibits prostaglandin synthesis by irreversibly acetylating a critical serine residue in cyclo-oxygenase, thereby blocking the formation of thromboxane A_2 (TxA_2). Since platelets cannot synthesize new enzymes, the inhibition is permanent for the lifespan of the platelet.
- Prolongs bleeding time.
- Inhibits collagen-induced platelet aggregation and secondary aggregation to weak agonists, such as ADP and epinephrine.
- Effects on aggregation and bleeding time last 4 to 7 days after a single oral dose.
- Inhibits the synthesis of the anticoagulant prostaglandin, PGI_2, in endothelial cells, but the inhibition is short lived since endothelium can synthesize new enzyme.
- A dose of aspirin which inhibits TxA_2 but not PGI_2 production has not been found, nor has the optimal dose of aspirin been defined for any specific indication.
- The dose used for a specific indication should take into account efficacy, as determined by clinical trials, and adverse effects, which

include, most importantly, gastrointestinal bleeding and hemorrhagic stroke.

Nonsteroidal Anti-inflammatory Drugs

• Appear to work by a mechanism similar to aspirin, but the effects are of much shorter duration.

Dipyridamole

• A phosphodiesterase inhibitor with vasodilator effects.
• Mechanisms of action may include increasing platelet cyclic AMP levels, or indirectly increasing the plasma levels of adenosine.
• Does not inhibit aggregation of platelet-rich plasma in vitro, but does inhibit aggregation of platelets in the presence of erythrocytes, as measured by whole blood aggregometry.

Ticlopidine

• Prolongs the bleeding time and inhibits aggregation induced by high shear force and by ADP.
• Mechanism of action unclear; may inhibit the ability of ADP to activate GP IIb/IIIa.
• Effective only when given orally and fully effective only after 3 to 5 days, implying activity due to a metabolite.
• Effects are irreversible for the lifespan of the platelet.
• Usual dose is 250 mg bid.
• Adverse effects include diarrhea and rash. Neutropenia, which may occur usually in the first 3 months of treatment, may be severe but is reversible.

Other Antiplatelet Agents

• PGI_2 (prostacyclin) and stable analogs, such as iloprost, are inhibitors of platelet aggregation as well as potent vasodilators.
• Dextran infusions increase the bleeding time and inhibit platelet function by unclear mechanisms which may involve alteration of platelet membranes or plasma proteins.
• Sulfinpyrizone is a weak inhibitor of platelet function when given at doses of 800 mg/day or higher. It may inhibit cyclo-oxygenase.
• Murine monoclonal antibodies against GP IIb/IIIa or chimeras of murine monoclonal antibodies with human antibody constant regions are potent inhibitors of platelet function and thrombus formation in animal models.
• Synthetic peptides containing arginine-glycine-asparagine sequences are also potent inhibitors of thrombosis in animal models.
• Omega-3 fatty acids (ω-3 fatty acids), which are found in high concentrations in fish oils, compete with arachidonic acid for cyclo-oxygenase and are converted into TxA_3, which is a much less potent

platelet agonist than TxA_2. Diets supplemented with these acids may prolong the bleeding time and decrease platelet aggregation.
- Nitrates, beta blockers, calcium channel blockers, beta-lactam antibiotics, serotonin antagonists, and suloctidil are other drugs with some degree of antiplatelet activity.

CLINICAL INDICATIONS FOR ANTIPLATELET THERAPY

Ischemic Heart Disease

- Aspirin therapy may be useful in the following situations:
  - Primary prevention in patients without previous cardiovascular events, but with risk factors including older age
  - Secondary prevention after previous myocardial infarction
  - Unstable angina
  - Acute myocardial infarction
  - As an adjunct to thrombolytic therapy, coronary angioplasty, or coronary artery bypass grafting
- Benefits of treatment have include significant reductions in nonfatal myocardial infarctions, nonfatal stroke, vascular death, and overall mortality.
- Doses of aspirin studied have ranged between 300 and 1500 mg/day, with no best dose defined.
- Aspirin does not affect the pattern of symptoms of chronic stable angina.
- Ticlopidine has also been shown to reduce the incidence of myocardial infarction and vascular death.

Valvular Heart Disease

- Oral anticoagulant therapy is generally recommended for patients with prosthetic heart valves, but the addition of aspirin or dipyridamole is recommended for patients who have systemic thromboembolism despite adequate anticoagulation.

Atrial Fibrillation

- Aspirin may be helpful in decreasing the incidence of stroke in patients with atrial fibrillation, but this approach should be reserved for patients unable to take oral anticoagulants or who are felt to have only mildly increased risk of thromboembolism.

Cerebrovascular Disease

- Trials of aspirin (300 to 1500 mg/day) in patients with cerebrovascular symptoms or previous myocardial infarction have shown a significant decrease in the incidence of stroke and vascular death. No further benefit was achieved by the addition of dipyridamole to aspirin.

- Other studies have shown ticlopidine to be effective in reducing stroke and death.
- Although the issue is not completely resolved, the benefits of aspirin seem to be comparable in men and women.

Peripheral Vascular Disease

- Aspirin treatment may decrease the need for vascular surgery without affecting the pattern of stable intermittent claudication, suggesting that antiplatelet therapy decreases the incidence of thrombotic complications without affecting the basic disease process.

Myeloproliferative Disorders

- Aspirin has been useful in controlling digital ischemia (erythromelalgia) in polycythemia vera.
- Its use in the prevention of thrombotic complications of myeloproliferative disorders is controversial, and the incidence of bleeding complications may be high.

Complications of Pregnancy

- Aspirin has been used in the treatment of pregnancy-induced hypertensive disorders such as eclampsia and preeclampsia. The prophylactic use of low-dose aspirin in patients at high risk for these disorders has been reported to lower the incidence of these conditions and their sequelae without obvious adverse effects.

Microangiopathic States

- Antiplatelet agents such as aspirin and dextran are often employed in the treatment of microangiopathic hemolytic anemic states, such as thrombotic thrombocytopenic purpura, though controlled trials are lacking.

Venous Thrombosis

- Although antiplatelet drugs are generally felt to be more useful in arterial thrombosis, and anticoagulants are generally used for venous thrombosis, aspirin may have some role in the prophylaxis of venous thrombosis in selected patients undergoing orthopedic surgery or with other forms of immobility.

For a more detailed discussion, see Harvey J. Weiss: Antiplatelet drugs and therapy, Chap. 145, p. 1550, in *Williams Hematology,* 5/e, 1995.

83 ANTICOAGULANT THERAPY

HEPARIN

Mechanism of Action

- Standard heparin consists of a heterogeneous mixture of sulfated glycosaminoglycans of different chain length with an average molecular mass of 15,000 daltons and an average chain length of 50 sugar residues.
- Heparin binds antithrombin III (AT III), forming a complex capable of both inhibiting the generation of thrombin and accelerating its decay.
- Heparin increases the efficiency of AT III's action on thrombin 1000-fold.
- The AT III–thrombin complex then dissociates from heparin and is cleared by the monocyte-macrophage system.
- The binding of AT III to heparin is dependent on a specific randomly distributed high-affinity pentasaccharide sequence within heparin.
- The enhancement of AT III activity against thrombin is dependent on the length of the heparin chains, which must be at least 18 sugar residues long.
- Heparin and AT III also inactivate other serine proteases of the coagulation cascade, especially factor Xa.
- For anti-Xa activity, binding of AT III to the high-affinity pentasaccharide is essential, but the heparin chain length is not.
- Heparin may also potentiate the extrinsic pathway inhibitor.

Pharmacokinetics

- Heparin pharmacokinetics are compatible with saturable binding (preferentially of high-molecular-weight species) to plasma proteins, endothelial cells, and monocytes, combined with unsaturable renal excretion.
- As the dose of heparin is increased, the anticoagulant response increases disproportionately, and the half-life lengthens from 30 to 150 min.
- Patients with pulmonary embolism have an accelerated rate of heparin clearance.

Route of Administration

- Continuous IV infusion of heparin is preferable to repeated IV boluses, because of a higher bleeding risk with boluses.
- Subcutaneous treatment is as effective as IV, but higher doses are needed.
- Subcutaneous treatment must be preceded by an IV loading dose when treating established thrombosis, to ensure prompt intravascular therapeutic levels via saturation of endothelial cell binding.

Laboratory Monitoring

- Standard heparin therapy is monitored by the activated partial thromboplastin time (aPTT).
- The usual therapeutic aPTT range is 1.5 to 2.5 times the upper limit of normal.
- A patient with a short aPTT can be monitored using the patient's own baseline aPTT as the control.
- A patient with a prolonged aPTT due to a lupus anticoagulant may be monitored with heparin levels determined by protamine neutralization (therapeutic range 0.2 to 0.4 U/ml) or chromogenic anti-Xa levels (range 0.3 to 0.6 U/ml).
- No laboratory monitoring is required for routine prophylactic subcutaneous heparin therapy at doses of 5000 U twice a day.

Heparin Therapy

- An acceptable schedule for full-dose IV heparin is a loading bolus of 5000 U followed by an infusion of 30,000 to 40,000 U per 24 h. Patients with standard bleeding risk should receive the higher dose and high-risk patients should receive less.
- The aPTT should be repeated 4 to 6 h after the bolus and doses adjusted to give an aPTT of 1.5 to 2.5 times normal.
- An additional bolus of 5000 U may be given if the aPTT is less than 1.2 times normal, and 2500 U given if its is 1.2 to 1.5 times normal.
- Failure to attain a therapeutic aPTT within the first 24 h, when treating a deep vein thrombosis or pulmonary embolism, has been associated with a substantial increase in repeated thromboembolic events.
- The dose required for therapeutic anticoagulation will often decrease after several days as the thrombotic process comes under control and oral anticoagulants take effect.
- For subcutaneous treatment, an initial IV bolus of 5000 U can be followed by 17,500 U subcutaneously every 12 h.
- Warfarin therapy is usually begun simultaneously with heparin. Use of this combination therapy is discussed below under Warfarin Therapy of Thrombosis.

Heparin Resistance

- Laboratory heparin resistance is defined as needing >35,000 U/24 h to achieve adequate anticoagulation.
- Such resistance may be caused by increased binding of heparin to plasma proteins such as vitronectin and platelet factor 4, or to monocytes and endothelial cells.
- An increasing heparin dose requirement during therapy may herald the development of heparin-induced thrombocytopenia.

- Clinical heparin resistance denotes ongoing thrombosis despite adequate anticoagulation as judged by laboratory tests, possibly due to the relative inability of heparin/AT III to neutralize fibrin-bound thrombin.

Adverse Effects

- Bleeding
  - The risk of a major bleeding episode is approximately 5 percent during a course of full dose heparin.
  - The risk of bleeding is higher in patients with a history of recent surgery or stroke, history of gastrointestinal or genitourinary tract bleeding, peptic ulcer disease, platelet counts less than 150,000, renal disease, advanced age, poor performance status, and concomitant use of antiplatelet or thrombolytic therapy.
  - Prophylactic low-dose heparin is not associated with an increase of major bleeding, but may be associated with an increase in minor bleeding.
- Heparin-induced thrombocytopenia
  - An idiosyncratic reaction which develops after 7 to 14 days of therapy but may occur sooner if the patient has been previously exposed to heparin.
  - It occurs more frequently with bovine than porcine heparin.
  - Bleeding is rare, but thrombosis, typically arterial, resulting from in vivo platelet activation may occur.
  - The diagnosis can be confirmed by laboratory studies based on ^{14}C-labeled serotonin release or platelet aggregations.
  - Discontinue heparin when heparin-induced thrombocytopenia is suspected.
  - Platelet counts usually normalize within 4 days after discontinuation of heparin.
  - Consider ancrod or hirudin for patients who need continued intravenous anticoagulation.
- Osteopenia
  - Heparin, when used in high doses (usually greater than 20,000 U/day) for 5 months or more, may induce osteopenia caused by potentiation of osteoclast action.
- Other side effects include hypoaldosteronism, priapism, hypersensitivity reactions, local skin necrosis, and hepatic transaminase elevations.

Reversal of Heparin Effects

- Standard heparin can be neutralized by protamine sulfate at a dose of 1 mg for each 100 U of heparin. Enough protamine should be given to neutralize one-half of the heparin given during the last hour.

- Protamine neutralizes the antithrombin effects but not the anti-Xa effects.

LOW-MOLECULAR-WEIGHT HEPARINS

- Low-molecular-weight (LMW) heparins have an average molecular mass of 6000 daltons and possess higher anti-Xa activity than antithrombin activity.
- LMW heparins do not prolong the aPTT. LMW heparin therapy may be monitored by chromogenic anti-Xa assays.
- LMW heparins have a longer half-life and a higher, more reliable bioavailability when administered intravenously or subcutaneously.
- LMW heparins have linear elimination kinetics, suggesting limited binding to proteins and cells.
- Half-life is prolonged in renal failure.
- Usually administered once daily, the dosage and anticoagulant profile depends on the particular LMW heparin preparation.
- One preparation, enoxaparin, is clinically available.
- Accumulating evidence suggests that LMW heparins are generally as safe and as effective as standard heparin.
- It is unknown if protamine reverses LMW heparins.
- LMW heparin has been reported to cause heparin-induced thrombocytopenia.

ORAL ANTICOAGULANTS

Mechanism of Action

- Coumarins act by inhibiting vitamin K–dependent posttranslational γ-carboxylation of glutamic acid residues in the Gla domains of coagulation factors II, VII, IX and X, as well as anticoagulant proteins C and S.
- γ-Carboxylation requires the reduced form of vitamin K as a cofactor. During γ-carboxylation, vitamin K is oxidized. The enzymes, vitamin K epoxide reductase, and vitamin K reductase are required to recycle vitamin K back to its reduced form. Coumarins inhibit these reductases, thus depleting reduced vitamin K.
- The absence of γ-carboxyglutamate residues results in coagulation factors with little or no activity because they are unable to bind calcium and undergo necessary conformation changes.
- The production of affected coagulation factors stops promptly, but the anticoagulant effect is delayed until the previously formed coagulation factors are removed from the circulation. Factor VII has the shortest half-life at 6 h, while the others range from 24 to 72 h.

Pharmacokinetics

- Warfarin, the most commonly used coumarin, has predictable oral absorption and a half-life of 36 to 48 h.

- It is highly protein-bound and only the free compound is active.
- Warfarin is metabolized by hydroxylation and conjugation in the microsomal enzymes of the liver, crosses the placenta, but is not excreted in breast milk.

Warfarin Administration

- Dosages required for adequate anticoagulation average 35 mg/week but vary widely, according to the rate of drug metabolism. It is usually administered in daily oral doses.
- An exaggerated response is seen in vitamin K deficiency (malabsorption, antibiotics, and starvation), liver disease, hypermetabolic states, and drug interactions.
- Warafarin resistance
  - May be hereditary due to increased metabolism or decreased binding of the drug to its hepatic receptor.
  - May be acquired due to pregnancy, poor absorption due to short bowel, or excessive intake of vitamin K.
- Many drugs interact with warfarin, and it is prudent to monitor anticoagulation closely whenever adding, stopping, or changing the dose of other drugs.
  - Drugs which displace warfarin from plasma proteins (chloral hydrate) increase the anticoagulant effect.
  - Drugs which retard its absorption (cholestyramine) or increase its metabolism through induction of the mixed oxidase enzymes (barbiturates, rifampin) decrease the anticoagulant effect.
  - Antibiotics may decrease the vitamin K available from gut flora.
  - Aspirin and NSAIDs increase the bleeding risk by causing platelet dysfunction and gastric erosions.

Laboratory Monitoring

- Warfarin therapy is monitored by the prothrombin time (PT).
- The sensitivity of the PT to anticoagulation varies with the source of thromboplastin in the assay.
- Interlab variation is corrected for by using the International Normalized Ratio (INR) instead of the PT ratio.
- The international sensitivity index (ISI) is a correction factor established for each thromboplastin. The INR is determined by the formula $INR = (patient\ PT/control\ PT)^{ISI}$.
- Current recommendations are to keep the INR between 2.0 and 3.0 for all indications except mechanical heart valve prophylaxis, for which it should be kept at 2.5 to 3.5.

Adverse Effects

- Bleeding is the major complication of warfarin therapy.
  - The annual risk of major bleeding episodes has been estimated at 5 percent and fatal bleeding episodes at 2 percent.

- The major determinants of bleeding risk are intensity of anticoagulation (an INR > 2.5 has higher risk), advanced age, history of gastrointestinal bleeding, hypertension, cerebrovascular disease, heart disease, severe anemia, and renal insufficiency.
- A risk benefit analysis needs to be done on patients with a high risk of bleeding and alternative strategies such as inferior vena cava interruption, aspirin, subcutaneous heparin, or no anticoagulation should be considered. It should be remembered that high-risk patients were often excluded from prospective trials which showed a benefit of anticoagulation.
- The most common sites of bleeding are gastrointestinal and genitourinary.
- Patients with gastrointestinal or genitourinary bleeding should undergo investigation to define the source of bleeding, since occult malignancy will be found in some of these patients.

Warfarin-Induced Skin Necrosis

- A rare condition in which painful and discolored areas of skin, usually over fatty areas such as the buttocks and breasts, appear between the third and eighth day of warfarin.
- Lesions progress to frank necrosis and eschar formation.
- It may be due to more rapid decline of protein C levels than other coagulation factors, thereby inducing a temporary hypercoagulable state.
- It is more common in females, in those with hereditary protein C deficiency, and in patients with ongoing venous thrombosis.
- Management strategies are anecdotal, but include immediate discontinuation of warfarin, and treatment with heparin, vitamin K, or fresh-frozen plasma.
- Subcutaneous heparin may be considered for long-term anticoagulation.
- The successful management of patients with previous skin necrosis who required futher warfarin therapy has been reported in which warfarin was initiated at low dose and slowly increased in combination with full-dose heparin therapy.

Other Side Effects of Warfarin

- Warfarin is a teratogen and is contraindicated in pregnancy, as it may induce nasal hypoplasia and stippled epiphysis in the fetus, if given during the 6th to 12th week, or CNS malformation if given at any time during gestation.
- Abnormalities in calcium metabolism and cholesterol embolization.

Reversal of Warfarin

- Discontinuation can reverse anticoagulation but will take at least 48 h because of the drug's half-life.

- Vitamin K given subcutaneously or intravenously may take up to 24 h to reverse anticoagulation.
- For asymptomatic over-anticoagulation, small doses of vitamin K should be administered (0.5 to 1.0 mg), as higher doses make re-anticoagulation difficult.
- Intravenous administration of vitamin K has been reported to cause anaphylaxis.
- For serious bleeding requiring immediate reversal of anticoagulation, fresh frozen plasma (15 ml/kg) can be transfused, or for extreme emergencies, prothrombin complex concentrates may be used, but carry a risk of thrombosis. Both carry some potential for viral transmission.

Warfarin Therapy of Thrombosis

- For acute thrombosis warfarin can be initiated with a loading dose of 10 mg daily for 2 days and then titrated according to the INR, which is tested daily until a stable dose is established.
- Heparin therapy should be employed until adequate anticoagulation with warfarin is achieved.
- Warfarin may be started at the same time as heparin, but the heparin should be continued for at least 48 to 72 h after attaining a therapeutic INR to ensure that factor II, IX, and X levels have declined.
- The PT should be repeated 6 h after stopping heparin to ensure that it remains therapeutic.
- In elective situations, warfarin may be started at its maintenance dose of 4 to 5 mg/day and the INR checked biweekly. A therapeutic dose is usually obtained after 1 week.

Perioperative Management of Anticoagulation

- For patients at low thrombotic risk such as atrial fibrillation warfarin is stopped 3 to 5 days prior to surgery and simply restarted when it is deemed prudent.
- For patients at higher thrombotic risk, such as recent DVT, full-dose heparinization should be substituted, and the heparin stopped 6 h prior to the procedure and restarted as soon as possible thereafter.
- Prosthetic heart valves carry an indeterminate risk.
- Minor procedures can often be done without reversing the anticoagulation by decreasing the intensity to an INR of 1.5.

For a more detailed discussion, see Louis Fiore, Daniel Deykin: Anticoagulant therapy, Chap. 146, p. 1562; Joseph P. Miletich: Prothrombin time, Chap. L33, p. L82; and Activated partial thromboplastin time, Chap. L34, p. L85, in *Williams Hematology,* 5/e, 1995.

- The aim of fibrinolytic therapy is to lyse thrombi rapidly and thereby decrease ischemic damage. All currently available thrombolytic agents activate the plasma zymogen plasminogen, which, in turn, converts fibrin into soluble fibrin degradation products.

STREPTOKINASE

- A single-chain polypeptide derived from β-hemolytic streptococci.
- It lacks intrinsic enzymatic activity but combines stoichiometrically with plasminogen to form a complex which possesses plasmin-like proteolytic activity.
- The streptokinase-plasminogen complex converts free plasminogen to plasmin.
- Partial proteolysis of the streptokinase-plasminogen complex, or the exposure of streptokinase to plasmin leads to the formation of a streptokinase-plasmin complex.
- Streptokinase-plasmin complex is more active in fibrin degradation than native plasmin and is relatively insensitive to the inhibitors of plasmin such as α_2-antiplasmin and α_2-macroglobulin.
- The activity of streptokinase is enhanced by fibrinogen, fibrin, and fibrin-degradation products.
- Circulating streptokinase-plasmin(ogen) complex leads to a systemic plasminemia and lytic state.
- The streptokinase-plasmin(ogen) complex is itself proteolytically degraded by plasmin.
- Allergic reactions to streptokinase, including fever, hypotension, urticaria, and bronchospasm may occur. Premedication with acetaminophen, diphenhydramine, and hydrocortisone is often recommended.
- Neutralizing antibodies are commonly induced after treatment with streptokinase, which abrogates response to further streptokinase therapy at standard doses.

ANISOYLATED PLASMINOGEN STREPTOKINASE ACTIVATOR COMPLEX (APSAC)

- A complex of chemically modified plasminogen noncovalently bound to streptokinase. The modified plasminogen has its active site protected by a covalently linked *p*-anisoyl group.
- After bolus administration deacylation of APSAC commences immediately and generates the active streptokinase-plasminogen complex.
- It has a longer half-life and greater lytic potency than streptokinase.
- APSAC may be given by rapid intravenous bolus administration without inducing hypotension.

UROKINASE

- A serine protease which directly activates plasminogen.
- In vivo it is present in single-chain form (scu-PA) that possesses low

levels of activity and serves as a zymogen, a high-molecular-weight two-chain form (HMW-tcu-PA), and a low-molecular-weight two-chain form (LMW-tcu-PA).

- The commercially available form in the United States is the LMW-tcu-PA.
- Urokinase induces a systemic lytic state.
- It does not commonly cause hypersensitivity reactions or induce antibody formation.

TISSUE PLASMINOGEN ACTIVATOR (t-PA)

- A serine protease synthesized by endothelial cells and commercially available as a recombinant product which activates plasminogen.
- t-PA binds to fibrin, which induces conformational changes in both t-PA and plasminogen that increase the catalytic efficiency of plasminogen activation several hundred-fold.
- The relative fibrin specificity of t-PA is a theoretical advantage over other fibrinolytic agents but may not be as clinically important as once believed. Effective treatment of arterial thrombosis entails rapid clot lysis, requiring t-PA doses high enough to provoke a systemic lytic state.
- t-PA does not provoke allergy or antibody formation, but is expensive.

THROMBOLYTIC REGIMENS

- Common therapeutic thrombolytic regimens are summarized in Table 84-1.

TABLE 84-1 Therapeutic Thrombolytic Regimens

Indication	Agent	Regimen
Acute myocardial infarction	Streptokinase	1,500,000 IU over 1 h
	t-PA*	100 mg over 3 h (60 mg/20 mg/20 mg)
	APSAC*	30 U over 5 min
Venous thromboembolism†	Streptokinase	250,000 IU loading dose, 100,000 IU/h for 24 h
	Urokinase	2000 IU/kg loading dose, 2000 IU/kg/h for 24–48 h
	t-PA	100 mg over 2 h

*t-PA, tissue-type plasminogen activator; APSAC; anisoylated plasminogen streptokinase activator complex.
†The use of thrombolytic therapy in the treatment of venous thromboembolism continues to be individualized.
Source: Table 147-2 of *Williams Hematology*, 5/e, p. 1589.

LABORATORY MONITORING OF FIBRINOLYTIC THERAPY

- The prothombin time, activated partial thromboplastin time, and thrombin time, as well as concentration of fibrin(ogen) degradation products, all increase with fibrinolytic therapy, and fibrinogen, plasmin, and α_2-antiplasmin concentrations are decreased.
- Routine monitoring of these parameters is not of clinical utility. However, demonstration of a systemic lytic state by these tests may occasionally be helpful in excluding antibody formation as the cause of clinical failure of streptokinase therapy.

LIMITATIONS OF FIBRINOLYTIC THERAPY

- The three major shortcomings of fibrinolytic therapy are hemorrhage, delayed time to lysis, and reocclusion.
- Bleeding complications occur in 5 percent of patients treated with streptokinase, and the incidence of severe hemorrhage is approximately 1 percent. Other agents have similar rates of bleeding complications.
- Bleeding can be minimized by avoidance of invasive procedures and by avoiding administration of thrombolytic agents over prolonged time periods.
- Contraindications to fibrinolytic therapy include cerebrovascular accidents, recent surgery, prolonged cardiopulmonary resuscitation, severe hypertension, active bleeding, or active peptic ulcer disease.
- The rate of reocclusion after successful lysis of arterial thrombosis is 30 to 40 percent.
- Reocclusion is decreased by the adjunctive use of anticoagulant therapy. The addition of aspirin (325 mg chewed immediately, then 325 mg orally daily) and full-dose intravenous heparin to the thrombolytic therapy of acute myocardial infarction are recommended.

For a more detailed discussion, see Joseph Loscalzo: Fibrinolytic therapy, Chap. 147, p. 1585, in *Williams Hematology,* 5/e, 1995.

STORAGE AND PRESERVATION OF BLOOD

- Erythrocytes are preserved by liquid storage at 4°C or by frozen storage at either −80 or −150°C.
- Preservative solutions for liquid storage all contain glucose, to provide energy, and citrate buffer at an acid pH to prevent coagulation by binding calcium and to counter the marked rise in pH which occurs when blood is cooled to 4°C.
- CPD-adenine is the preservative solution most used now in the United States. It contains *c*itrate, *p*hosphate, and *d*extrose (glucose). Adenine is added to help maintain intracellular levels of ATP.
- Stored blood develops the so-called storage lesion, characterized in part by reduced levels of ATP, which interfere with glucose metabolism and reduce cell viability. In addition, 2,3-bisphosphoglycerate levels are reduced, which increase the oxygen affinity of hemoglobin and thereby decrease the effectiveness of reinfused red cells.
- Potassium also leaks rapidly from stored cells.
- Preparation of components of whole blood requires removal of most of the plasma and preservative solution. The remaining red cells may be preserved by adding a nutrient solution containing glucose, adenine, and mannitol. Mannitol is included because it prevents hemolysis by some unknown mechanism.
- Frozen storage requires a cryoprotective agent to avoid hemolysis during freezing and thawing. Glycerol is the most frequently used agent. With proper technique over 80 percent of erythrocytes will survive frozen storage and function normally after transfusion.
- Frozen erythrocytes must be extensively washed after thawing, which introduces the possibility of bacterial contamination and makes it necessary to use such erythrocytes within 24 h.

WHOLE BLOOD PREPARATIONS

- A unit of whole blood contains 435 to 500 ml of blood and 14 to 15 ml of preservative-anticoagulant solution for each 100 ml. Thus, if 450 ml of blood is collected, stored, and transfused, the patient will receive about 515 ml of total fluid.
- Blood collected in CDPA-1 (CDP with adenine) may be used after storage up to 35 days.

FRESH BLOOD

- When blood is stored, viable platelets are depleted within 48 h, and the activity of coagulation factors V, VIII, and IX falls significantly.

413

- Thrombocytopenia and deficiency of the labile coagulation factors may occur in patients who receive transfusions of banked blood equal to their total blood volume in 24 h.
- Fresh blood is often requested in an effort to avoid administration of blood deficient in these hemostatic components.
- It is better to treat such patients with a combination of packed red cells, fresh-frozen plasma, and platelet concentrates.
- Whole blood less than 5 to 7 days old may be transfused to patients with severe renal or hepatic disease, or in newborns receiving exchange transfusion, in order to avoid infusing excess free potassium.
- Patients who require massive transfusion should be given at least part of the transfusion as blood less than a few days old in order to avoid oxygen release problems due to depletion of red cell 2,3-bisphosphoglycerate.
- Patients with chronic transfusion-dependent anemia should probably receive blood less than 10 days old in order to maximize the interval between transfusions.

PACKED RED BLOOD CELLS

- Packed red blood cells can be prepared from stored blood any time before the expiration date by centrifugation and removal of plasma to give a hematocrit of 60 to 90 percent.
- Red cells packed to an hematocrit of less than 80 percent can be stored until the expiration date of the original blood.
- Red cells, rather than whole blood, should be used for replacement of a red cell deficit.
- Packed red cells and electrolyte solutions are as effective as whole blood in replacing surgical blood loss.

LEUKOCYTE-POOR BLOOD

- Best prepared by passing blood or packed cells through a special filter which removes the leukocytes.
- Used to prevent or avoid febrile reactions to leukocytes or platelets in previously sensitized patients; to minimize transmission of viral diseases, such as HIV or cytomegalovirus infections; and perhaps in patients awaiting kidney transplant.

WASHED RED CELLS

- Obtained from whole blood by centrifugation techniques.
- Must be used within 24 h of preparation because of the danger of bacterial contamination.
- Indicated for patients who are hypersensitive to plasma.
- Sometimes used in neonatal transfusions to reduce the amount of anticoagulant, extracellular potassium, etc., infused.

FROZEN RED CELLS

- May be stored for years but cost two to three times as much as stored liquid blood.
- Somewhat leukocyte poor and almost free of plasma.
- May be used for autotransfusion, to ensure a supply of rare blood, or to reduce sensitization to histocompatibility antigens in potential transplant patients.

INDICATIONS FOR TRANSFUSION THERAPY

- Informed consent should be obtained and documented before transfusion therapy is given.

Hemorrhage and Shock

- Volume support is of primary concern, but replacement of red cells is also necessary with larger losses of blood.
- Packed red cells with crystalloids or albumin are as effective as whole blood in replacing volume loss.
- Blood of any age within the storage limits is suitable.

Surgery

- Blood loss (even >1000 ml) may be safely replaced with crystalloids.
- Because of the hazards of blood transfusion (see below) every effort should be made to minimize the use of blood for volume replacement in surgery.

Burns

- Severe burns require extensive volume replacement in the first 24 h.
- Plasma loss occurs over the next 5 days and can be replaced with plasma and colloids.
- Anemia can be treated with packed red cells.

Anemia

- Patients with stable anemia with a hemoglobin level above 7 g/dl should not be transfused unless they are elderly or have cardiac or pulmonary disease.
- Attempts to improve the efficiency of transfusion by using young red cells ("neocytes") have had limited success.

MODE OF ADMINISTRATION

- *It is essential that the person administering blood or a blood component read the label to ensure that the unit to be used was selected by the laboratory for the particular patient.*

- Usually blood does not need to be warmed unless amounts greater than 3 liters are to be given at greater than 100 ml/min. At the usual rate of administration, the aggregates that may develop in patients with high-titer cold agglutinins are dispersed when the blood reaches body temperature.
- Blood should be given slowly in the first 30 min to minimize an adverse reaction.
- Drugs or medications should not be added to blood or blood components.

SPECIAL SITUATIONS

Autologous Transfusion

- Minimizes the probability of adverse reactions to transfusion, such as transmission of disease or alloimmunization.
- May be achieved by preoperative collection and storage of blood, immediate preoperative phlebotomy and hemodilution with postoperative return of the blood, or reinfusion of blood collected intraoperatively.
- In some patients erythropoietin has been given to permit increasing the amount of blood taken preoperatively.
- Autologous donation is ideal for patients with rare blood types or with antibodies that make cross-matching difficult or impossible.

Directed or Designated Donations

- Donors recruited from among family or friends appear to be no safer than volunteer blood donors. Graft-vs.-host disease is a greater risk if blood is donated by family members.

TRANSFUSION REACTIONS

- Majority of fatal transfusion reactions are due to management–clerical errors.
- Up to 20 percent of all transfusions may lead to some type of adverse reaction.

Immediate Reactions

Acute Hemolytic Reactions

- May occur intravascularly, usually due to ABO incompatibility, or extravascularly.
- Intravascular hemolysis may lead to disseminated intravascular coagulation (DIC) or to ischemic necrosis of tissues, particularly the kidney.
- Patients may develop fever, low-back pain, sensation of chest compression, hypotension, nausea, or vomiting.

- The transfusion should be terminated immediately when an acute reaction is suspected, and measures to control hemorrhage, if present, and to prevent renal damage instituted promptly.
- Renal damage may be prevented by hydration with addition of a diuretic if necessary to maintain urinary flow > 100 ml/h. Mannitol may be used at an initial dose of 100 ml of a 20 percent solution given intravenously over 5 min. Furosemide in a dose of 40 to 80 mg intravenously may be more effective. If oliguria occurs, standard measures for acute renal failure should be instituted.
- Laboratory diagnosis is based on evidence of hemolysis (hemoglobinemia, methemalbuminemia, hemoglobinuria) and detection of a blood group incompatibility.
- The risk of sequelae is dependent on the amount of incompatible blood given. Severe complications rarely occur if less than 200 ml of red cells have been transfused.

Febrile Reactions

- Fever may be due to a hemolytic reaction, sensitivity to leukocytes or platelets, bacterial pyrogens, or unidentified causes.
- 30 percent of all transfusion reactions are nonhemolytic, febrile reactions.
- A febrile reaction of itself is not an indication for termination of the transfusion, but one should not hesitate to stop if there is any doubt about the cause.
- Chills may indicate a more serious situation, but there are no reliable guidelines.
- Sensitization to leukocyte or platelet antigens is a common cause of febrile reactions.
- At least seven transfusions are usually required for sensitization, but previously pregnant women may be sensitized after only one or two.
- Clinical findings are primarily fever, which may continue to rise for 2 to 6 h after the transfusion is stopped and may continue for 12 h.
- Diagnosis depends on demonstration of antibodies to leukocyte or platelet antigens. Most reactions are due to antibodies to granulocytes.
- Treatment is supportive.
- Many reactions can be prevented by use of a leukocyte filter.

Pulmonary Hypersensitivity Reaction (Noncardiogenic Pulmonary Edema)

- Leukocyte incompatibility may also cause acute respiratory distress, chills, fever, and tachycardia due to pulmonary edema.
- Donor leukocytes may react with recipient antibodies, or donor antibodies may react with recipient leukocytes.

- Almost 25 percent of multiparous women have antibodies which can cause this reaction.
- Can occur with transfusion of platelets, plasma, whole blood, or packed red cells.
- Onset is usually within 4 h of transfusion.
- Chest films show bilateral diffuse, patchy pulmonary densities without cardiac enlargement.
- Treatment is supportive.
- In a healthy individual symptoms subside in less than 24 h, and the pulmonary infiltrates disappear within 4 days.

Allergic Reactions

- Transfusion may result in generalized pruritus and urticaria, and occasionally there may be bronchospasm, angioedema, or anaphylaxis.
- The cause is poorly understood, but may be hypersensitivity to plasma proteins or other substances in the administered product.
- These reactions are usually mild and respond to antihistamine drugs, but epinephrine may be required in some cases.

Anti-IgA in IgA-Deficient Recipient

- Severe anaphylactic reactions may occur in IgA-deficient patients who have formed anti-IgA antibodies.
- Deficiency or absence of IgA occurs in about 1 in several hundred people.
- IgA in the transfused product reacts with circulating antibody in the recipient. Less than 10 ml plasma can cause a reaction.
- Symptoms are dyspnea, nausea, chills, abdominal cramps, emesis, diarrhea, and profound hypotension. There is no fever.
- Diagnosis depends on demonstration of IgA deficiency and anti-IgA antibodies in the recipient.
- Reactions can usually be prevented by using washed red cells. Platelet or granulocyte transfusions for sensitized patients should be from donors with absent IgA.

Bacterial Contamination

- Blood may be contaminated by cold-growing organisms (*Pseudomonas* or coli-aerogenes group) which utilize citrate and may therefore lead to formation of visible clots.
- Infusion of blood containing large numbers of gram-negative organisms leads to endotoxin shock, with fever, hypotension, abdominal pain, vomiting, diarrhea, and vascular collapse, beginning 30 min or more after the infusion.
- Diagnosis may be made by examining a Gram stain of plasma obtained by low-speed centrifugation of some of the transfused

blood. If the blood is heavily contaminated, organisms should be seen in every oil immersion field.

- Bacterial contamination of blood is uncommon if disposable plastic blood bags are used, but contamination may be a significant hazard with platelet concentrates stored at room temperature.

Circulatory Overload

- Congestive heart failure with pulmonary edema may develop following transfusion in patients with cardiovascular compromise. Treatment is primarily with diuretics.
- Patients with severe chronic anemia may also develop congestive heart failure if transfused rapidly. Diuretics should be given and the transfusion limited to 2 ml/kg/h.

Microaggregates in Blood

- Particles of 13 to 100 μm in size ("microaggregates") and consisting largely of platelets and fibrin in banked blood are not removed by the usual filters in transfusion sets.
- Such particles can cause pulmonary insufficiency when massive transfusion of banked blood is given using standard filters, but this can be prevented with microaggregate filters.

Citrate Intoxication

- Blood transfused into adults at a rate greater than 1 liter in 10 min will cause significant reduction in ionized calcium concentrations and lead to myocardial depression and ECG changes.
- Can be prevented by giving 10 ml of 10 percent calcium gluconate IV for every liter of citrated blood administered.

Delayed Reactions

Delayed Hemolytic Reaction

- Previously undetected alloantibodies may appear 4 to 14 days after transfusion and cause destruction of the transfused cells.
- Usually an anamnestic response to a previous immunization from prior transfusion or pregnancy.
- Clinical findings are jaundice, falling hemoglobin level, and a positive direct antiglobulin reaction (Coombs test).
- Delayed hemolytic reactions may be mild and probably are frequently undetected.

Posttransfusion Purpura

- Thrombocytopenia due to antibodies to a platelet-specific antigen may develop shortly after transfusion (see Chap. 67).

Transmission of Disease

- The greatest risk are viral agents such as hepatitis B or C or HIV.

Graft-vs.-Host Disease

- An uncommon complication of transfusion, preventable by administering irradiated blood.
- Iron overload occurs in patients receiving many transfusions.
- Alloimmunization to antigens not included in routine cross matching occurs in immunocompetent patients receiving multiple transfusions and creates a major problem in obtaining blood for some patients with chronic anemia.

For a more detailed discussion, see Loni Calhoun, Lawrence D. Petz: Erythrocyte antigens and antibodies, Chap. 148, p. 1595; and Ernest Beutler, S. P. Masouredis: Preservation and clinical use of erythrocytes and whole blood, Chap. 151, p. 1622, in *Williams Hematology,* 5/e, 1995.

---

86 PRESERVATION AND CLINICAL USE OF PLATELETS

The development of both *plastic equipment* to permit sterile separation of platelets and *effective storage methods* for platelet concentrates has allowed for the safe and widespread use of platelet transfusions.

PLATELET PRODUCTS FOR TRANSFUSION

- Random donor platelets are prepared by centrifugation techniques that yield from 7 to 10×10^{10} platelets per unit of blood.
- Platelets so obtained are suspended in citrated autologous plasma and are significantly contaminated with leukocytes. Several units of platelets are pooled to provide sufficient platelets for transfusion (4 to 6 U for an adult).
- Single-donor platelets are prepared from a single individual by plateletpheresis. Each plateletpheresis contains approximately 3 to 4×10^{11} platelets, significantly contaminated with leukocytes.
- Fresh whole blood is used for platelet transfusion in children less than 2 years old who have undergone open-heart surgery.

STORAGE OF PLATELET CONCENTRATES

- Platelet suspensions may be stored with continuous agitation for 5 days at 20 to 24°C in plastic containers which allow for adequate diffusion of oxygen.
- In vivo function of stored platelets appears to be normal.
- Platelets may be stored frozen in plasma containing dimethylsulfoxide (DMSO).
- Viability of thawed platelets is 50 percent that of fresh platelets.
- Frozen storage is usually done to provide autologous platelets for use in patients who are refractory to allogeneic platelet transfusions.

CHOICE OF PLATELET PREPARATION

- Platelet transfusion may begin with random donor pooled platelets.
- ABO-compatible platelets should be used whenever possible.

CLINICAL RESPONSE AND COMPLICATIONS OF PLATELET TRANSFUSION

- The response to infusion of random donor platelets can be evaluated by calculating the *corrected count increment P*:

$$P = \frac{C \times S}{U} \qquad \text{platelets}/\mu l$$

where C = measured platelet increase (platelets/μl)
S = measured body surface area in m^2
U = number of units of platelets given

- Average corrected count increment is 10,000/μl.
- The 20-h increment is two-thirds of the 1-h increment.
- In a single-donor plateletpheresis product there are about the same number of platelets as in five random donor units.
- Factors that lower the corrected count increment are
  - allosensitization
  - loss of platelet viability in storage
  - splenomegaly
  - consumptive coagulopathy
  - fever
  - infection
  - marrow transplantation
  - amphotericin therapy
- Alloimmunization frequently develops in patients receiving random-donor platelet transfusions.
- Alloimmunization should be considered if two to three consecutive random donor transfusions produce a corrected count increment of less than 3000/μl.
- Alloimmunization is usually due to development of antibody against HLA antigen on the platelet surface. Leukocyte depletion of platelet products may reduce alloimmunization.
- Alloimmunized patients may respond to single-donor platelets from either family members or unrelated individuals selected by matching for the HLA-A and -B antigens.
- Graft-vs.-host disease may occur in immunosuppressed patients given unirradiated platelet transfusions.
- Rh-negative recipients may become sensitized to Rh-positive red cells contaminating infused platelets.
- During and after platelet transfusion chills and fever may occur from alloantibodies against contaminating leukocytes. Leukocyte depletion may reduce the frequency of chills and fever.
- Febrile reactions may be due to allergic reactions to some component(s) of the suspending plasma
- Platelet transfusion can transmit viruses, e.g., hepatitis B and C and HIV.

INDICATIONS FOR PLATELET TRANSFUSION

- Platelet counts of 20,000 to 50,000/μl are adequate to protect patients against life-threatening spontaneous bleeding.
- Invasive procedures require raising the platelet count to 60,000 to 100,000/μl.
- ε-Aminocaproic acid (3 to 5 g orally q6h) can reduce mucosal bleeding in thrombocytopenic patients.

  Thrombocytopenia Due to Underproduction

  - Platelets should be transfused prophylactically for a platelet count of 5000/μl or less.

- The decision whether to transfuse platelets in the range of 5000 to 20,000/µl must be made on an individual basis using clinical considerations such as
  - presence of fever and sepsis
  - presence of gastrointestinal ulceration or bleeding
  - administration of drugs which interfere with platelet function
  - abnormalities of coagulation factors
  - high leukocyte counts

Thrombocytopenia due to Platelet Loss, Sequestration, or Destruction

- Massive red blood cell transfusion does not require prophylactic platelet transfusion unless there is abnormal bleeding.
- Prophylactic platelet transfusion is not indicated for the thrombocytopenia that develops after cardiopulmonary bypass unless there is abnormal bleeding.
- Thrombocytopenia from splenomegaly and sequestration of platelets does not usually require prophylactic platelet transfusion unless an invasive procedure is to be done.
- Idiopathic thrombocytopenic purpura (ITP) does not usually require platelet transfusion.
  - If bleeding is life-threatening, 3 to 6 U of random donor platelets/m^2 body surface area may raise the platelet count for 12 to 48 h.
  - The same considerations apply for other disorders with accelerated destruction of platelets, e.g., thrombotic thrombocytopenic purpura, disseminated intravascular coagulation.
- Transfusion of washed maternal platelets to an infant is indicated in neonatal alloimmune thrombocytopenia.

Qualitative Platelet Disorders

- Platelet transfusion is not indicated for extrinsic platelet disorders, e.g., uremia, von Willebrand disease, hyperglobulinemia.
- Inherited intrinsic platelet disorders are often mild and do not require platelet transfusion except for severe bleeding and surgery.
- Acquired intrinsic platelet disorders usually do not require platelet transfusion unless the patient is thrombocytopenic.

For a more detailed discussion, see Scott Murphy: Preservation and clinical use of platelets, Chap. 153, p. 1643, in *Williams Hematology,* 5/e, 1995.

87 THERAPEUTIC HEMAPHERESIS: INDICATIONS, EFFICACY, COMPLICATIONS

- Therapeutic apheresis is the application of blood cell separation techniques to treat certain clinical conditions.
  - *Cytapheresis* refers to removal of a blood cell element, e.g., leukapheresis, plateletpheresis, red blood cell exchange.
  - *Plasmapheresis* refers to removal of plasma.

LEUKAPHERESIS

- In acute or chronic leukemia a single therapeutic leukapheresis will reduce the leukocyte count by 25 to 50 percent.
- The rate of mobilization of cells and the rate of cell proliferation dictate the frequency of therapeutic leukapheresis.
- Leukostasis may be prevented or treated by leukapheresis with rapid cytoreduction in patients with AML whose leukocyte count is greater than 100,000/μl; patients with ALL with leukocyte count above 200,000/μl; or patients with CML with leukocyte count above 300,000/μl.
- Therapeutic leukapheresis prior to chemotherapy reduces tumor burden and may minimize metabolic abnormalities due to tumor lysis.
- Therapeutic leukapheresis may be used in lieu of chemotherapy to treat chronic myelogenous leukemia, e.g., in pregnancy, to allow for delay in starting chemotherapy.
- Therapeutic leukapheresis can lower the white cell counts, reduce organomegaly, and reduce tumor burden in chronic lymphocytic leukemia, Sézary syndrome, and hairy cell leukemia.

PLATELETPHERESIS

- Plateletpheresis is useful for temporary reduction of the platelet count.
  - Reduction in the platelet count of about 50 percent may be achieved per procedure
  - The platelet count returns to pretreatment value in a few days.
- Plateletpheresis is indicated for symptomatic thrombocytosis.
- Cytotoxic therapy should be administered at the same time as plateletpheresis in patients with thrombocythemia due to myeloproliferative disorders.

ERYTHROCYTAPHERESIS

- Red cell exchange carries all the hazards of blood transfusion.
- Indications for red cell exchange in sickle cell disease include pria-

pism, unremitting painful crises, prior to surgery, during pregnancy, and prior to radiographic studies requiring contrast medium.
- Acute neurologic symptoms have occurred in sickle cell anemia patients undergoing red cell exchange for priapism.

PLASMA EXCHANGE THERAPY

- Plasma exchange is used in disorders in which there is a known or presumed abnormal plasma constituent.
- Therapeutic plasma exchange removes pathologic material in the plasma.
- An exchange of 1 plasma volume reduces the abnormal plasma constituent by approximately 65 percent.
- An exchange of 2 plasma volumes reduces the abnormal plasma constituent by approximately 88 percent.
- Alterations in plasma components after plasma exchange:
  - Levels of coagulation factors are reduced after large volume exchange and replacement with albumin and crystalloid, but bleeding is rare.
  - Serum immunoglobulin levels are decreased after repeated 1-volume plasma exchanges and replacement with albumin.
- Mortality associated with plasma exchange is 3 in 10,000 procedures.
- Disorders for which plasma exchange may be useful are:
  - thrombotic thrombocytopenic purpura
  - hyperviscosity syndrome due to paraproteins
  - cold agglutinin disease with life-threatening hemolysis not responding to other measures
  - cryoglobulinemia
  - renal failure associated with multiple myeloma
  - pure red cell plasma
  - removal of coagulation factor inhibitors
  - recipients of ABO-incompatible marrow transplants prior to transplantation
  - posttransfusion purpura
  - myasthenia gravis
  - acute and chronic inflammatory demyelinating polyradiculoneuropathy.

For a more detailed discussion, see Jacob Nusbacher: Therapeutic hemapheresis: indications, efficacy, complications, Chap. 155, p. 1663, in *Williams Hematology*, 5/e, 1995.

INDEX

ISBN 0-07-070394-9

90000

9 780070 703940